DORLAND'S

Gastroenterology
WORD BOOK

for Medical
Transcriptionists

Series Editor
SHARON B. RHODES, CMT, RHIT

Edited & Reviewed by:
Marge Parker, CMT

W.B. SAUNDERS COMPANY
A Harcourt Health Sciences Company

Philadelphia   London   New York   St. Louis   Sydney   Toronto

W.B. Saunders Company
A Harcourt Health Sciences Company

The Curtis Center
Independence Square West
Philadelphia, Pennsylvania 19106

616.3 DORLAND 2002

Dorland's gastroenterology word book for medical

Library of Congress Cataloging-in-Publication Data

Dorland's gastroenterology word book for medical transcriptionists / Sharon B. Rhodes, editor; edited & reviewed by Marge Parker.

p. cm.

ISBN 0-7216-9389-X

1. Gastroenterology—Terminology.   2. Medical transcription—Terminology.   I. Title: Gastroenterology word book for medical transcriptionists.   II. Rhodes, Sharon B.   III. Parker, Marge.

RC802.D673 2002

616.3'3'014—dc21   2001034391

Dorland's Gastroenterology Word Book for
Medical Transcriptionists   ISBN 0-7216-9389-X

Printed in the United States of America.

Last digit is the print number: 9 8 7 6 5 4 3 2 1

DORLAND'S

Gastroenterology
WORD BOOK

for Medical
Transcriptionists

PREFACE

I am proud to present the *Dorland's Gastroenterology Word Book for Medical Transcriptionists*—one of the ongoing series of word books being compiled for the professional medical transcriptionist. For over one hundred years, W. B. Saunders has published the *Dorland's Illustrated Medical Dictionary*. With the advent of medical transcription, it became the dictionary of choice for medical transcriptionists.

When I was approached in the fall of 1999 to help develop a new series of word books for W. B. Saunders, I have to admit the thought absolutely overwhelmed me. The *Dorland's Illustrated Medical Dictionary* was one of my first book purchases when I began my transcription career over thirty years ago. To be invited to participate in this project is an honor I could never have imagined for myself!

Transcriptionists need and will continue to need trusted up-to-date resources to help them research difficult terms quickly. In developing the *Dorland's Gastroenterology Word Book for Medical Transcriptionists*, I had access to the entire *Dorland's* terminology database for the book's foundation. In addition to this immense database, a context editor, Marge Parker, CMT, a recognized leader in the field of medical transcription, was selected to review the material from the database, to contribute new and unique terms, and to remove outdated and obsolete ones. With Marge's extensive research and diligent work, I believe this to be the most up-to-date word book for the field of gastroenterology.

In developing the gastroenterology word book, I wanted the size to be manageable so the book would be easy to handle, provide a durable long-lasting binding, and use a type font large enough to read while providing extensive terminology.

Anatomical plates were added as well as identification of anatomical landmarks. Additionally, a list of the most frequently prescribed drugs has been included.

Although I have tried to produce the most thorough word book for gastroenterology available to medical transcriptionists, it is difficult to include every term as the field of medicine is constantly evolving. As you discover new terms, please feel free to share them with me for inclusion in the next edition of *the Dorland's Gastroenterology Word Book for Medical Transcriptionists.*

I may be reached at the following e-mail address: Sharon@TheRhodes.com.

SHARON B. RHODES, CMT, RHIT
Brentwood, Tennessee

A
A bile
A ring
A ring of esophagus

α
α adrenoreceptor
α-agonist
α₁-antitrypsin disease

AAA
abdominal aortic aneurysm
aromatic amino acid

AAC
antibiotic-associated colitis

AAG
antral atrophic gastritis

AAH
atypical adenomatous hyperplasia

AAL
anterior axillary line

AAPBDS
anomalous arrangement of pancreaticobiliary ductal system

Aaron sign

AATD
α₁-antitrypsin disease
AATD-related emphysema

AAV
adeno-associated virus

abate

Abbe operation

Abbott
A. esophagogastroscopy
A. esophagogastrostomy
A. HCV E1A 2nd generation kit
A. HCV 2.0 test kit
A. IMx PSA assay

Abbott *(continued)*
A. LifeCare pump
A. Lifeshield needleless system
A. TDx monoclonal fluorescence polarization immunoassay
A. tube
A.-Miller tube
A. -Rawson double-lumen gastrointestinal tube
A.-Rawson tube

ABC
alkaline phosphatase Vectastain ABC
ABC reagent

abdomen
acute a.
acute surgical a.
boardlike rigidity of a.
boat-shaped a.
carinate a.
diffusely tender a.
distended a.
doughy a.
dull to percussion a.
exquisitely tender a.
flabby a.
flat a.
flat plate of a.
hyperresonant a.
navicular a.
nondistended a.
a. obstipum
pendulous a.
plain film of a.
protuberant a.
resonant a.
rigid a.
rotund a.
scaphoid a.
silent a.
soft a.
splinting of a.
surgical a.
tight a.
tympanitic a.

abdominal
- a. abscess
- a. angina
- a. apoplexy
- a. aorta
- a. aortic aneurysm
- a. aortography
- a. apron
- a. bruits
- a. canal
- a. cavity
- a. colectomy
- colicky a. pain
- a. compression belt
- a. contents
- deep a. ring
- a. desmoid tumor
- a. distention
- a. dropsy
- a. ectopic pregnancy
- a. esophagus
- external a. ring
- a. fasciocutaneous flap
- a. fat
- a. fat pad
- a. fistula
- a. fluid wave
- a. fullness
- a. girth
- a. guarding
- a. hernia
- hydraulic a. concussion
- a. incision dehiscence
- internal a. fascia
- internal a. ring
- a. kidney
- a. laparotomy pad
- a. lavage
- a. mass
- a. membrane
- a. migraine
- a. muscle deficiency syndrome
- a. nephrectomy
- a. nephrotomy
- a. pad
- a. pain
- a. paracentesis

abdominal *(continued)*
- a. part of esophagus
- a. patch electrode
- a. partitioning
- a. patch electrode
- a.-perineal resection
- a. peritoneum
- a. pool
- posterior a. wall
- a. pressure
- a. pressure technique
- a. procedure
- a. pulse
- a. rectopexy
- a. regions
- a. rigidity
- a. ring
- a. section
- a. situs inversus
- a. stoma
- superficial a. ring
- a. surgery
- a. tap
- a. testis
- a. tympany
- a. typhoid
- a. ultrasonography
- a. ultrasound
- a. vascular accident
- a. viscus
- a. wall
- a. wall hernia
- a. wall mass
- a. wall venous pattern
- a. zone

abdominalis
- pulsus a.

abdominis
- angina a.
- diastasis recti a.
- rectus a.

abdominocentesis

abdominocystic

abdominogenital

abdominopelvic
- a. cavity
- a. orocecal transit time

abdomino-Peña pull-through procedure

abdominoperineal
a. excision
a. resection (APR)

abdominoscopy

abdominoscrotal
a. hydrocele

abdominothoracic

abdominovaginal

abdominovesical

abenteric

aberrant
inferior a. ductule
a. obturator vein
a. pancreas
superior a. ductule
a. umbilical stomach

aberration
a's by scintigraphy

ABG
arterial blood gas

A bile

ablation
carbon dioxide laser plaque a.
cold forceps a.
cold snare a.
cryogenic a.
cryosurgical a.
homogeneous a.
laser a.
tumor a.
valve a.
visual laser a.

ablative laser therapy

abluminal

abnormality
amino acid a.
chromosomal a.

abnormality *(continued)*
clotting a.
diminished branching a.
electrolyte a.
hematologic a.
hepatic a.
a. of the hepatic artery
immunologic a.
mucosal a.
vascular a.

ABO
ABO barrier
ABO-incompatible

AB/PAS
alcian blue and periodic acid-Schiff

Abrikosov tumor

abrogate

abrupt pulse

abscess
abdominal a.
amebic a.
anorectal a.
appendiceal a.
appendicular a.
bile duct a.
biliary a.
cavernosal a.
cholangitic a.
crypt a.
cuff a.
deep interloop a.
diaphragmatic a.
Douglas a.
echinococcal a.
echinococcal liver a.
Entamoeba histolytica a.
enteroperitoneal a.
epiploic a.
fecal a.
a. formation
fungal a.
fungal liver a.
gallbladder wall a.
gas a.
hepatic a.

abscess *(continued)*
high intermuscular a.
horseshoe a.
interloop a.
intermesenteric a.
ischiorectal a.
intersphincteric perirectal a.
intra-abdominal a.
intrahepatic a.
intramesenteric a.
intraperitoneal a.
ischiorectal perirectal a.
kidney a.
lacunar a.
liver a.
midabdominal a.
non–gas-forming liver a.
pancreatic a.
pancreatic pseudocyst a.
paracolic a.
parafrenal a.
paranephric a.
pararectal a.
pelvic a.
pelvirectal a.
perianal a.
perianal fistula a.
pericecal a.
pericholecystic a.
pericolic a.
pericolonic a.
perinephric a.
perirenal a.
peritoneal a.
peritoneal cavity a.
periureteral a.
phlegmonous a.
pilonidal perirectal a.
postoperative a.
psoas a.
pyogenic a.
rectal a.
renal cortical a.
retrocecal a.
retroperitoneal-iliopsoas a.
root a.
spermatic a.

abscess *(continued)*
splenic a.
stercoraceous a.
stercoral a.
subacute a.
subcapsular hepatic a.
subdiaphragmatic a.
subhepatic a.
subperitoneal a.
subphrenic a.
suprahepatic a.
supralevator perirectal a.
urethral a.
urinary a.

absent
a. bowel sounds
a. gag reflex
a. peristalsis

Absidia
A. corymbifera
A. ramosum

absolute
a. alcohol
a. alcohol sclerosant
a. dehydration
a. diet
a. erythrocytosis

absorbable
a. clip
a. gelatin sponge
a. sponge
a. suture

absorptiometry
dual-energy x-ray a.
dual-photon a.

absorption
alcohol a.
dual-energy x-ray a. (DEXA)
enteral a.
gastrointestinal a.
impaired gastric a.
internal a.
intestinal a.
paracetamol a.
reservoir mucosal a.

absorptive
    a. cell
    a. hypercalciuria
    a. hyperoxaluria
    intestinal a. cell

abuse
    alcohol a.
    ethanol (ETOH) a.
    intravenous drug a.
    ipecac a.
    laxative a.
    phencyclidine a.
    salicylate a.
    substance a.

AC
    adenylate cyclase

ACA
    adenocarcinoma
    anticardiolipin antibody

acalculous
    acute a. cholecystitis
    a. cholecystitis
    a. gallbladder disease

acanthosis
    glycogenic a.
    a. nigricans

Acarbose

acathectic

acathexia

ACBE
    air contrast barium enema

accelerated
    a. hypertension
    a. transplant rejection

accelerator
    a. urinae

access
    arteriovenous a.
    hemodialysis a.
    hemodialysis vascular a.
    peritoneal a.

access *(continued)*
    vascular a.
    venovenous a.

accessorium
    pancreas a.

accessory
    a. adrenal
    a. adrenal gland
    a. diaphragm
    a. duct of Luschka
    a. duct of Santorini
    a. pancreas
    a. pancreatic duct
    a. parotid gland
    a. portal system of Sappey
    a. saphenous vein
    a. superior colic artery
    a. thyroid gland
    a. trocar
    a. vessel

accident
    abdominal vascular a.

accumulation
    gamma-aminobutyric
        acid a.
    glycoprotein a.
    tubular iron a.

AccuSharp endoscope

Accuson-128 color flow Doppler
    machine

ACE
    angiotensin-converting en-
        zyme
    antegrade continuous en-
        ema procedure

ACEI
    angiotensin-converting en-
        zyme inhibitor

acetaldehyde

acetaminophen
    a. hepatotoxicity
    a. overdose

acetate
  calcium a.
  cortisone a.
  cyproterone a. (CPA)
  free a.
  goserelin a.
  hydrocortisone a.
  leuprolide a.
  medroxyprogesterone a.
  megestrol a.
  methylprednisolone a.
  octreotide a.
  phorbol myristate a. (PMA)
  uranyl a.

acetic acid

acetohydroxamic acid
  a. a. irrigation

acetowhite
  a. lesion

acetylcholine

acetylcholinesterase

acetyl-Co-hypoglycin A

acetylcysteine

acetylsalicylic acid
  5-a. a.

ACG
  American College of Gas-
    troenterology

ACGE
  American Society for Gas-
    trointestinal Endoscopy

achalasia
  a. balloon dilation
  a. cardia
  classic a.
  cricopharyngeal a.
  a. dilator
  esophageal a.
  idiopathic a.
  pelvirectal a.
  secondary a.
  sphincteral a.
  vigorous a.

achalasialike esophagus

ache
  stomach a.

Achiever
  A. balloon dilation catheter
  A. balloon dilator

achlorhydria
  gastric a.
  histamine-resistant a.
  medically-induced a.

achlorhydric

acholangic biliary cirrhosis

acholia

acholic
  a. stool

acholuria

acholuric
  a. jaundice

achoresis

achromaturia

Achromycin
  A. V

achylia
  a. gastrica
  a. pancreatica

achylous

achymia

achymosis

acid
  acetic a.
  acetohydroxamic a.
  acetylsalicylic a.
  5-acetylsalicylic a.
  amino a.
  aminocaproic a.
  p-aminohippuric a.
  5-aminosalicylic a. (5-ASA)
  arachidonic a.
  aromatic amino a. (AAA)

acid *(continued)*
    ascorbic a.
    a.-ash diet
    a.-base imbalance
    bile a. (BA)
    branched-chain amino a.
      (BCAA)
    caustic a.
    a. cells
    chenodeoxycholic a. (CDCA)
    cholic a. (CA)
    a. clearance test (ACT)
    complementary deoxyri-
      bonucleic a. (cDNA)
    conjugated bile a.
    diethylenetriamine penta-
      acetic a. (DTPA)
    diisopropyl iminodiace-
      tic a. (DISIDA)
    a. dyspepsia
    epsilon-aminocaproic a.
    esophageal a. infusion test
    essential amino a.
    essential fatty a.
    esterified fecal a.
    ethacrynic a.
    fatty a.
    fecal bile a. (FBA)
    folic a.
    folinic a.
    free fatty a.
    free fecal bile a.
    gamma-aminobutyric a.
    gastric a.
    a. glands
    glutamic a.
    a. hemolysis test
    hepato-iminodiacetic a.
      (HIDA)
    homovanillic a. (HVA)
    hyaluronic a.
    hydrochloric a. (HCl)
    a. indigestion
    a. ingestion
    a. injury
    keto a.
    lactic a.
    luminal a.
    mucosal fatty a.

acid *(continued)*
    oral bile a. (OBA)
    pantothenic a.
    a. peptic ulcer
    a. perfusion test
    polyglycolic a.
    a. pump
    a. reflux
    a. reflux test
    a. regurgitation
    renal messenger ribonu-
      cleoprotein a.
    reptilase a.
    ribonucleic a. (RNA)
    serum uric a.
    short-chain fatty a. (SCFA)
    sulfuric a.
    a. suppression
    tannic a.
    taurocholic a.
    Travasol amino a.
    uric a.
    valproic a.

acid-base
    a.-b. balance
    a.-b. disturbance
    a.-b. equilibrium

acidemia
    a. defect
    a. of stool test

acidity
    circadian gastric a.
    gastric a.
    intracellular a.
    intragastric a.
    urinary a.

acid-labile

acidophilic
    a. body
    a. PAS-positive granule

acidophilus
    a. capsule
    Lactobacillus acidophilus
    a. milk

acidosis
    acute a.
    chronic metabolic a.

acidosis *(continued)*
    congenital lactic a.
    distal renal tubular a.
      (dRTA)
    generalized distal renal
      tubular a.
    high anion-gap metabolic a.
    hyperchloremic metabol-
      ic a.
    hypokinetic renal tubular a.
    lactic a.
    non−anion-gap metabolic a.
    proximal renal tubular a.
    renal hyperchloremia a.
    renal tubular a. (types 1−4)
    respiratory a.
    uremic a.
    winter a.

acidotic

acid-pepsin reflux esophagitis

acid-peptic
    a.-p. condition
    a.-p. disease
    a.-p. esophagitis
    a.-p. juice

acid-provoked spasm

acid-suppressed stomach

acid-suppression therapy

Acidulin

acinar
    a. adenocarcinoma
    a. cell
    a. cell carcinoma
    a. gradient
    pancreatic a. cell
    pancreatic a. cell carci-
      noma
    a. tissue

Acinetobacter calcoaceticus

acini (*plural of* acinus)

acinic
    a. cell

aciniform

acinose

acinotubular

acinous
    a. adenoma
    a. cell

acinus *pl.* acini
    liver a.
    pancreatic a.
    a. renalis [malpighii]
    a. renis [malpighii]

AcipHex

ackee fruit poisoning

ACLA
    anticardiolipin antibody

ACMI
    ACMI endoscope
    ACMI fiberoptic colono-
      scope
    ACMI fiberoptic esophago-
      scope
    ACMI gastroscope
    ACMI Martin endoscopy
      forceps
    ACMI ulcer measuring de-
      vice

acoprosis

acoprous

acorn
    a.-tipped bougie
    a.-tipped catheter
    a. treatment

acquired
    a. cystic kidney disease
      (ACKD)
    a. diverticulosis
    a. functional megacolon
    a. gastric ectopy
    a. hernia
    a. hyperlipoproteinemia
    a. hyperoxaluria
    a. immunodeficiency
    a. immunodeficiency syn-
      drome (AIDS)

acquired *(continued)*
  a. lactose deficiency
  a. megacolon
  a. pancreatitis

acrobystiolith

acrobystitis

acromegalic
  a. gigantism

acromegaly

acroposthitis

acrosomal granule

ACT
  acid clearance test

ACTH
  adrenocorticotropic hormone

Actigall

actin
  a. filament
  smooth muscle isoform a.

Actinomyces

actinomycosis
  biliary a.
  gastric a.

actinomycotic appendicitis

action
  cytolytic a.
  immunomodulatory a.
  viruslike a. (VLA)

activated
  a. alkaline glutaraldehyde
  a. charcoal
  CH-40 a. charcoal
  a. partial thromboplastin time
  a. thromboplastin time

activation
  complement a.
  very late a. (VLA)

activator
  plasminogen a. (PA)

activator *(continued)*
  tissue plasminogen a. (TPA)
  tissue-type plasminogen a. (t-PA)
  urokinase plasminogen a.
  vascular plasminogen a. (v-PA)

active
  a. bowel sounds
  a. chronic gastritis
  a. chronic hepatitis
  a. congestion
  a. duodenal ulcer
  a. renin
  a. source of bleeding
  a. systemic bacterial infection

Active Living
  A. L. incontinence pad
  A. L. incontinence shield

actively bleeding varix

activity
  adenosine deaminase a.
  ATPase a.
  brush-border enzyme a.
  brush-border hydrolase a.
  complement hemolytic a.
  fibrinolytic a.
  gastric myoelectrical a.
  gastric urease a.
  intrinsic enzymatic a.
  mitotic a.
  motor a.
  myoelectric a.
  opsonic a.
  plasma renin a. (PRA)
  protein serine/threonine kinase a.
  serum cholinesterase a.
  specific a.
  spike-burst electrical a.
  sympathetic nervous system a.
  tyrosine kinase a.

AcuClip endoscopic multiple clip applier

acuity

acuminatum *pl.* acuminata
  condyloma a.
  esophageal condyloma a.

acupuncture

AcuSnare

acute
  a. abdomen
  a. abdominal vascular disease
  a. acalculous cholecystitis
  a. acidosis
  a. alcohol hepatitis
  a. appendicitis
  a. catarrhal cystitis
  a. cellular rejection
  a. cholecystitis
  a. diverticulitis
  a. drug-induced cholestasis
  a. erosive gastritis (AEG)
  a. fatty liver
  a. fatty liver of pregnancy (AFLP)
  a. flank pain syndrome
  a. focal bacterial nephritis (AFBN)
  a. gallstone pancreatitis
  a. gastric anisakiasis
  a. gastric mucosal lesion
  a. gastroenteritis (AGE)
  a. glomerulonephritis
  a. graft-versus-host disease
  a. hemorrhagic gastritis
  a. hemorrhagic pancreatitis
  a. hepatic coma
  a. hepatic failure
  a. hepatic rupture
  a. hepatic toxicity
  a. hepatitis (AH)
  a. hepatocellular degeneration
  a. hydramnios
  a. idiopathic inflammatory bowel disease
  a. infectious colitis

acute *(continued)*
  a. infectious diarrhea
  a. infectious gastroenteritis
  a. infectious nonbacterial gastroenteritis
  a. intermittent porphyria (AIP)
  a. interstitial nephritis
  a. intrinsic renal failure
  a. juvenile cirrhosis
  a. lead poisoning
  a. leukopenia
  a. megacolon
  a. mercury poisoning
  a. mononucleosis-like hepatitis
  a. myelomonocytic leukemia
  a. nephritic syndrome
  a. nephritis
  a. nephrosis
  a. nonocclusive bowel infarction
  a. nonvariceal upper gastrointestinal hemorrhage
  a. obstructive cholangitis
  a. obstructive suppurative cholangitis (AOSC)
  a. pancreatitis
  a. pancreatitis prevention
  a. parenchymatous hepatitis
  a. polycystic disease
  a. porphyria
  a. proctitis
  a. pyelonephritis
  a. recurrent pancreatitis (ARP)
  a. rejection of liver transplant
  a. relapsing pancreatitis
  a. renal failure (ARF)
  a. renal transplant vasculopathy
  a. sclerosing hyaline necrosis
  a. scrotum
  a. self-limited colitis (ASLC)

acute *(continued)*
    a. self-limited hepatitis
    a. suppurative cholangitis (ASC)
    a. suppurative nephritis
    a. surgical abdomen
    a. tubular necrosis
    a. urate nephropathy
    a. uric acid nephropathy
    a. vac rejection
    a. vascular rejection
    a. viral hepatitis (AVH)
    a. yellow atrophy

acyclovir
    a. sodium

acystia

acystinervia

acystineuria

ADA
    American Diabetes Association
        ADA diet

Adair-Allis forceps

Adalat CC

adapter
    camera a.
    c-mount a.
    Cook plastic Luer lock a.
    friction-fit a.
    Olympus a.
    Polaroid XS-70 with ACMI a.
    Touhy-Borst a.

adaptor *(variant of* adapter*)*

ADCC
    antibody-dependent cell-mediated cytotoxicity

ADD
    angled delivery device

Addis count

Addison
    A. clinical planes
    A. disease

Addison *(continued)*
    A. planes
    A. point
    A. syndrome

adductor
    a. brevis muscle
    a. longus muscle

Aden fever

adenitis
    mesenteric a.

adenoacanthoma

adeno-associated virus (AAV)

adenocarcinoma (ACA)
    acinar a.
    annular a.
    appendiceal a.
    clear cell a.
    colloid-producing a.
    colonic a.
    colorectal a.
    ductal a. of the prostate
    duodenal a.
    esophageal a.
    exophytic a.
    gastric a.
    giant cell a.
    hepatoid a.
    infiltrating a.
    a. in situ
    invasive a.
    a. of kidney
    metastatic a.
    mucinous a.
    mucin-producing a.
    mucosal a.
    papillary a.
    peritoneal a.
    prostatic a.
    renal a.
    scirrhous a.
    a. of the stomach
    ulcerating a.
    urachal a.

adenoid cystic carcinoma

adenofibromyoma

adenolysis

adenoma *pl.* adenomas, adeno-
mata
    acinous a.
    aggressive a.
    bile duct a. (BDA)
    Brunner gland a.
    a.-carcinoma sequence
    colonic a.
    colorectal villous a.
    cortical a's
    depressed a.
    a. destruens
    duodenal a.
    embryonal a.
    flat a.
    gastric a.
    hepatic a.
    hepatocellular a. (HCA)
    a.-hyperplastic polyp ratio
    incidental a.
    islet cell a.
    a's of kidney
    Leydig cell a.
    liver cell a.
    metachronous a.
    moderately differentiated a.
    monopolypoid a.
    mucinous a.
    nephrogenic a.
    a.-nonadenoma ratio
    papillary a.
    Pick testicular a.
    Pick tubular a.
    poorly differentiated a.
    prostatic a.
    rectal villous a.
    renal cortical a.
    a. sebaceum
    sessile a.
    synchronous a's
    testicular tubular a.
    tubulovillous a.
    undifferentiated a.
    villoglandular a.
    villous a.

adenoma *(continued)*
    villous colorectal a.
    well-differentiated a.

adenomatoid tumor

adenomatosis
    multiple endocrine a. type I
    multiple endocrine a. type
      II

adenomatous
    a. colorectal polyp
    a. epithelium
    a. gastric polyp
    a. hyperplasia (AH)
    a. polyp (AP)
    a. polyp–cancer sequence
    a. polyp of the colon (APC)
    a. polyposis
    a. polyposis coli
    a. polyposis coli gene
    a. polyp of the stomach

adenomyoma
    a. of gallbladder

adenomyomatosis

adenomyosarcoma
    embryonal a.

adenomyosis

adenopapillomatosis
    gastric a.

adenopathy
    axillary a.
    inguinal a.
    lymph node a.
    palpable a.
    paraductal a.

adenosine

adenosine deaminase activity

adenosis
    sclerosing a.

adenosquamous carcinoma

adenovirus
    a. colitis
    enteric a.

adenovirus *(continued)*
    human a. 12
    a. infection
    a.-12 viral protein

adenylate cyclase (AC)

ADF
    aortoduodenal fistula

ADH
    alcohol dehydrogenase
    antidiuretic hormone

adherence
    bacterial a.

adherent clot

adhesion
    antigen-independent a.
    attic a.
    bacterial a.
    banjo-string a.
    cell–cell a.
    coronal a.
    dense a.
    a. dyspepsia
    filmy a.
    a. formation
    freeing up of a's
    hard a.
    hepatic a.
    intra-abdominal a.
    intraperitoneal a.
    lysis of a's
    a. molecule
    omental a.
    pelvic a.
    perihepatic a.
    peritoneal a.
    postcholecystitis a.
    postoperative a.
    taking down of a's
    T cell a.
    thick a.
    thin a.
    tight a.
    violin-string a.

adhesive
    a. band
    Comfeel skin a.

adhesive *(continued)*
    a. dressing
    fibrin tissue a.
    a. ileus
    a. peritonitis
    a. protein receptor
    a. tape
    Uro-Bond skin a.

Adipex-P

adipocele

adipohepatic

adipose
    a. arteries of kidney
    a. capsule of kidney
    a. tissue

adiposis
    a. hepatica

adiposus
    ascites a.

adjuvant
    anesthesia a.
    a. chemotherapy
    Freund's a.

adminiculum *pl.* adminicula
    a. lineae albae

adnexa
    hepatocellular a.

adnexal
    a. tenderness

adrenal
    accessory a.
    accessory a. gland
    a. gland
    middle a. artery
    a. rest
    a. rest tumor

adrenergic
    alpha-a.

adrenocorticotropic hormone
    (ACTH)

adrenogenital syndrome

adrenoreceptor
α a.

adult
a. celiac disease
a.-onset diabetes mellitus
a.-onset obesity
a. polycystic liver disease (APLD)
a. respiratory distress syndrome (ARDS)

Advanced surgical suture applier

advanced therapeutic endoscopy

advancement
a. of rectal flap

advance to regular diet

adventitious cyst

adynamic
a. ileus
a. intestinal obstruction

AEG
acute erosive gastritis

AER
atheroembolic renal disease

aerocystoscope

aerocystoscopy

aerodigestive

aerogastria
blocked a.

Aeromonas
A.-associated enterocolitis
A. diarrhea

aerourethroscope

aerourethroscopy

AFBN
acute focal bacterial nephritis

afferent
a. fiber
a. glomerular arteriole
a. limb
a. loop
a. loop syndrome
a. vessel of glomerulus

AFLP
acute fatty liver of pregnancy

African
A. hemochromatosis

aganglionic megacolon

agastria

agastric

AGE
acute gastroenteritis

agent
anticholinergic a.
antidiarrheal a.
antifungal a.
antihypertensive a.
antimicrobial a.
antimotility a.
antimuscarinic a.
antisecretory a.
antispasmodic a.
5-ASA a.
azole antifungal a.
beta-sympathomimetic tocolytic a.
bulking a.
carbon dioxide–trapping a.
central adrenergic a.
chemotherapeutic a.
contrast a.
cytotoxic a.
embolic a.
hemostatic a.
iodinated contrast a.
mucolytic a.
parasympathomimetic a.
peripheral adrenergic a.
progestational a.
prokinetic a.

agent *(continued)*
    sclerosing a.
    thrombolytic a.
    virucidal a.

ageusia

ageusic

agglutinin
    febrile a's

aggregate

aggregation
    erythrocyte a.
    familial a.

aggressive
    a. adenoma
    chronic a. hepatitis

aglutition

agonic intussusception
    aggregated lymphatic folli-
      cles of Peyer

agonist
    α-a.
    adrenergic-cholinergic a.
    alpha$_2$-adrenergic a.
    beta-adrenergic a.
    dopamine a.
    5-HT4 a.
    muscarinic cholinergic a.
    nicotinic a.

Agoral

agranulocytic ulcer

AH
    acute hepatitis
    adenomatous hyperplasia

AIDS
    acquired immunodeficiency
      syndrome
        AIDS-related complex
          (ARC)

AIP
    acute intermittent por-
      phyria

air
    biliary a.
    blood gas on room a.
    a. contrast barium enema
      (ACBE)
    a. cyst
    a.-filled loop
    free a.
    a. insufflation
    intramural colonic a.
    intraperitoneal a.
    a. pressure enema reduc-
      tion
    a. swallowing
    a. thermometer

airway
    a. epithelium
    a. obstruction
    patent a.

AJCC
    American Joint Committee
      on Cancer
        AJCC TNM tumor clas-
          sification

AJCC/UICC
    American Joint Committee
      on Cancer/International
      Union against Cancer
        AJCC/UICC staging sys-
          tem

Åkerlund
    diverticulum of Å.

alba
    linea a.

Albarrán
    A. gland
    A. tubules

Albert suture

albiduria

albinuria

Albright solution

albuginea
    a. penis

albugineotomy

albuminoid liver

alcian blue and periodic acid-Schiff (AB/PAS)

alcohol
  absolute a.
  a. absorption
  a. abuse
  a. cooling bath
  a. consumption
  a.-fixed gastric biopsy
  glyceryl a.
  a. dehydrogenase (ADH)
  graded a.
  glycyl a.
  isoamyl a.
  pantothenyl a.
  polyvinyl a.
  a. sclerosis

alcoholic
  chronic a. cirrhosis
  chronic a. pancreatitis
  a. cirrhosis
  decompensated a. cirrhosis
  a. fatty liver
  a. fibrosis
  a. hemorrhagic gastritis
  a. hepatitis
  a. hyalin
  a. liver disease
  a. pancreatitis
  a. prognostic factor
  a. varix

alcohollike hepatitis

alcoholism

Alden loop gastric bypass

alder buckthorn

aldosterone

alfa-2a
  interferon a.-2a
  recombinant interferon a.-2a

alfa-2b
  interferon a.-2b

alfa-n1
  interferon a.-n1

alfa-n3
  interferon a.-n3

algoid cells

alimentary
  a. apparatus
  a. bolus
  a. canal
  a. diabetes
  a. glycosuria
  a. hyperinsulinism
  a. obesity
  a. system
  a. tract
  a. tract duplication

alimentation
  central venous a.
  enteral a.
  forced a.
  parenteral a.
  peripheral intravenous a.
  rectal a.
  total parenteral a.

aliquot

alkali
  caustic a.
  a. ingestion

alkaline
  a.-ash diet
  a. injury
  a. milk drip
  a. phosphatase (ALP, AP)
  a. phosphatase test
  a. phosphatase Vectastain ABC
  a. reflux esophagitis
  a. reflux gastritis

alkalinization
  a. test

Alka-Mints

alkane
  breath a.

Alka-Seltzer

allergen
  food a.

allergic
  a. colitis
  a. cystitis
  a. enteropathy
  a. gastroenteropathy
  a. interstitial nephritis
  a. proctitis
  a. prostatitis
  a. purpura
  a. vasculitis

allergy
  cow's milk a.
  food a.
  latex a.
  medication a.

Allis
  A. catheter
  A. clamp
  A. forceps
  A. inhaler
  A. tooth grasper

allogeneic
  a. fetus
  a. kidney transplant
  a. liver perfusion
  a. transplantation

allogenic (see allogeneic)

allograft
  hepatic a.
  kidney a.
  a. parenchyma
  a. rejection
  renal a.
  a. survival rate

allopurinol

allotransplantation

allowance
  recommended daily a.
    (RDA)

aloin

alpha
  a.-adrenergic
  a.-adrenergic antagonist
  a.-amylase
  a. blockade
  a.-chain disease
  a. fetoprotein (AFP)
  a.-gliadin fraction
  a.-glucosidase inhibitor
  a. heavy-chain disease
  a.-hemolytic streptococcus
  a. interferon
  a. interferon therapy
  a. interferon treatment
  a.-receptor antagonist
  a. *Streptococcus viridans*
  a. sympathetic blockade

alpha$_1$
  a.$_1$-adrenergic receptor
  a.$_1$-antitrypsin
  a.$_1$ blocker

alpha$_2$
  a.$_2$ adrenergic agonist
  a.$_2$ globulin
  a.$_2$-beta$_1$ integrin cell-surface collagen

alteration
  genetic a.
  molecular genetic a.
  nuclear matrix a.

alternate-day treatment

alternating calculus

aluminum
  a. aminoacetate
  basic a. carbonate
  basic a. carbonate gel
  colloidal a. hydroxide
  dried a. hydroxide gel
  a. glycinate

aluminum *(continued)*
    a. hydrate
    a. hydroxide
    a. hydroxide gel
    a. phosphate
    a. phosphate gel

Amanita
    A. mushroom
    A. mushroom hepatotoxic-
       ity

Amaryl

ambulatory
    chronic a. peritoneal dialy-
       sis
    a. hemorrhoidectomy
    a. monitoring
    a. pH monitoring
    a. probe

amebiasis
    hepatic a.
    intestinal a.

amebic
    a. abscess
    a. appendicitis
    a. balanitis
    a. colitis
    a. dysentery
    a. granuloma
    a. hepatitis

ameboma

American
    A. ACMI (S3565, TX-915)
       flexible fiberoptic sig-
       moidoscope
    A. Anorexia/Bulimia Associ-
       ation
    A. College of Gastroenterol-
       ogy (ACG)
    A. Diabetes Association
       (ADA)
    A. Dilation System dilator
    A. Endoscopy automatic re-
       processor
    A. Endoscopy dilator

American *(continued)*
    A. Joint Commission on
       Cancer/International Un-
       ion against Cancer (AJCC/
       UICC)
    A. Society for Gastrointesti-
       nal Endoscopy (ACGE)
    A. trypanosomiasis
    A. Type Culture Collection
       (ATCC)

Am factor

amiloride
    a. hydrochloride

Amin-Aid

amino
    a. terminus

amino acid
    a. a. abnormality
    aromatic a. a. (AAA)

aminocaproic acid

p-aminohippuric acid

5-aminosalicylic acid (5-ASA)

ammonia
    blood a.

ammonium
    a. chloride
    a. muriate

amniotic umbilicus

Amphojel

ampulla *pl.* ampullae
    biliaropancreatic a.
    a. biliaropancreatica
    a. ductus deferentis
    duodenal a.
    a. duodeni
    Henle a.
    hepatopancreatic a.
    a. hepatopancreatica
    Lieberkühn a.
    phrenic a.
    rectal a.
    a. recti

ampulla *(continued)*
    a. of vas deferens
    a. of Vater

ampullar

ampullary
    a. carcinoma
    a. granulation tissue
    a. hamartoma
    a. stenosis
    a. stone
    a. tumor

ampullitis

ampulloma

ampullopancreatic
    a. carcinoma

Amussat operation

amylase
    ascitic a.
    a. concentration
    measurement of a. in So-
      mogyi units
    pancreatic a.
    P-type a.
    salivary a.
    serum a.
    S-type a.
    a. unit
    urinary a.

amyloid
    a. kidney
    a. liver
    a. nephrosis

amyloidosis
    dialysis a.
    familial a.
    hemodialysis-associated a.
    hepatic a.
    hereditary a.
    heredofamilial a.
    rectal a.
    renal a.
    secondary a.

anabolic
    a. steroid

anabolic *(continued)*
    a. steroid treatment

anacidic
    a. stomach

anacidity
    gastric a.

anaerobic
    a. culture
    a. glycolysis

anal
    a. anastomosis
    a. atresia
    a. bulging
    a. canal
    8-channel cross-sectional a.
      sphincter probe
    cloacogenic a. carcinoma
    a. columns
    a. condyloma
    a. crypts
    a. cryptitis
    a. dilatation
    a. dilation
    a. dilator
    a. discharge
    a. disk
    a. effluent
    a. electrical stimulation
    a. encirclement
    a. endoscopy
    external a. sphincter
    a. fascia
    a. fissure
    a. fistula
    a. foreign body
    a. glands
    a. ileostomy with preserva-
      tion of sphincter
    internal a. sphincter
    a. intersphincteric groove
    a. intramuscular gland
    a. lesion
    a. manometry
    a. mapping
    a. pit
    a. pitting

anal *(continued)*
   a. plate
   a. pouch
   a. pressure
   a. procidentia
   a. prolapse
   a. protrusion
   a. region
   a. sinuses
   a. sphincter
   a. sphincter contraction
   a. sphincter dysfunction
   a. sphincter function
   a. sphincter reconstruction
   a. sphincter repair
   a. sphincter squeeze pressure
   a. sphincter tone
   a. stenosis
   a. stricture
   a. transition zone
   a. ulceration
   a. valves
   a. verge
   a. wart
   a. wound

analeptic enema

analgesic
   a. nephropathy

analogue
   folic acid a.

analysis
   anthropometric a.
   bioelectrical impedance a.
   body composition a.
   cineradiographic a.
   cytogenetic a.
   electrophoresis immuno-
      blot a.
   fecal a.
   fluid a.
   gastric a.
   heteroduplex a.
   histochemical-ultrastruc-
      tural a.
   image a.
   Northern blot a.

analysis *(continued)*
   pentagastrin-stimulated a.
   regression a.
   sequencing a.
   Southern blot a.
   spectral a.
   spectrophotometric a.
   trace-gas a.
   Western blot a.
   x-ray a.

analyzer
   Hamilton-Thorn motility a.

anapepsia

anaphylactic reaction

anaphylactoid
   a. food sensitivity
   a. purpura

anaphylaxis

anaplasia

anaplastic
   a. seminoma

Anaprox

anasarca

anascitic

Anaspaz

anastomose

anastomosis *pl.* anastomoses
   anal a.
   antecolic a.
   antiperistaltic a.
   arteriovenous a.
   biliodigestive a.
   Billroth I a.
   Billroth II a.
   biodigestive a.
   Brackin ureterointestinal a.
   Braun a.
   Carrel aortic patch a.
   Coffey ureterointestinal a.
   coloanal a. (CAA)
   colocolonic a.
   Couvelaire ileourethral a.
   curved end-to-end a.

anastomosis *(continued)*
    dog-ear a.
    end-to-end a.
    end-to-side a.
    esophagocolic a.
    extravesical a.
    Hofmeister a.
    Hofmeister-Polya a.
    Horsley a.
    H-shaped ileal pouch–anal a.
    ileal pouch–anal a.
    ileal pouch–distal rectal a.
    ileoanal a.
    ileoanal pull-through a.
    ileorectal a.
    ileovesical a.
    ileotransverse colon a.
    ileovesical a.
    intestinal a.
    isoperistaltic a.
    intravesical a.
    J-shaped ileal pouch–anal a.
    Kocher a.
    mesocaval a.
    mucosa-to-mucosa a.
    Parks ileoanal a.
    portal-systemic a.
    portosystemic a.
    primary a.
    pyeloileocutaneous a.
    rectosigmoid a.
    right-angled end-to-side a.
    Roux-en-Y a.
    Schoemaker a.
    side-to-side a.
    splenorenal venous a.
    S-shaped ileal pouch-anal a.
    State end-to-end a.
    sutureless bowel a.
    tension-free a.
    transureteroureteral a.
    two-layer a.
    ureterocolonic a.
    ureteroileal a.
    ureteroileocutaneous a.
    ureterosigmoid a.

anastomosis *(continued)*
    ureterotubal a.
    ureteroureteral a.
    urethrocecal a.
    vascular a.
    vesicourethral a.
    W-shaped ileal pouch–anal a.

anastomotic
    a. leakage
    a. material
    a. recurrence
    a. stoma
    a. stricture
    a. suture
    a. ulcer
    a. ulceration

anatomy
    anomalous a.
    congenitally altered a.
    peritoneal a.

anatrophic nephrotomy

Ancef

anchoring suture

anchovy sauce pus

Anderson
    A. classification
    A. disease
    A. gastric tube

androblastoma

androcyte

androgone

andrology

anechoic

anemia
    autoimmune hemolytic a.
    B_{12} a.
    a. of chronic disease
    a. of chronic renal failure
    deficiency a.
    febrile pleomorphic a.
    folate a.
    hemolytic a.

anemia *(continued)*
    homozygous sickle cell a.
    hypovolemic a.
    iron-deficiency a.
    megaloblastic a.
    pernicious a.
    posthepatitis aplastic a.
    sickle cell a.

anephric

anepiploic

anesthesia
    a. adjuvant
    general a.
    general endotracheal a.
    local a.
    pharyngeal a.
    Ponka technique for lo-
      cal a.
    preperitoneal a.
    topical a.
    topical oropharyngeal a.

anesthetic
    Cetacaine topical a.
    EMLA a.
    a. hepatitis
    a. hepatotoxicity
    lidocaine topical a.
    topical a.
    Xylocaine topical a.

aneurysm
    abdominal aortic a.
    aortic a.
    arterial a.
    arteriosclerotic a.
    bilobate false a.
    Dieulafoy cirsoid a.
    dissecting abdominal a.
    hepatic artery a.
    mycotic a.
    perforating a.
    renal a.
    renal artery a.
    ruptured a.
    saccular a.

aneurysmal
    a. dilatation

aneurysmectomy

Angelchik
    A. antireflux prosthesis
    A. prosthesis
    A. ring prosthesis

angina
    abdominal a.
    a. abdominalis
    a. abdominis
    a. dyspeptica
    intestinal a.

anginal
    a. attack

anginiform

anginose

anginous

angioaccess

angiocatheter

angiocholecystitis

angiocholitis

angiodysplasia
    bleeding colonic a.
    diffuse a.

angiodysplastic
    a. lesion

angioedema
    hereditary a.

angiofibroma
    nasopharyngeal a.

angiogenesis
    tumor a.

Angiografin

angiogram
    celiac a.
    cystic duct a.
    splenic a.

angiographic
    a. embolization
    a. end-hole catheter

angiographic *(continued)*
    a. intervention
    a. portacaval shunt
    a. variceal embolization

angiographically

angiography
    a. catheter
    celiac a.
    diagnostic a.
    digital subtraction a.
    dynamic fluorescein a.
    fluorescence a.
    intra-arterial digital subtraction a.
    intraoperative ultrasonography and a.
    magnetic resonance a.
    mucosal a.
    renal a.
    selective mesenteric a.
    subtraction a.
    superior mesenteric a.
    therapeutic a.

angioinfarction

angiolipoleiomyoma

angioma *pl.* angiomas, angiomata
    bleeding a.
    cherry a.
    gastric a.
    petechial a.
    spider a.
    telangiectatic a.
    umbilicated a.
    UGI angiomata
    upper gastrointestinal angiomata

angiomatoid tumor

angiomatosis
    hepatic a.

angiomatous
    a. lymphoid hamartoma

Angiomed
    A. blue stent
    A. Puroflex stent

angiomyolipoma
    gastric a.

angioneurotic
    a. anuria
    a. edema

angioneurectomy

angioplasia

angioplasty
    a. balloon
    a. balloon catheter
    percutaneous transluminal renal a.

angiosarcoma
    hepatic a.
    radiation-induced a.

angiotensin (I, II, III)
    a.-converting enzyme (ACE)
    a.-converting enzyme inhibitor (ACEI)
    a. II infusion test

angle
    anopouch a.
    anorectal a.
    anterior vesicourethral a.
    cardiodiaphragmatic a.
    cardiohepatic a.
    cardiophrenic a.
    epigastric a.
    hepatorenal a.
    a. of His
    a. of incidence
    inferior a. of duodenum
    mesangial a.
    posterior vesicourethral a.
    splenorenal a.
    superior a. of duodenum
    vesicourethral a.

angled
    a. delivery device (ADD)
    a. dissecting forceps

angular
    a. incisure of stomach
    a. notch of stomach
    a. sulcus

angularis
    a. body
    incisura a.

angulation

angulus *pl.* anguli
    a. of the lesser curve
    a. of stomach

anhaustral colonic gas pattern

anhemolytic strep

anhepatic
    a. stage of liver transplantation

anhydrochloric

ani (*genitive of* anus)
    levator a.
    pruritus a.

anicteric
    a. hepatitis
    a. sclera
    a. skin
    , a. viral hepatitis

aniline cancer

anion
    a. exchange resin
    a. gap

anionic
    a. ferritin
    a. IgG 4 fraction

anisakiasis
    acute gastric a.
    gastric a.

anismus

anisuria

ankylostomiasis

ankylurethria

anlage *pl.* anlagen
    a. of pancreas
    prepancreatic anlagen
    splenic a.

Ann Arbor
    A. A. cancer staging
    A. A. classification

annexin

annular
    a. adenocarcinoma
    a. esophageal stricture
    a. pancreas

annulorrhaphy

annulus *pl.* annuli
    a. abdominalis
    a. abdominis
    a. femoralis
    a. inguinalis profundus
    a. inguinalis superficialis
    a. lymphaticus cardiae
    a. urethralis

ano (*ablative of* anus)
    fissure in a.
    fissura in a.
    fistula in a.

anococcygeal
    a. raphe

anocutaneous
    a. line
    a. reflex
    a. stimulation

anoderm

anomalous
    a. anatomy
    a. arrangement of pancreaticobiliary ductal system (AAPBDS)
    a. genitalia
    a. pancreaticobiliary communication
    a. pancreaticobiliary duct (APBD)
    a. pancreaticobiliary ductal union (APBDU)

anoperineal

anoplasty
    chronic a. treatment

anoplasty *(continued)*
    cutback a.
    House advancement a.
    House flap a.
    Martin a.
    a. treatment
    Y-V a.

anopouch angle

anorchia

anorchid

anorchidic

anorchidism

anorchism

anorectal
    a. abscess
    a. angle
    a. atresia
    a. band
    a. carcinoma
    a. disease
    a. dysgenesis
    a. fistula
    a. flexure of rectum
    a. foreign body
    a. inhibitory reflex
    a. junction
    a. line
    a. malformation
    a. manometry
    a. measurement
    a. myectomy
    a. physiology
    a. physiology testing
    a. ring
    a. sensorimotor dysfunction
    a. sepsis
    a. space
    a. sphincter
    a. stenosis
    a. surgery
    a. test
    a. varix

anorectic
    a. drug

anorectitis

anorectocolonic

anorectoplasty
    Laird-McMahon a.

anorectum

anorexia
    a. nervosa
    a.-cachexia syndrome

anorexiant

anorexigenic

anoscope
    Bacon a.
    Hirschmann a.
    slotted a.

anoscopic

anoscopy

anoscrotal fascia

anosigmoidoscopic

anosigmoidoscopy

anospinal
    a. center

anovesical

anoxia
    chemical a.
    gastric a.

ANP
    atrial natriuretic peptide

ansa *pl.* ansae
    a. nephroni
    a. pancreatica

Ansaid

antacid

antagonist
    alpha-adrenergic a.
    alpha-receptor a.
    beta-adrenergic a.
    calcium a.
    calcium channel a.

antagonist *(continued)*
 cytokine a.
 histamine$_2$ receptor a.
 hormone a.
 H$_2$ receptor a.
 opiate a.
 potassium canrenoate a.
 serotonin a.

antalgesic

antecardium

antecedent pancreatic injury

antecolic
 a. anastomosis
 a. long-loop isoperistaltic gastrojejunostomy

antecubital arteriovenous fistula

anteflexed uterus

antegrade
 a. approach
 a. continuous enema procedure (ACE)
 a. contrast study
 a. enema

antepartum constipation

anteprostate

anteprostatic gland

anteprostatitis

anterior
 a. abdominal wall
 a. abdominal wall syndrome
 a. approach
 a. axillary line
 a. band of colon
 a. border of body of pancreas
 a. border of pancreas
 a. cord syndrome
 a. crus of anterior inguinal ring
 a. duodenal ulcer
 a. exenteration

anterior *(continued)*
 a. fecal incontinence
 a. gastric wall
 a. hemiblock
 a. iliac artery
 a. inferior segment
 a. inferior segmental artery of kidney
 a. inguinal ligament
 a. innominate osteotomy
 a. ligament of colon
 a. margin of testis
 a. mediastinal arteries
 a. mediastinal cavity
 a. nephrectomy
 a. opening of stomach
 a. pelvic exenteration
 a. rectopexy
 a. rectus fascia
 a. rectus sheath
 a. renal fascia
 a. resection
 a. segmental artery of liver
 a. superior pancreaticoduodenal artery
 a. superior segment
 a. superior segmental artery of kidney
 a. surface of kidney
 a. surface of pancreas
 a. surface of stomach
 a. transabdominal approach
 a. true ligament of bladder
 a. urethra
 a. urethral valve
 a. vesicourethral angle
 a. wall antral ulcer
 a. wall of stomach

anteroinferior surface of body of pancreas

antero-oblique position

anterosuperior surface of body of pancreas

anthracene-type laxative

anthrax
 intestinal a.

anthropometric
  a. analysis
  a. measurement

anti-actin antibody

antibiotic
  a.-associated colitis
  a.-associated diarrhea
  a.-associated enterocolitis
  broad-spectrum a.
  a.-induced diarrhea
  a.-induced enterocolitis
  intraoperative a.
  perioperative a.
  postoperative a.
  preoperative a.
  prophylactic a.
  a. prophylaxis
  a. therapy
  topical a.

antibody
  anti-actin a.
  anticardiolipin a. (ACA, ACLA)
  anticolonic a.
  antidelta IgM a.
  antiendomysial a.
  antiendothelial a.
  antigliadin a.'s
  anti-HA a.
  anti-HAV IgM a.
  anti-HB a.
  anti-HBc IgM a.
  anti-HBe a.
  anti-HBs a.
  anti-HCV core a.
  anti-HD a.
  anti-HGF a.
  antimitochondrial a.
  antineutrophil cytoplasmic a. (ANCA)
  antinuclear a.
  antiphospholipid a.
  antiphospholipid/anticardiolipin a.
  antirotavirus a.
  anti–smooth muscle a.
  anti-somatostatin a.

antibody *(continued)*
  a.-dependent cell-mediated cytotoxicity (ADCC)
  a. feedback
  ferritin conjugated a.
  fluorescent a.
  Forssman a.
  gamma globulin a.'s
  HBe a.
  HCV a.
  a. to hepatitis C virus
  a. to hepatitis D virus
  IgM anti-HAV a.
  IgM anti-HBc a.
  IgM-HA a.
  islet cell a.
  liver-kidney microsomal a.
  milk protein a.
  PBC-associated a.
  serum virus a.

anticardium

anticholelithogenic

anticholinergic
  a. agent
  a. drug

anticolonic antibody

anticonvulsant agent hepatotoxicity

antidelta IgM antibody

antidepressant drug hepatotoxicity

antidiabetic agent hepatotoxicity

antidiarrheal
  a. agent
  opioid a.

antidiarrheic

antidiuresis

antidiuretic
  a. hormone (ADH)

antiemetic
  a. drug

antiendomysial antibody

antiendothelial antibody

antiflatulent

antifol
  Baker a.

antifungal
  a. agent
  a.-resistant opportunistic
    infection
  azole a. agent

anti-GBM antibody disease

antigen
  a.-independent adhesion
  carcinoembryonic a. (CEA)
  Forssman a.
  hepatitis B a. (HBAg)
  hepatitis B core a. (HBcAg)
  hepatitis Be a. (HBeAG)
  hepatitis B surface a.
  hepatitis B virus–enco-
    ded a.
  hepatitis D a. (HDAg)
  histocompatibility a.
  HLA a's
  liver membrane a.
  liver-specific a.
  pancreatic oncofetal a.
  prostate-specific a.
  prostate-specific membra-
    ne a.
  soluble liver a.

antigliadin antibodies

anti–glomerular basement
  membrane antibody disease

anti-HA
  anti–hepatitis A
    anti-HA antibody

anti-HAV
  anti–hepatitis A virus
    IgM anti-HAV
    anti-HAV IgM antibody
    anti-HAV-positive

anti-HB
  antibody to hepatitis B
    anti-HB antibody

anti-HBc
  antibody to hepatitis B
    core antigen
      anti-HBc IgM antibody
      monoclonal anti-HBc

anti-HBe
  antibody to hepatitis B e
    antigen

anti-HBs
  antibody to hepatitis B sur-
    face antigen

anti-HCV
  antibody to hepatitis C vi-
    rus
      anti-HCV core antibody

anti-HD
  antibody to hepatitis D an-
    tigen

anti-HDV
  antibody to hepatitis D vi-
    rus

anti–*Helicobacter pylori* IgM

anti–*Helicobacter pylori* treatment

anti–hepatitis A–IgM immuno-
  logical study

anti-HGF
  antibody to hepatocyte
    growth factor

anti-HSV
  antibody to herpes simplex
    virus
      anti-HSV IgM Ab titer

antihypertensive agent

anti-icteric

antilipemic
  a. drug

anti–liver microsomal antibody
detection

antimesenteric
a. border
a. border of distal ileum
a. enterotomy
a. fat pad
a. pad

antimesocolic
a. side of the cecum

antimicrobial agent

antimitochondrial antibody

antimotility
a. agent
a. drug

antimuscarinic
a. agent

antinatriuresis

antinauseant

antineoplastic drug hepatotoxicity

antinephritic

antineutrophil cytoplasmic antibody (ANCA)

antinuclear antibody

antinucleoprotein factor

antiperistalsis

antiperistaltic
a. anastomosis

antiphospholipid antibody

antiphospholipid/anticardioli-
pin antibody

antipsychotic drug hepatotoxicity

antireflux
Cohen a. procedure
Collis a. operation

antireflux *(continued)*
a. double-J stent
a. flap-valve mechanism
a. operation
a. procedure
a. prosthesis
a. regimen
a. surgery
a. therapy

antirefluxing colonic conduit

antirotavirus antibody

antiruminant

antisecretory
a. agent

anti–smooth muscle antibody

anti-somatostatin antibody

antispasmodic
a. agent
biliary a.
a. drug

antithyroid hepatotoxicity

antitrypsin
alpha$_1$-a.
α_1-a. disease

antiurolithic

antral
a. atrophic gastritis
a. biopsy
a. D-cell
a. diaphragm
a. EC-cell
a. edema
a. gastric cell
a. gastrin
a. gastrin cell hyperfunction
a. gastritis
a. G-cell hyperplasia
a. membrane
a. mucosa
a. peptide
a. polyp
a.-predominant gastritis

antral *(continued)*
a. pressure transducer
a. somatostatin
a. stasis
a. stenosis
a. stricture
a. ulcer
a. vascular ectasia
a. web

antroduodenal

antrectomy
Roux-en-Y biliary bypass
with a.

antroduodenectomy

antropyloric

antrostomy

antrotomy

antrum *pl.* antrums, antra
cardiac a.
a. cardiacum
gastric a.
a. gastritis
prepyloric a.
a. pylori
pyloric a.
a. pyloricum
retained a.
a. of stomach
a. of Willis

anulus *(variant of* annulus)

anuresis

anuretic

anuria
angioneurotic a.
calculous a.
obstructive a.
postrenal a.
prerenal a.
renal a.
suppressive a.

anuric

anus
artificial a.

anus *(continued)*
ectopic a.
imperforate a.
patulous a.
prolapse of a.
a. vesicalis
a. vestibularis
vulvovaginal a.

anusitis

Anusol
A.-HC
A.-HC-1

anvil portion of EEA stapler

anxiety-related diarrhea

Anzemet

aorta
abdominal a.
a. abdominalis
a. descendens
descending a.
paravisceral a.
supraceliac a.
a. thoracalis
thoracic a.
a. thoracica
thoracoabdominal a.

aortic
a. aneurysm
a. dissection
a. graft
a. patch
a. punch
a. stenosis
a. suprarenal artery
a. valvular stenosis

aortoduodenal
a. fistula (ADF)

aortoenteric
a. fistula
a. graft

aortoesophageal
a. fistula

aortogastric
a. fistula

aortograft duodenal fistula

aortography
 abdominal a.

aortohepatic arterial graft

aortoiliac

aortorenal
 a. bypass
 a. reimplantation

aortosigmoid fistula

AP
 adenomatous polyp
 alkaline phosphatase

apancrea

apancreatic

apatite
 a. calculus

APBD
 anomalous pancreaticobiliary duct

APBDU
 anomalous pancreaticobiliary ductal union

APC
 adenomatous polyposis coli

aperient

aperistalsis

aperistaltic
 a. esophagus

apertura
 a. pelvica inferior
 a. pelvica superior
 a. pelvis inferior
 a. pelvis superior
 aperturae superior et inferior fossae axillaris
 a. thoracis inferior
 a. thoracis superior

aperture
 inferior thoracic a.

aperture *(continued)*
 superior thoracic a.

apex *pl.* apexes, apices
 a. of bladder
 a. of duodenal bulb
 a. of external ring
 a. prostatae
 a. of prostate gland
 a. vesicae
 a. vesicalis

aphagia
 a. algera

aphasia

apheresis

aphtha *pl.* aphthae

aphthoid
 a. proctocolitis
 a. ulcer

aphthous
 a. gastropathy
 a. stomatitis
 a.-type lesion
 a. ulcer

apical
 a. canaliculus
 a. duodenal ulcer
 a. sound
 a. thickening

aplasia
 germinal cell a.

apocrine
 a. gland

aponeurosis *pl.* aponeuroses
 Denonvilliers a.
 external oblique a.
 a. of external oblique
 internal oblique a.
 a. of internal oblique
 ischiorectal a.
 a. of superior surface of levator ani muscle

apoplexy
 abdominal a.

apoplexy *(continued)*
    mesenteric a.
    pancreatic a.
    renal a.

aposthia

apparatus *pl.* apparatus, appa-
   ratuses
    alimentary a.
    biliary a.
    digestive a.
    GIA autosuture a.
    juxtaglomerular a.
    a. urogenitalis
    Wangensteen a.

appearance
    cobblestone-like a.
    collar-button a. in colon
    ground-glass a.
    hose-pipe a. of terminal il-
      eum
    picket fence a.
    stack of coins a.
    tadpole-like a.

appendage
    cecal a.
    a. of epididymis
    epiploic a's
    fibrous a. of liver
    testicular a.
    a. of the testis
    vermicular a.

appendagitis
    epiploic a.

appendectomy
    colonoscopic a.
    emergency a.
    emergent a.
    incidental a.
    interval a.
    inversion a.
    a. tape

appendiceal
    a. abscess
    a. adenocarcinoma
    cutaneous a. conduit
    a. intussusception

appendiceal *(continued)*
    a. mass
    a. opening
    a. orifice
    a. perforation
    a. stump

appendicectomy

appendicitis
    actinomycotic a.
    acute a.
    amebic a.
    chronic a.
    a. by contiguity
    foreign-body a.
    fulminating a.
    gangrenous a.
    helminthic a.
    left-sided a.
    lumbar a.
    a. obliterans
    nonperforated a.
    obstructive a.
    pelvic a.
    perforated a.
    perforating a.
    perforative a.
    protective a.
    purulent a.
    recurrent a.
    relapsing a.
    retrocecal a.
    retroileal a.
    segmental a.
    skip a.
    stercoral a.
    subperitoneal a.
    suppurative a.
    traumatic a.
    verminous a.

appendicocecostomy

appendicocele

appendicocystostomy
    continent cutaneous a.
    dismembered reimplan-
      ted a.
    nonplicated a.
    orthotopic a.

appendicocystostomy *(continued)*
   plicated a.
   reversed reimplanted a.

appendicoenterostomy

appendicolithiasis

appendicolysis

appendicopathy

appendicostomy

appendicular
   a. abscess
   a. artery
   a. colic
   a. dyspepsia
   a. lithiasis
   a. lobe
   a. vein

appendicovesicostomy
   Mitrofanoff a.

appendix *pl.* appendixes, appendices
   base of a.
   cecal a.
   a. dyspepsia
   a. epididymidis
   epiploic a.
   appendices epiploicae
   a. fibrosa
   a. fibrosa hepatis
   gangrenous a.
   hot a.
   indurated a.
   inflamed a.
   a. mass
   Morgagni a.
   nonperforated a.
   normal a.
   omental appendices
   appendices omentales
   opening of vermiform a.
   paracecal a.
   perforated a.
   preileal a.
   retrocecal a.
   retroileal a.
   ruptured a.

appendix *(continued)*
   subcecal a.
   suppurative a.
   a. testis
   a. vermicularis
   vermiform a.
   a. vermiformis
   xiphoid a.

appendolithiasis

apple-core lesion

apple-peel bowel syndrome

appliance
   external a.
   external cooling a.
   Karaya ring ileostomy a.
   ostomy a.

application
   laparoscopic clip a.

applicator

applier
   AcuClip endoscopic multiple clip a.
   Advanced surgical suture a.
   Stone clamp a.

Appolito suture

approach
   antegrade a.
   anterior a.
   anterior transabdominal a.
   fascial sling a.
   gasless laparoscopic a.
   peroral a.
   retroperitoneal a.
   transmural a.
   transpapillary a.

appy
   appendectomy

APR
   abdominoperineal resection

aproctia

apron
   abdominal a.

apron *(continued)*
    fatty omental a.
    a. skin incision

A-4 protein

arachidonic acid

arachnoid fibrosis

Arantius ligament

ARC
    AIDS-related complex

arch
    arterial a's of kidney
    deep crural a.
    tendinous a. of levator ani
      muscle
    venous a's of kidney

archiform fibers

architecture
    hepatic a.
    lobular a. of liver

arciform veins

arcuate
    a. arteries of kidney
    a. renal tubule
    a. veins of kidney

arcus *pl.* arcus
    a. tendineus musculi levatoris ani

ardor
    a. urinae

ARDS
    adult respiratory distress syndrome

area *pl.* areae, areas
    bare a. of liver
    cell surface a.
    cribriform a. of renal papilla
    a. cribrosa papillae renalis
    areae gastricae
    midepigastric a.
    midrectal a.

area *(continued)*
    a. nuda hepatis
    subhepatic a.

areflexic bladder

ARF
    acute renal failure

argentaffinoma
    a. syndrome

argon laser

Armanni
    A.-Ebstein cells
    A.-Ebstein change
    A.-Ebstein degeneration
    A.-Ebstein kidney
    A.-Ebstein lesion

aromatic
    a. amino acid (AAA)
    a. bitters
    a. cascara fluidextract
    a. castor oil

ARP
    acute recurrent pancreatitis

arrangement
    anomalous a. of pancreaticobiliary ductal system (AAPBDS)

arteria *pl.* arteriae
    a. adrenalis media
    a. appendicularis
    arteriae arciformes renis
    arteriae arcuatae renis
    a. ascendens ileocolica
    a. caecalis anterior
    a. caecalis posterior
    arteriae capsulares
    a. cecalis anterior
    a. cecalis posterior
    a. colica dextra
    a. colica media
    a. colica sinistra
    a. cremasterica
    a. cystica
    a. deferentialis

arteria *(continued)*
- a. ductus deferentis
- a. epigastrica inferior
- a. epigastrica superficialis
- a. epigastrica superior
- a. gastrica dextra
- a. gastrica posterior
- a. gastrica sinistra
- a. gastroduodenalis
- a. gastroepiploica dextra
- a. gastroepiploica sinistra
- a. gastroomentalis dextra
- a. gastroomentalis sinistra
- a. haemorrhoidalis inferior
- a. haemorrhoidalis media
- a. haemorrhoidalis superior
- a. hepatica communis
- a. hepatica propria
- a. hypogastrica
- arteriae ileae
- arteriae ileales
- arteriae ilei
- a. ileocolica
- a. iliaca communis
- a. iliaca externa
- a. iliaca interna
- a. iliolumbalis
- arteriae interlobulares hepatis
- arteriae interlobares renis
- arteriae intestinales
- arteriae intrarenales
- arteriae jejunales
- a. lienalis
- arteriae lumbales
- a. marginalis coli
- a. mesenterica inferior
- a. mesenterica superior
- a. pancreatica dorsalis
- a. pancreatica inferior
- a. pancreatica magna
- arteriae pancreaticoduodenales inferiores
- a. pancreaticoduodenalis superior anterior
- a. pancreaticoduodenalis superior posterior

arteria *(continued)*
- a. perinealis
- a. perinei
- arteriae perirenales
- a. prepancreatica
- a. rectalis inferior
- a. rectalis media
- a. rectalis superior
- a. renalis
- arteriae retroduodenales
- arteriae sacrales laterales
- a. sacralis mediana
- a. segmenti anterioris hepatici
- a. segmenti anterioris inferioris renalis
- a. segmenti anterioris superioris renalis
- a. segmenti inferioris renalis
- a. segmenti lateralis hepatici
- a. segmenti medialis hepatici
- a. segmenti posterioris hepatici
- a. segmenti posterioris renalis
- a. segmenti superioris renalis
- arteriae sigmoideae
- a. splenica
- a. supraduodenalis
- a. suprarenalis inferior
- a. suprarenalis media
- arteriae suprarenales superiores
- a. transversa colli
- a. umbilicalis
- a. urethralis
- a. vesicalis inferior
- arteriae vesicales superiores

arterial
- a. aneurysm
- a. arches of kidney
- a. blood gas
- a. embolization

arteriogram
   hepatic a.

arteriola *pl.* arteriolae
   a. glomerularis afferens
   a. glomerularis efferens
   arteriolae rectae renis
   arteriolae rectae spuriae
   arteriolae rectae verae

arteriolar nephrosclerosis

arteriole
   afferent glomerular a.
   efferent glomerular a.
   false straight a's of kidney
   postglomerular a.
   preglomerular a.
   straight a's of kidney
   true straight a's of kidney

arteriolitis
   hyperplastic a.
   necrotizing a.

arteriolosclerosis
   hyaline a.

arteriosclerotic
   a. aneurysm
   a. kidney
   a. nephritis

arteriovenous (AV)
   a. access
   a. anastomosis
   a. fistula
   a. graft
   a. malformation
   a. shunt

artery
   abnormality of the hepatic a.
   accessory superior colic a.
   adipose a's of kidney
   anterior iliac a.
   anterior inferior segmental a. of kidney
   anterior mediastinal a's
   anterior segmental a. of liver

artery *(continued)*
   anterior superior pancreaticoduodenal a.
   anterior superior segmental a. of kidney
   aortic suprarenal a.
   appendicular a.
   arcuate a's of kidney
   ascending ileocolic a.
   caudal a.
   central a's of spleen
   colic a.
   common hepatic a.
   common iliac a.
   cremasteric a.
   cystic a.
   deep external pudendal a.
   dorsal pancreatic a.
   a. of ductus deferens
   efferent a. of glomerulus
   external iliac a.
   funicular a.
   gastroduodenal a.
   gastroepiploic a.
   gonadal a's
   great pancreatic a.
   hepatic a.
   hypogastric a.
   ileal a's
   ileocolic a.
   a's of ileum
   iliac a.
   iliolumbar a.
   inferior epigastric a.
   inferior hemorrhoidal a.
   inferior mesenteric a.
   inferior pancreatic a.
   inferior pancreaticoduodenal a's
   inferior rectal a.
   inferior right colic a.
   inferior segmental a. of kidney
   inferior suprarenal a.
   inferior vesical a.
   inguinal a's
   interlobar a's of kidney
   interlobular a's of kidney
   interlobular a's of liver

artery *(continued)*
    internal iliac a.
    internal pudendal a.
    intestinal a's
    intrarenal a's
    jejunal a's
    lateral sacral a's
    lateral segmental a. of liver
    left colic a.
    left gastric a.
    left gastroepiploic a.
    left inferior gastric a.
    left gastro-omental a.
    a's of kidney
    lumbar a's
    medial segmental a. of liver
    median sacral a.
    middle adrenal a.
    middle capsular a.
    middle colic a.
    middle hemorrhoidal a.
    middle rectal a.
    middle suprarenal a.
    perineal a.
    perirenal a's
    posterior gastric a.
    posterior mediastinal a's
    posterior pelvic a.
    posterior segmental a. of
      kidney
    posterior segmental a. of
      liver
    posterior superior pancrea-
      ticoduodenal a.
    prepancreatic a.
    proper hepatic a.
    pubic a.
    pyloric a.
    radiate a's of kidney
    renal a.
    retroduodenal a's
    right colic a.
    right gastric a.
    right gastroepiploic a.
    right gastro-omental a.
    right inferior gastric a.
    sacrococcygeal a.
    short gastric a's
    sigmoid a's

artery *(continued)*
    small iliac a.
    splenic a.
    straight a's of kidney
    superficial epigastric a.
    superficial external puden-
      dal a.
    superior epigastric a.
    superior hemorrhoidal a.
    superior mesenteric a.
    superior rectal a.
    superior segmental a. of
      kidney
    superior suprarenal a's
    superior vesical a's
    supraduodenal a.
    umbilical a.
    urethral a.
    vermiform a.

arthritis *pl.* arthritides
    enteropathic a.

artificial
    a. anus
    a. bezoar
    a. gut
    a. hepatic support
    a. kidney
    a. organ
    a. sphincter

aryepiglottic
    aryepiglottic fold

arytenoid cartilage

ASA
    aminosalicylic acid
      ASA-induced gastric ul-
        ceration

5-ASA
    5-aminosalicylic acid
      5-ASA agent
      5-ASA enema

ASC
    acute suppurative cholangi-
      tis

ascending
    a. cholangitis

ascending *(continued)*
 a. colon
 a. ileocolic artery
 a. limb
 a. lumbar vein
 thick a. limb
 thin a. limb

ascites
 a. adiposus
 bile a.
 biliary a.
 blood-tinged a.
 bloody a.
 chyliform a.
 a. chylosus
 chylous a.
 cirrhotic a.
 cloudy a.
 culture-negative neutrocytic a.
 demeclocycline-induced a.
 dialysis-related a.
 a. drainage tube
 eosinophilic a.
 exudative a.
 fatty a.
 gelatinous a.
 hemodialysis-associated a.
 hemorrhaged a.
 hemorrhagic a.
 hydremic a.
 idiopathic a.
 malignant a.
 milky a.
 myxedema a.
 narrow albumin gradient a.
 nephrogenic a.
 neutrocytic a.
 nonchylous a.
 pancreatic a.
 pseudochylous a.
 refractory a.
 resistant a.
 straw-colored a.
 tense a.
 transudative a.
 urinary a.
 wide albumin gradient a.

ascitic
 a. amylase
 chylous a. fluid
 a. fluid
 a. fluid total protein

ascitogenous

ascorbic acid

Aselli's gland

Asiatic
 A. cholera
 A. schistosomiasis

ASLC
 acute self-limited colitis

Aspergillus
 A. fumigatus
 A. infection

aspergillosis
 a. esophagitis

aspermatism

aspermatogenesis

aspermia

aspirate
 gastric a.
 heme-positive NG (nasogastric) a.
 nasogastric a.
 NG (nasogastric) a.

aspiration
 a. biopsy
 CT-guided fine-needle a.
 CT-guided needle-a. biopsy
 fine-needle a.
 gastric a.
 gastric a. tube
 silent a.

aspirator

aspirin
 enteric-coated a.
 a.-induced gastritis

assay
  Abbott IMx PSA a.
  fluorescent antibody
    (FA) a.
  fluorescent antigen a.

assessment
  endoscopic a.
  endoscopic color Dop-
    pler a.

assistant
  gastrointestinal a. (*see* GIA)

asterixis

asthenospermia

astrovirus gastroenteritis

asymptomatic
  a. gallstone
  a. mass

Atarax

ATCC
  American Type Culture Col-
    lection

atheroembolic renal disease
  (AER)

atherosclerotic stenosis

Atkinson scoring system for
  dysphagia

Atlantic ileostomy catheter

atonic
  a. bladder
  a. constipation
  a. dyspepsia
  a. esophagus
  a. neurogenic bladder

atony
  gastric a.
  intestinal a.
  primary ureteral a.
  sphincter a.

ATPase activity

atresia
  anal a.
  anorectal a.
  a. ani
  biliary a.
  duodenal a.
  esophageal a.
  extrahepatic biliary a.
    (EBA)
  follicular a.
  gastric a.
  intestinal a.
  prepyloric a.
  pyloric a.

atretogastria

atretostomia

atreturethria

atrial
  a. natriuretic factor
  a. natriuretic peptide
    (ANP)

atriopeptin

atrophia
  a. testiculi

atrophic
  chronic a. duodenitis
  chronic a. gastritis
  a. cirrhosis
  diffuse corporal a. gastritis
  a. gastritis
  a.-hyperplastic gastritis
  a. kidney

atrophy
  acute yellow a.
  fundic gland a.
  gastric a.
  granular a. of kidney
  healed yellow a.
  red a.
  skin a.
  splenic a.
  subacute a. of liver
  subchronic a. of liver

atrophy *(continued)*
    Sudeck a.
    villous a.
    yellow a.

atropine
    a. oxide hydrochloride
    a. sulfate

Atropisol

attack
    anginal a.

attenuated tubule

attic adhesion

atypia
    cellular a.
    hepatocellular a.

atypical
    a. adenomatous hyperplasia
    a. ductular cell
    a. gallbladder disease

Auerbach
    A. and Meissner plexus
    A. mesenteric plexus

augmentation
    bladder a.
    a. cystoplasty
    demucosalized a. with gastric segment
    gastroileac a.
    gastroileal a.

augmented histamine test

auscultation of bowel sounds

auscultatory sound

autocholecystectomy

autocystoplasty

autodigestion

autodrainage

autoimmune
    chronic a. hepatitis
    a. cirrhosis

autoimmune *(continued)*
    a. connective tissue disorder
    a. deficiency syndrome
    a. disease
    a. gastritis
    a. hemolytic anemia
    a. hepatitis
    idiopathic a. cholangitis

autolavage

autologous liver cell

automated endoscopic system for optimal positioning (AESOP)

automatic bladder

autonephrectomy

autonephrotoxin

autonomic
    a. bladder
    a. neuropathy

autonomous bladder

autoplasty
    peritoneal a.

autosuture
    GIA a. apparatus
    GIA a. device

autotoxic cyanosis

autotransplantation
    colostomy pyloric a.
    posttraumatic a.
    pyloric a.
    a. of splenic fragment

AV
    arteriovenous
        AV fistula

avascular
    a. necrosis

avenolith

AVH
    acute viral hepatitis

avulsion
    splenic a.

axial
    a. hiatal hernia
    a. plane

Axid

axis *pl.* axes
    bowel a.
    brain-gut a.
    cardiopyloric a.
    celiac a.
    a. deviation
    renal a.
    renin-aldosterone a.

axis *(continued)*
    renin-angiotensin a.

axillary adenopathy

azole antifungal agent

azoospermatism

azoospermia

azotemia
    extrarenal a.
    postrenal a.
    prerenal a.
    renal a.

azotemic
    a. nephritis

B₁₂
    B$_{12}$ anemia
B5
    B5 tumor marker
bacillary
    b. dysentery
    b. peliosis
backflow
    pyelovenous b.
Bacon anoscope
bacterascites
    monomicrobial non-neutro-
        cytic b.
    polymicrobial b.
bacteria (*plural* of bacterium)
bacterial
    b. adherence
    b. adhesion
    b. biofilm
    b. cast
    b. cholangitis
    chronic b. enteropathy
    b. cirrhosis
    b. colitis
    b. cystitis
    b. endotoxin
    b. enterocolitis
    b. esophagitis
    b. flora
    b. food poisoning
    b. infection
    b. metabolism in intestines
    b. mucosal infiltration
    b. nephritis
    b. overgrowth
    b. overgrowth syndrome
    b. peritonitis
bacteriospermia
bacterium *pl.* bacteria
    coliform bacteria
    colonic bacteria
    gram-negative bacteria
    gram-positive bacteria

bacterium *(continued)*
    human gut bacteria
    intestinal bacteria
    mesophilic bacteria
    pathogenic bacteria
    pyogenic bacteria
    spiral bacteria
    toxigenic bacteria
Baehr-Löhlein lesion
Baermann
    B. stool filter
    B. stool test
bag
    bile b.
    Biohazard b.
    bowel b.
    colostomy b.
    DeRoyal Surgical grab b.
    EndoMate grab b.
    Hagner b.
    Hollister urostomy b.
    ileostomy b.
    intestinal b.
    Lahey liver transplant b.
    Le B.
    micturition b.
    ostomy b.
    perfusate b.
    Perry b.
    Petersen b.
    Pilcher b.
    Plummer b.
    pneumatic b.
    stomal b.
    Vacutainer b.
    Whitmore b.
Bainbridge intestinal clamp
Baker
    B. antifol
    B. intestinal decompres-
        sion tube
    B. jejunostomy tube
Bakes common duct dilator
baking soda

Balance lavage solution

balance
acid-base b.
chloride b.
electrolyte b.
equal fluid b.
metabolic b.
negative nitrogen b.
nitrogen b.
positive nitrogen b.
potassium b.
sodium b.
vagosympathetic b.

balanced
b. diet
b. electrolyte solution

balanic
b. epispadias
b. hypospadias

balanitic
b. epispadias
b. hypospadias

balanitis
amebic b.
b. circinata
b. circumscripta plasmacellularis
b. diabetica
erosive b.
Follmann b.
b. gangraenosa
gangrenous b.
phagedenic b.
plasma cell b.
b. plasmacellularis
b. xerotica obliterans

balanocele

balanoplasty

balanoposthitis
chronic circumscribed
plasmocytic b.
b. chronica circumscripta
plasmocellularis
specific gangrenous and ulcerative b.

balanoposthomycosis

balanopreputial

balanorrhagia

balantidial
b. colitis
b. dysentery

balantidiasis

balantidiosis

balantidosis

balanus

Balkan
B. nephritis
B. nephropathy

Balfour
B. abdominal retractor
B. gastroenterostomy
B. retractor
B. self-retaining retractor

Ball valves

ball
food b.
fungal b.

balloon
achalasia b. dilation
angioplasty b.
banana-shaped b.
barostat b.
biliary b. dilator
Bilisystem stone removal b.
b. cholangiogram
b. decompression
b. defecation
b. dilation
b. dilation of the papilla
b. dilator
dissecting b.
endoscopic papillary b. dilation
esophageal b.
esophageal b. dilator
esophageal b. distention
esophageal b. tamponade

balloon *(continued)*
    b. esophagoscope
    French Swan-Ganz b.
    Gan gastric b.
    Garren-Edwards b.
    gastric b.
    intragastric b.
    occlusion b.
    b. occlusion cholangiography
    Percival gastric b.
    percutaneous b. dilation
    b. proctogram
    rectal b.
    Rigiflex achalasia b.
    Rigiflex TTS b.
    Sengstaken-Blakemore esophageal b.
    stone retrieval b.
    b. tamponade
    Taylor gastric b.
    through-the-scope b.
    Wilson-Cook dilating b.
    Wilson-Cook esophageal b.
    Wilson-Cook gastric b.
    windowed esophageal b.

ballooning
    b. degeneration of hepatocytes
    eosinophilic b.
    hepatocellular b.

ballotable liver

ballottement
    renal b.
    b. tenderness

Balser fatty necrosis

banana-shaped balloon

bananas, rice cereal, applesauce, tea, and toast (BRATT)

bananas, rice cereal, applesauce and toast (BRAT)

band
    adhesive b.
    anorectal b.

band *(continued)*
    anterior b. of colon
    dysgenetic fibrous b.
    free b. of colon
    Harris b.
    Henle b.
    Ladd b's
    Lane b's
    b. ligation
    longitudinal b's of colon
    Marlex b.
    mesocolic b.
    omental b.
    omphalodiverticular b.
    peritoneal b.
    retention b.

banding
    esophageal b.
    hemorrhoid b.
    hemorrhoidal b.

B_{12} anemia

banjo-string adhesion

bar
    b. of bladder
    cricopharyngeal b.
    intersymphyseal b.
    median b.
    Mercier b.
    symphyseal b.
    b.-type esophageal varix

barbaloin

Barcoo
    B. vomit
    B. vomitus

Bard
    B. gastrostomy catheter
    B. gastrostomy feeding tube
    B. PEG
    B. PEG tube
    B. protective barrier

bare area of liver

bariatric
    b. operation
    b. surgery

Baricon
  B. contrast medium

barium
  air contrast b. enema
    (ACBE)
  b. bezoar
  b. burger
  b. contrast radiography
  double-contrast air b. en-
    ema
  double-contrast b. enema
  b. enema (BE)
  b. enema reduction
  b. enema with air contrast
  b. esophagram
  flexible b. enema
  full-column b. enema
  b. granuloma
  b.-impregnated marshmal-
    low
  b. meal
  b. peritonitis
  puddling on b. enema
  residual b.
  retained b.
  b. retention
  retrograde flow on b. en-
    ema
  single-contrast b. enema
  b. study
  b. sulfate
  b. suspension
  b. swallow

bark
  bearberry b.
  buckthorn b.
  chittem b.
  Purshiana b.
  sacred b.

Baroflave
  B. contrast medium

baroreceptor-mediated mesenteric arterial vasoconstriction

Barosperse
  B. contrast medium

barostat balloon

Barr
  B. fistula hook
  B. fistula probe
  B. rectal retractor
  B. rectal speculum
  B.-Shuford rectal speculum

Barrett
  B. carcinoma
  B. disease
  B. dysplasia
  B. epithelium
  B. esophagitis
  B. esophagus (BE)
  B. intestinal forceps
  B. metaplasia
  B. syndrome
  B. ulcer

barrier
  ABO b.
  Bard protective b.
  blood-testis b.
  blood-urine b.
  filtration b.
  gastric mucosal b.

Barron
  B. ligation
  B. rubber band ligator

Barth hernia

Bartter syndrome

baruria

basal
  b. anal canal pressure
  b. anal sphincter pressure
  b. cell carcinoma
  b. diet
  b. interferon-gamma
  b. metabolic rate
  b. pelviprostatic ligament
  b. pressure
  b. renal excretion
  b. renal vascular resistance

Basaljel

basaloid
  b. carcinoma

bascule
    cecal b.

base
    b. of appendix
    b. excess
    b. of prostate
    ulcer b.

baseplate

bas-fond

basic
    b. aluminum carbonate
    b. aluminum carbonate gel
    b. bismuth carbonate

basis *pl.* bases
    b. prostatae
    b. pyramidis renalis

basket
    Dormia b.
    b. extractor
    Gemini paired wire heli-
        cal b.

Bassini
    B. inguinal hernia repair
    B. inguinal herniorrhaphy
    B. operation

bath
    alcohol cooling b.
    HydraClense sitz b.
    sitz b.

bathroom privileges

battery-powered endoscope

Battle operation

Bauhin valve

B bile

BBS
    brown bowel syndrome

BCAA
    branched-chain amino acid

B cell
    B c. growth factor

B cell *(continued)*
    noncleaved B c.

BDA
    bile duct adenoma

BDL
    bile duct ligation

BE
    barium enema
    Barrett esophagus

beaded hepatic duct

Beale
    sacculi of B.

bearberry
    b. bark

bear claw ulcer

Beardsley esophageal retractor

Bearn
    B.-Kunkel syndrome
    B.-Kunkel-Slater syndrome

bearwood

BEB
    blind esophageal binding

Beck
    B. gastrostomy
    B. method

Béclard hernia

bed
    gallbladder b.
    graft b.
    hepatic b.

beef tapeworm

behavior
    binge-purge b.

Behçet
    B. colitis
    B. disease
    B. syndrome

Behrend cystic duct forceps

belch

belching

Bell muscle

bell
  b.-shaped orifice

Belladenal

belladonna
  b. extract
  b. tincture

Bellergal-S

Bellini
  B. duct
  B. tubule

belly
  drum b.
  wooden b.

bellyache

Belsey
  B. Mark IV antireflux operation
  B. Mark IV 240-degree fundoplication
  B. Mark IV fundoplication
  B. Mark IV operation
  B. Mark IV repair
  B. partial fundoplication
  B. two-thirds wrap fundoplication

Belt technique

belt
  abdominal compression b.
  b. test

Belzer
  B. machine
  B. solution
  B. UW liver preservation solution

Bence Jones cylinders

Benchekroun
  B. hydraulic valve
  B. ileal valve
  B. pouch

Benchekroun *(continued)*
  B. stoma

Benedict gastroscope

benign
  b. adenomatous polyp
  b. anorectal disease (BAD)
  b. arteriolar nephrosclerosis
  b. bile duct stricture
  b. biliary stricture
  b. cystic mesothelioma
  b. cystic teratoma
  b. duodenocolic fistula
  b. familial hematuria
  b. familial icterus
  b. gastric ulcer
  b. glycosuria
  b. hyperplastic gastropathy
  b. mesothelioma of genital tract
  b. mucous membrane pemphigoid
  b. neoplastic precursor
  b. nephrosclerosis
  b. papillary stenosis
  b. paroxysmal peritonitis
  b. pneumatic colonoscopy complication
  b. pneumatic problem
  b. pneumoperitoneum
  b. postoperative jaundice
  b. prostatic hyperplasia
  b. prostatic hypertrophy
  b. recurrent hematuria
  b. recurrent intrahepatic cholestasis
  b. stenosis
  b. stricture
  b. tumor
  b. ulcer

Benson pylorus separator

Bentyl

benzodiazepine
  b. conscious sedation
  b.-induced hypoventilation

benzoin
  tincture of b.

Berci-Shore choledochoscope

Berens esophageal retractor

Berger disease

Bernard
  B. duct
  B. glandular layer

Bernstein
  B. acid perfusion test
  B. gastroscope

berry
  buckthorn b.

Bertin
  columns of B.

Best
  B. bite block
  B. gallstone forceps
  B. right-angle colon clamp

beta
  b.-HCG
  b. interferon
  interferon b.
  b.-lactam−associated diar-
    rhea
  b.-sympathomimetic toco-
    lytic agent

beta-adrenergic antagonist

Bevan
  B. abdominal incision
  B. gallbladder forceps
  B. operation
  B. orchiopexy

bezoar
  artificial b.
  barium b.
  fungal b.
  gastric b.
  medication b.
  persimmon b.

BIB
  biliointestinal bypass

BICAP
  BICAP Hemorrhoid System

BICAP *(continued)*
  BICAP Hemostatic System
  BICAP Probe
  BICAP Silver ACE Hemosta-
    sis Probe

bicarbonate
  saliva b.
  b. of soda

Bicitra

bicornuate uterus

bicoudate catheter

bidirectional ligation

bifid tongue

bifurcation
  b. of common bile duct
  b. tumor

Bigelow operation

bilabe

bilateral
  b. lithotomy
  b. pudendal artery emboli-
    zation
  b. subcostal incision
  b. transabdominal incision

bile
  A b.
  b. acid (BA)
  b. acid breath test
  b. acid−EDTA solution
  b. acid malabsorption
  b. acid measurement
  b. acid pool
  b. acid therapy
  b. acid tolerance test
  b. ascites
  B b.
  b. bag
  C b.
  b. canaliculi
  b. capillaries
  cloudy b.
  b. concretion
  cystic b.
  gallbladder b.

bile *(continued)*
   inspissated b.
   b. lake
   b. leakage
   limy b.
   lithogenic b.
   milk of calcium b.
   obstruction of b. flow
   b. papilla
   b. peritonitis
   b. pigment
   b. pleuritis
   b. plug
   b. pulmonary embolism
   b. reflux
   b. reflux gastritis
   b. salts
   b. salt diarrhea
   b. salt–losing enteropathy
   b. salt–phospholipid ratio
   b. solubility test
   stagnant b.
   b. stasis
   thick b.
   b. thrombus
   turbid b.
   b. vessels
   viscid b.
   viscous b.
   white b.

bile duct
   b. d. abscess
   b. d. adenoma (BDA)
   bifurcation of common
     b. d.
   b. d. brushing
   b. d. calculus
   b. d. canaliculus
   b. d. cancer
   b. d. cannulation
   b. d. carcinoma
   common b. d. (CBD)
   common b. d. exploration
     (CBDE)
   common b. d. obstruction
   common b. d. stent
   common b. d. stone
   common b. d. varices
   Crile b. d. forceps

bile duct *(continued)*
   b. d. cystadenoma
   dilated b. d.
   distal b. d.
   b. d. dyskinesia
   b. d. epithelial cell
   extrahepatic b. d.
   glands of b. d.
   b. d. hypoplasia
   infected b. d.
   infundibulum of b. d.
   interlobular b. d's
   intrahepatic b. d.
   intrapancreatic b. d.
   Kron b. d. dilator
   b. d. ligation
   b. d. lumen
   Moynihan b. d. probe
   b. d. paucity
   b. d. pressure
   b. d. proliferation
   sphincter muscle of b. d.
   b. d. stone
   b. d. stricture
   terminal b. d.
   b. d. trauma
   b. d.–type cytokeratin

bile ductules

bile-laden macrophage

bile salt–binding resin

bile-stained
   b.-s. fluid
   b.-s. vomitus

bile-tinged fluid

bilharzial
   b. carcinoma
   b. dysentery

biliaropancreatic
   b. ampulla

biliary
   b. abscess
   acholangic b. cirrhosis
   b. actinomycosis
   b. air
   b. antispasmodic

biliary *(continued)*
- b. apparatus
- b. ascites
- b. atresia
- b. balloon catheter
- b. balloon dilator
- b. balloon probe
- b.-bronchial fistula
- b. calculus
- b. canaliculi
- b. cannulation
- cannulation of the b. tree
- b. carcinoma
- cholangitic b. cirrhosis
- b. cholesterol secretion
- b. cirrhosis
- b. cirrhotic liver
- b. clonorchiasis
- b. colic
- b.-cutaneous fistula
- b. cycle
- b. cyst
- b. decompression
- b. dilatation
- b. dilation
- b. diverticulum
- b. drainage
- b. duct
- b. ductules
- b.-duodenal fistula
- b. dyskinesia
- b. dyspepsia
- b. dyssynergia
- b. echinococcosis
- b. endoprosthesis
- b.-enteric fistula
- b. excretion
- b. fibroadenomatosis
- b. fistula
- focal b. cirrhosis
- b. glands
- b. hypercholesterolemia xanthomatosis
- b. infestation
- b. instrumentation
- interlobular b. canals
- intralobular b. canals
- b. leakage
- b. lipid

biliary *(continued)*
- b. lithotripsy
- malignant b. obstruction
- b. manometry
- b. microhamartoma
- b. mud
- obstructive b. cirrhosis
- b. pain
- b. pancreatitis
- b. passages
- b. peritonitis
- b. piecemeal necrosis
- b. plexus
- b. pore
- primary b. cirrhosis
- b. prosthesis
- b. radicle
- b. saturation index
- b. scintiscan
- b. sclerosis
- secondary b. cirrhosis
- b. sepsis
- b. sludge
- b. sphincter
- b. sphincterotomy
- b. stasis
- b. steatorrhea
- b. stent
- b. stenting
- b. stent patency
- b. stricture
- b. tract
- b. tract disease
- b. tract obstruction
- b. tract pressure
- b. tract stricture
- b. xanthomatosis

biliary-bronchial fistula

biliary-cutaneous fistula

biliary-duodenal
- b.-d. fistula
- b.-d. pressure gradient

biliary-enteric fistula

biliary-like

bilicyanin

bilifaction *(also* bilification)

biliferous
   b. tubule

biliflavin

bilifuscin

biligenesis

biligenetic

biligenic

Biligrafin
   B. contrast medium

bilihumin

bilin

biliodigestive anastomosis

bilioduodenal prosthesis

bilioenteric
   b. bypass
   b. fistula

biliointestinal bypass (BIB)

biliopancreatic
   b. bypass
   b. diversion
   b. shunt

bilious
   b. colic
   b. diarrhea
   b. emesis
   b. remittent fever
   b. remittent malaria
   b. stool
   b. vomit
   b. vomiting

biliousness

biliprasin

bilirachia

bilirubin
   conjugated b.
   direct b.
   b. encephalopathy
   fat-soluble b.
   fractionation of b.

bilirubin *(continued)*
   indirect b.
   b. pigment gallstone
   serum b.
   b. test
   total b.
   unconjugated b.
   urine b.
   water-soluble b.

bilirubinate

bilirubinemia

bilirubinic

bilirubinuria

Biliscopin
   B. contrast medium

Bilisystem
   B. ERCP cannula
   B. stone removal balloon
   B. wire-guided papillotome

bilitherapy

biliverdin

biliverdinate

Bilivist
   B. contrast medium

Billingham-Bookwalter rectal
  fenestrated blade

Billroth
   B. I anastomosis
   B. II anastomosis
   B. forceps
   B. gastrectomy
   B. I gastrectomy
   B. II gastrectomy
   B. I gastroenterostomy
   B. II gastroenterostomy
   B. II gastrojejunostomy
   B. hypertrophy
   B. operation
   B. I reconstruction
   B. II reconstruction

bilobar
   b. hyperplasia
   b. hypertrophy

bilobate false aneurysm

bilobed
b. gallbladder
b. polypoid lesion

bilocular stomach

biloma

Bilopaque
B. contrast medium

Biloptin
B. contrast medium

Biltricide

binding
blind esophageal b. (BEB)

binge

bingeing

binge-purge behavior

bioartificial liver support device

biocompatibility

biodigestive anastomosis

bioelectrical impedance analysis

biofilm
bacterial b.

biofragmentable anastomotic ring

Biohazard bag

Biolab
Malakit *Helicobacter pylori* B.

biopsy
alcohol-fixed gastric b.
antral b.
aspiration b.
bite b.
blind percutaneous liver b.
bone marrow b.
brush b.
brush and b.
b. capsule

biopsy *(continued)*
b. channel
CLO b.
cold b.
cold cup b.
colonoscopic b.
colorectal b.
core needle b.
corporal b.
CT-guided liver b.
CT-guided needle-aspiration b.
cytologic b.
digitally guided b.
direct vision liver b.
endoscopic b.
endoscopic small bowel b.
ERCP-guided b.
esophageal b.
exploratory b.
fine-needle b.
fine-needle aspiration b.
b. forceps
b. of gastric mucosa
guided transcutaneous b.
guillotine needle b.
b. gun
hot b.
ileal b.
incisional b.
b. instrument
laparoscopic b.
large-particle b.
lift-and-cut b.
liver b.
mucosal b.
multiple b.
native renal b.
needle b.
open b.
percutaneous b.
percutaneous fine-needle pancreatic b.
percutaneous liver b.
percutaneous native renal b.
percutaneous pancreas b.
peritoneal b.
pouch b.

biopsy *(continued)*
    b. punch
    punch b.
    rectal b.
    renal b.
    saucerized b.
    scan-directed b.
    shave b.
    skinny-needle b.
    small-bowel b.
    snap-frozen b.
    snare excision b.
    snare loop b.
    sonoguided b.
    strip b.
    suction b.
    systematic sextant b.
    tangential b.
    transcutaneous b.
    transgastric fine-needle aspiration b.
    transitional zone b.
    transjugular liver b.
    transpapillary b.
    transrectal ultrasound-guided–sextant b.
    transvenous liver b.
    Tru-Cut b.
    Tru-Cut needle b.
    ultrasound-guided b.
    Vim-Silverman technique for liver b.
    Watson capsule b.
    wedge hepatic b.

bisacodyl
    b. tannex

bisegmentectomy

bishop cap

bismuth
    basic b. carbonate
    b. benign bile duct stricture classification
    b. compound
    b.-free triple therapy
    b. salt
    b. subcarbonate
    b. subgallate

bismuth *(continued)*
    b. subnitrate
    b. subsalicylate

bismuth, metronidazole, tetracycline (BMT)

bite biopsy

bite block
    Best b. b.
    OB-10 Comfort b. b.

bitter
    aromatic b's
    b. tonic

Bittorf reaction

bizarre leiomyoma

black
    b. hairy tongue
    b. jaundice
    b. liver disease
    b. pigment gallstone
    b. pigment stone
    b. tarry stool
    b. vomit
    b. vomitus

bladder
    areflexic b.
    atonic b.
    atonic neurogenic b.
    b. augmentation
    automatic b.
    autonomic b.
    b. carcinoma
    cord b.
    denervated b.
    double b.
    fasciculated b.
    ileal b.
    ileocecal b.
    ileocolonic b.
    irritable b.
    motor paralytic b.
    b. neck
    nervous b.
    neurogenic b.
    nonneurogenic neurogenic b.

bladder *(continued)*
    nonreflex b.
    opening of b.
    orthotopic b.
    b. outlet
    paralytic b.
    b. prolapse
    reflex b.
    b. reflex
    sacculated b.
    schistosomal b. carcinoma
    sensory paralytic b.
    spastic b.
    b. stone
    string b.
    tabetic b.
    b. training
    uninhibited neurogenic b.
    urinary b.
    ileal b.
    autonomous b.

blade
    Billingham-Bookwalter rectal fenestrated b.
    Bookwalter-Cook anal rectal b.
    Bookwalter malleable retractor b.
    Bookwalter-Mayo b.
    Bookwalter-Parks anal sphincter b.
    Bovie b.
    knife b.
    malleable b.
    razor b.
    scalpel b.

Blake gallstone forceps

bland
    b. diet
    b. food
    b. thrombosis

bleb

bleed
    gastrointestinal (GI) b.
    herald b.
    postgastrectomy b.
    postpolypectomy b.

bleeder

bleeding
    b. acid-peptic disease
    active source of b.
    b. angioma
    b. colonic angiodysplasia
    colorectal b.
    b. control
    diverticular b.
    duodenal b.
    dysfunctional b.
    esophageal variceal b.
    esophagogastric variceal b.
    excessive b.
    functional b.
    gastric b.
    gastric b. time
    gastric variceal b.
    b. gastritis
    gastrointestinal b.
    GI (gastrointestinal) b.
    b. hemorrhoid
    jetlike b.
    b. lesion
    lower GI (gastrointestinal) b.
    occult b.
    occult GI (gastrointestinal) b.
    pancreatitis-related b.
    b. peptic ulcer
    b. per rectum
    b. point
    b. polyp
    rectal b.
    b. site
    b. site localization
    b. time
    b. tumor
    upper gastrointestinal b. (UGIB)
    vaginal b.
    variceal b.

blenderized diet

blennemesis

blind
    b. cautery
    b. enema

blind *(continued)*
  b. esophageal binding (BEB)
  b. esophageal brushing
  b. gut
  b. intestine
  b. limb
  b. lithotripsy
  b. loop
  b. loop syndrome
  b. percutaneous liver biopsy
  b. stump
  b. technique
  b. upper esophageal pouch

blindgut

Blocadren

block
  Best bite b.
  OB-10 Comfort bite b.

blockade
  alpha b.
  alpha sympathetic b.
  renal b.

blocked aerogastria

blocker
  alpha$_1$ b.
  H$_2$ receptor b.
  proton pump b.
  starch b.

Blom
  B.-Singer esophagoscope
  B.-Singer tracheoesophageal fistula

blood
  b. admixed with stool
  b. ammonia
  bright red b.
  b. calculus
  b. cast
  b. clot
  clotted b.
  crossmatched b.
  b. culture
  frank b.
  frank b. in stool

blood *(continued)*
  b. gas on oxygen
  b. gas on room air
  gastroepiploic b. vessel
  b. glucose
  ileal b. vessel
  nonhemolyzed b.
  nostril b.
  occult b.
  oozing b.
  b. passed with stool
  b. pressure
  stool for occult b.
  b. in stool
  b. stream infection
  b. on surface of stool
  b. vessel

blood-testis barrier

blood-tinged ascites

blood-urea clearance

blood-urine barrier

bloody
  b. ascites
  b. diarrhea
  b. discharge
  b. peritoneal fluid
  b. stool
  b. vomitus

blow-hole ileostomy

Blumberg
  inguinal ligament of B.
  B. sign

Blumer rectal shelf

blunt
  b. abdominal trauma
  b. dissection
  b. liver trauma
  b. needle
  b. pancreatic trauma
  b. probe
  b. and sharp dissection
  b. trauma

blunting
  costophrenic b.
  haustral b.

blunting *(continued)*
    b. of valve

blunt-tipped obturator

BM
    bowel movement

BMT
    bismuth, metronidazole,
        tetracycline (BMT)

boardlike
    b. rigidity
    b. rigidity of abdomen

Boari flap

Boas
    B. point
    B. sign
    B. test

boat-shaped abdomen

Bochdalek hernia

body
    acidophilic b.
    anal foreign b.
    angularis b.
    anorectal foreign b.
    cavernous b. of penis
    b. composition analysis
    crystalloid b.
    b. of epididymis
    esophageal foreign b.
    foreign b.
    b. of gallbladder
    gastric b.
    b. habitus
    b. of Highmore
    Jaworski b's
    Lallemand b's
    Lallemand-Trousseau b's
    Lieutaud b.
    Mallory b's
    malpighian b's of kidney
    Michaelis-Gutmann b's
    Nothnagel b's
    b. of pancreas
    paranephric b.
    pararenal fat b.
    rectal foreign b.

body *(continued)*
    spongy b. of male urethra
    spongy b. of penis
    b. of stomach
    Trousseau-Lallemand b's
    vermiform b's

Boerema anterior gastropexy

Boerhaave syndrome

bolster suture

bolus
    alimentary b.
    b. dressing
    b. feeding
    food b.
    food b. impaction
    food b. obstruction
    marshmallow b.
    solid b. challenge

bone marrow biopsy

bony tenderness

Bookwalter
    B. malleable retractor
        blade
    B.-Cook anal rectal blade
    B.-Mayo blade
    B.-Parks anal sphincter
        blade

BOR
    branchio-oto-renal
        BOR syndrome

borborygmus *pl.* borborygmi

border
    anterior b. of body of pan-
        creas
    anterior b. of pancreas
    antimesenteric b.
    antimesenteric b. of distal
        ileum
    b. cells
    fundopyloric mucosal b.
    inferior b. of body of pan-
        creas
    inferior b. of liver
    inferior b. of pancreas

border *(continued)*
    superior b. of body of pancreas
    superior b. of pancreas

boring pain

Borrmann gastric cancer classification

Bouchard disease

bougie
    b. à boule
    acorn-tipped b.
    bulbous b.
    conic b.
    cylindrical b.
    dilating b.
    b. dilator
    elastic b.
    elbowed b.
    filiform b.
    French b.
    fusiform b.
    Hegar b.
    Hurst b's
    Jackson esophageal b.
    large-diameter b.
    Maloney b's
    olive-tipped b.
    Trousseau esophageal b.
    wax-tipped b.
    whip b.

bougienage
    transgastric esophageal b.

bout
    recurrent b's of vomiting

Bouveret syndrome

Bovie blade

bovine graft

bowel
    aganglionic b.
    b. axis
    b. bag
    b. bypass
    b. bypass syndrome
    Child-Phillips b. plication

bowel *(continued)*
    Colonlite b. prep
    b. contents
    b. continuity
    dead b.
    b. dilatation
    dilated loops of b.
    b. dilation
    Dulcolax b. prep
    Emulsoil b. prep
    Evac-Q-Kit b. prep
    Evac-Q-Kwik b. prep
    fluid-filled small b.
    b. function
    functional b. disorder (FBD)
    functional b. distress
    b. gas
    GoLYTELY b. prep
    b. habits
    high-pitched b. sounds
    hyperactive b. sounds
    inadequate b. prep
    incarcerated b.
    infarcted b.
    ischemic b.
    b. intussusception
    kink in b.
    large b.
    large b. carcinoma
    b. loop
    musical b. sounds
    b. necrosis
    b. obstruction
    b. perforation
    b. plate
    pleating of small b.
    b. prep
    b. preparation
    b. preparation complication
    prolapsed b.
    b. pseudo-obstruction
    b. refashioning procedure
    b. resection
    b. rest
    small b.
    b. sounds
    b. stoma

bowel *(continued)*
    strangulated b.
    b. tone
    b. training
    b. wall

bowel prep
    bowel preparation

Bower PEG tube

Bowman
    B. capsule
    B. space

Boyce sign

Boyden
    sphincter of B.

Braasch bulb catheter

brachiocephalic fistula

brachiosubclavian bridge graft
    fistula

brachyesophagus

Brackin
    B. technique
    B. ureterointestinal anasto-
        mosis

Bradley disease

bradygastria

bradypepsia

bradyphagia

bradyspermatism

bradystalsis

bradyuria

brain-gut axis

brain metastasis
    bran

branched-chain amino acid
    (BCAA)

branchio-oto-renal
    b. syndrome

brash
    water b.

BRAT diet

BRATT diet

Braun
    B. anastomosis
    B. stent
    B.-Jaboulay gastroenteros-
        tomy

breakbone fever

breakfast
    Ewald b.

breath
    b. alkane
    liver b.

breathing
    diaphragmatic b.

Brescia-Cimino fistula

Brewer
    B. infarcts
    B. point

Bricker
    B. operation
    B. pouch
    B. ureteroileostomy
    B. urinary diversion

bridge
    agar b.
    colostomy b.
    loop ostomy b.
    mucosal b.
    ureteric b.

bridging necrosis

Bright
    B. disease
    B. granulations

bright red
    b. r. blood
    b. r. blood per rectum
    b. r. vomitus

brightic

brightism

brim
    pelvic b.

brimstone liver

Brinkerhoff
    B. rectal speculum
    B. speculum

Brinton disease

broad-based
    b.-b. gait
    b.-b. polyp

broad ligament of liver

broad-spectrum antibiotic

Brödel white line

Brodie sign

Broesike fossa

Broncho-Cath double-lumen endotracheal tube

bronchoesophageal
    b. muscle
    b. fistula

bronchoesophagology

bronchoesophagoscopy

Brooke ileostomy

brown
    b. bowel syndrome (BBS)
    b. stool

Browne operation

Brown-Séquard paralysis

Bruening esophagoscope

bruit
    abdominal b's

Brunn epithelial nests

Brunner
    B. glands

Brunner (continued)
    B. gland adenoma
    B. gland hamartoma

Brunschwig operation

brush
    b. biopsy
    b. and biopsy
    stomach b.

brush-border
    b.-b. enzyme activity
    b.-b. hydrolase activity

brushing
    bile duct b.

brushite
    b. calculus

B5 tumor marker

bubble
    Garren gastric b.
    Garren-Edwards gastric b.
    gastric air b.
    GEG b.
    intragastric b.
    b. therapy

bubble-free

bubonocele

buccal
    b. mucosa
    b. mucosal patch graft

bucket-handle incision

Buck fascia

buckthorn
    alder b.
    b. bark
    b. berry
    cascara b.
    common b.

bud
    b. of urethra

Budd
    B. cirrhosis

Budd (continued)
    B. disease
    B. jaundice
    B.-Chiari syndrome

buffer solution

Buie
    B. clamp
    B. fistula probe
    B. forceps
    B. pile clamp
    B. pile forceps
    B. position
    B. rectal scissors
    B. rectal suction tip
    B. rectal suction tube
    B. suction tip

Build Up enteral feeding

bulb
    apex of duodenal b.
    b. of corpus spongiosum
    b. deformity
    duodenal b.
    b. of penis
    b. of urethra

bulbar
    b. colliculus
    b. peptic ulcer

bulbitis

bulbocavernosus
    bulbocavernous gland
    bulbocavernous muscle

bulbospongiosus

bulbourethral
    b. gland

bulbous bougie

bulbus pl. bulbi
    b. corporis spongiosi
    b. penis
    b. urethrae

bulge
    inguinal b.

bulging
    anal b.
    b. flank

bulimia nervosa

bulk
    b. cathartic
    b.-forming laxative
    high b., low fat diet
    b. laxative

bulkage

bulking agent

bulk laxative

bulky stool

bullous edema

bull's eye lesion

bumetanide

bundle
    fiber b.
    fiberoptic b.

burbulence

Burch culposuspension

Burkitt lymphoma

burning pain

bursa pl. bursae
    omental b.
    b. omentalis
    b. of testes

bursitis
    omental b.

Buselmeier shunt

butter stool

button
    b. drainage
    b. gastrostomy
    gastrostomy b.
    Jaboulay b.
    Murphy b.

button *(continued)*
    One-Step gastric b.
    peritoneal b.

buttonhole incision

buttress
    fascia lata b.

bypass
    Alden loop gastric b.
    aortic/superior mesenteric
      artery b.
    aortorenal b.
    bilioenteric b.
    biliointestinal b. (BIB)
    biliopancreatic b.
    bowel b.
    bowel b. syndrome
    duodenoileal b.

bypass *(continued)*
    gastric b.
    b. graft
    Greenville gastric b.
    Griffen Roux-en-Y b.
    Hallberg biliointestinal b.
    hepatorenal b.
    iliorenal b.
    intestinal b.
    jejunal b.
    jejunoileal b.
    mesenterorenal b.
    partial ileal b.
    Roux-en-Y biliary b. with
      antrectomy
    Roux-en-Y gastric b.
    splenorenal b.

Bywaters syndrome

C
C bile

CA
cholic acid

cacation

cacatory

Cacchi-Ricci disease

cachectic
c. diarrhea
c. fever

cachexia
malignant c.
uremic c.

cadaver
c. kidney
c. renal preservation

cadaveric
c. renal transplant
c. liver transplant
c. transplant

caecum

caecus
c. minor ventriculi

caffeine, alcohol, peppery,
spicy foods (CAPS)

CAG
chronic atrophic gastritis

CAGEIN
catheter-guided endo-
scopic intubation

CAH
chronic active hepatitis
chronic aggressive hepatitis
congenital adrenal hyper-
plasia

Cajal
interstitial cells of C.

cake kidney

calcareous pancreatitis

calcification
dystrophic c.
pancreatic c.

calcific pancreatitis

calcified
c. enterolith
c. gallstone

calcifying
chronic c. pancreatitis
c. pancreatitis

Calcijex

calcipyelitis

calcium
c. acetate
c. antagonist
c. carbonate
c. channel antagonist
c. citrate
docusate c.
c. oxalate
c. oxalate calculus
c. phosphate calculus
c. polycarbophil
precipitated c. carbonate
prepared c. carbonate

calculogenesis

calculous
c. anuria
c. cholecystitis
c. cirrhosis
c. formation
c. gallbladder disease
c. pyelitis

calculus *pl.* calculi
alternating c.
apatite c.
bile duct c.
biliary c.
blood c.
brushite c.
calcium oxalate c.

calculus *(continued)*
- calcium phosphate c.
- caliceal diverticular c.
- cholesterol c.
- c. cirrhosis
- combination c.
- coral c.
- cystine c.
- decubitus c.
- c. disease
- encysted c.
- fibrin c.
- fusible c.
- gallbladder c.
- gastric c.
- gonecystic c.
- hemp seed c.
- hepatic c.
- impacted c.
- indigo c.
- infection c.
- intestinal c.
- matrix c.
- metabolic c.
- c. migration
- mulberry c.
- nephritic c.
- oxalate c.
- pancreatic c.
- pocketed c.
- preputial c.
- primary renal c.
- prostatic c.
- renal c.
- secondary renal c.
- shellac c.
- spermatic c.
- staghorn c.
- stomach c.
- stomachic c.
- struvite c.
- submucosal c.
- triple phosphate c.
- urethral c.
- uric acid c.
- urinary c.
- urostealith c.
- vesical c.
- vesicoprostatic c.

calculus *(continued)*
- Volkmann spoon for pancreatic c.
- weddellite c.
- whewellite c.
- whitlockite c.
- xanthic c.

caliceal
- c. diverticular calculus
- c. diverticulum

calicectasis

calicectomy

calicivirus gastroenteritis

caliectasis

caliectomy

calix *pl.* calices
- greater renal calices
- major renal calices
- minor renal calices
- renal calices
- calices renales
- calices renales majores
- calices renales minores

calorie
- high c. diet
- low c. diet

Calot triangle

calyceal
- c. diverticulum
- c. fistula

calycectasis

calycectomy

calyx *pl.* calyces
- calyces renales
- calyces renales majores
- calyces renales minores

camera adapter

Cameron
- C. gastroscope
- C. omni-angle gastroscope

Camey
- C. enterocystoplasty

Camey *(continued)*
    C. enterocystoplasty urinary diversion
    C. ileocystoplasty
    C. neobladder
    C. procedure
    C. urinary pouch

Camper
    fascia of C.
    C. ligament

camphorated opium tincture

Campylobacter
    C. enteritis

Canada-Cronkhite syndrome

Canadian repair

canal
    abdominal c.
    alimentary c.
    anal c.
    connecting c.
    digestive c.
    c. of epididymis
    gastric c.
    Henle c.
    c's of Hering
    hernial c.
    inguinal c.
    interlobular biliary c's
    intralobular biliary c's
    intestinal c.
    c. of Nuck
    pancreatobiliary c.
    paraurethral c's of male urethra
    portal c.
    pyloric c.
    Santorini c.
    seminal c.
    sheathing c.
    spermatic c.
    c. of stomach
    urogenital c's
    Velpeau c.
    ventricular c.
    c. of Wirsung

canalicular
    c. cholestasis

canaliculus *pl.* canaliculi
    apical c.
    bile canaliculi
    bile duct c.
    biliary canaliculi
    intracellular canaliculi of parietal cells
    pseudobile c.

canalis *pl.* canales
    c. alimentarius
    c. analis
    c. gastricus
    c. inguinalis
    canales paraurethrales urethrae masculinae
    c. pyloricus
    c. ventricularis
    c. ventriculi

canalization

cancer
    aniline c.
    bile duct c.
    Borrmann gastric c. classification
    colorectal c.
    duodenal c.
    dye workers c.
    esophageal c.
    extrahepatic c.
    extrahepatic bile duct c.
    gastric c.
    gastrointestinal c.
    hypoechoic c.
    intramucosal c.
    liver c.
    metastatic c.
    nonpolyposis colorectal c.
    ovarian c.
    pancreatic c.
    rectal c.
    recurrent colorectal c.
    restaging of c.
    schistosomal bladder c.

cancer *(continued)*
    c. screening
    staging of c.

cancerous

cancrum
    c. pudendi

Candida
    C. esophagitis
    C. peritonitis

candidal
    c. cellulitis
    c. esophagitis
    c. infection

candidiasis
    esophageal c.

candiduria

canker sore

cannula
    Bilisystem ERCP c.
    contour ERCP c.
    Fluoro Tip ERCP c.
    Hasson c.
    Hasson open laparoscopy c.
    laparoscopy c.
    large-bore c.
    nasal c.
    Teflon ERCP c.
    Veress c.

cannulate

cannulation
    bile duct c.
    biliary c.
    c. of the biliary tree
    endoscopic retrograde c.
    endoscopic transpapillary c.
    ERCP c.
    postsphincterotomy ERCP c.
    retrograde c.
    selective c.
    selective ductal c.

cannulation *(continued)*
    transpapillary c.

cannulization

canrenoate potassium

Cantor tube

cap
    bishop c.
    ConvaTec Active Life stoma c.
    duodenal c.
    pyloric c.

capacity
    gastric c.
    maximal tubular excretory c.

capillary
    bile c's
    c. drainage
    glomerular c.
    c. wall

capistration

capita *(plural of* caput*)*

capotement

capreolary

capreolate

CAPS
    caffeine, alcohol, peppery, spicy foods
        CAPS-free diet

capsula *pl.* capsulae
    c. adiposa renis
    c. fibrosa [Glissoni]
    c. fibrosa hepatis
    c. fibrosa perivascularis
    c. fibrosa renis
    c. glomeruli
    c. pancreatis
    c. prostatica
    capsulae renis

capsular
    c. cirrhosis of liver

capsular *(continued)*
   c. epithelium
   inferior c. artery
   middle c. artery
   c. nephritis
   pelviprostatic c. ligament
   c. space
   c. tear

capsule
   acidophilus c.
   adipose c. of kidney
   biopsy c.
   Bowman c.
   Crosby c.
   fatty c. of kidney
   fibrous c. of corpora cavernosa of penis
   fibrous c. of kidney
   fibrous c. of liver
   fibrous c. of testis
   Gerota c.
   Glisson c.
   glomerular c.
   c. of glomerulus
   hepatic c.
   hepatobiliary c.
   liver c.
   malpighian c.
   Müller c.
   müllerian c.
   c. of pancreas
   pelvioprostatic c.
   perinephric c.
   perirenal fat c.
   c. of prostate
   radiotelemetering c.
   renal c.
   telemetering c.

capsulectomy
   renal c.

capsulitis
   hepatic c.

capsulotomy
   renal c.

caput *pl.* capita
   c. epididymidis
   c. gallinaginis

caput *(continued)*
   c. pancreatis
   c. penis

carbamazepine hepatotoxicity

carbohydrate
   high c. diet

carbon dioxide
   c. d. laser
   c. d. laser plaque ablation
   c. d. trapping agent

carbuncle
   renal c.

Carcassone
   C. ligament
   perineal ligament of C.

carcinoembryonic antigen (CEA)

carcinogenesis
   colorectal c.
   oncogene-induced c.

carcinogenic

carcinogenicity

carcinoid
   duodenal c.
   gastric c.
   gastroduodenal c.
   hindgut c.
   c. syndrome
   c. tumor

carcinoma *pl.* carcinomas, carcinomata
   acinar cell c.
   adenoid cystic c.
   adenosquamous c.
   ampullary c.
   ampullopancreatic c.
   anorectal c.
   Barrett c.
   basal cell c.
   basaloid c.
   bile duct c.
   bilharzial c.
   biliary c.
   cholangiocellular c.

carcinoma *(continued)*
  cholangitis c.
  clear cell c.
  clear cell hepatocellular c.
  clear cell nonpapillary c.
  cloacogenic anal c.
  colon c.
  colorectal c.
  ductal c. of the prostate
  Dukes classification of c.
  Edmondson grading system
    for hepatocellular c.
  embryonal c.
  encephaloid gastric c.
  esophageal c.
  esophageal squamous
    cell c.
  excavated gastric c.
  extrahepatic bile duct c.
  familial medullary thy-
    roid c.
  familial medullary thyroid
    c.-pheochromocytoma
    syndrome
  fibrolamellar c.
  gallbladder c.
  gastric c.
  germ cell c.
  hepatocellular c. (HCC)
  hereditary nonpolyposis
    colorectal c.
  hypernephroid c.
  infantile embryonal c.
  intrahepatic bile duct c.
  intramucosal c.
  islet cell c.
  juvenile embryonal c.
  Kulchitsky-cell c.
  large bowel c.
  laryngeal c.
  Lauren gastric c. classifica-
    tion
  metastatic c.
  Ming gastric c. classifica-
    tion
  mutated colorectal c.
  non–germ cell c.
  oat cell c.
  obstructing c.

carcinoma *(continued)*
  oropharyngeal c.
  ovarian c.
  pancreatic c.
  pancreatic acinar cell c.
  pancreatic islet cell c.
  papillary gastric c.
  papillary transitional cell c.
  perforated c.
  periampullary c.
  rectal c.
  renal cell c.
  schistosomal bladder c.
  sclerosing hepatic c.
  secondary metastatic c.
  sessile nodular c.
  splenic flexure c.
  superficial esophageal c.
  superficial gastric c.
  supraglottic squamous
    cell c.
  TNM classification of c.
  transitional cell c.
  transthoracic resection of
    esophageal c.
  ulcerating c.
  unresectable hepatocellu-
    lar c.
  WHO gastric c. classifica-
    tion
  yolk sac c.
carcinomatosis
  peritoneal c.
carcinosarcoma
  embryonal c.
  gastric c.
cardia
  achalasia c.
  crescent gastric c.
  gastric c.
  patulous c.
  c. of stomach
cardiac
  c. antrum
  c. cirrhosis
  c. glands
  c. impression

cardiac *(continued)*
    c. incisure of stomach
    c. notch of stomach
    c. opening
    c. orifice
    c. part of stomach
    c. sphincter
    c. stomach

cardial
    c. notch
    c. part of stomach

cardialgia

cardiectomy

cardiochalasia

cardiodiaphragmatic
    c. angle

cardiodilatin

cardiodilator

cardiodiosis

cardioesophageal
    c. junction
    c. sphincter

cardiofundic gastropathy

cardiohepatic
    c. angle
    c. triangle

cardiohepatomegaly

cardiomyotomy
    Heller c.

cardionatrin

cardionephric

cardiophrenic
    c. angle

cardioplasty

cardiopyloric
    c. axis

cardiorenal

cardiospasm

cardiotomy

cardiovascular drug hepatotoxicity

carinate abdomen

Carlsbad salt

carminative

Caroli disease

Carrel aortic patch anastomosis

caruncle
    major c. of Santorini
    Morgagni c.
    morgagnian c.
    urethral c.

cascara
    c. amarga
    c. sagrada
    c. sagrada fluidextract

caseous nephritis

Cassia
    C. acutifolia
    C. angustifolia

cast
    bacterial c.
    blood c.
    coma c.
    epithelial c.
    false c.
    fibrinous c.
    granular c.
    hair c.
    hemoglobin c.
    hyaline c.
    Külz c.
    leukocyte c.
    mucous c.
    pus c.
    red cell c.
    renal c.
    spiral c.
    spurious c.
    spurious tube c.
    tube c.
    urate c.
    urinary c.

cast *(continued)*
    waxy c.

Castle intrinsic factor

castor oil
    aromatic c. o.

castrate

castration
    male c.

catarrhal
    acute c. cystitis
    c. dysentery
    c. dyspepsia
    c. gastritis
    c. jaundice

cathartic
    bulk c.
    c. colitis
    lubricant c.
    saline c.
    stimulant c.

catheter
    Achiever balloon dilation c.
    acorn-tipped c.
    Allis c.
    angiographic end-hole c.
    angiography c.
    angioplasty balloon c.
    Atlantic ileostomy c.
    Bard gastrostomy c.
    bicoudate c.
    c. bicoudé
    biliary balloon c.
    biliary dilator c.
    Braasch bulb c.
    cholangiocath c.
    cholangiographic c.
    conical c.
    c. coudé
    c. à demeure
    de Pezzer c.
    double-current c.
    double-lumen c.
    elbowed c.
    Eliminator nasal biliary c.
     set
    end-hole c.

catheter *(continued)*
    endoscopic nasobiliary c.
     drainage
    endoscopic transpapillary
     catheterization of the gall-
     bladder
    female c.
    fiberoptic c.
    filiform-tipped c.
    Foley c.
    French Cope loop nephros-
     tomy c.
    Gouley c.
    c.-guided endoscopic intu-
     bation (CAGEIN)
    Hickman c.
    indwelling c.
    large-bore c.
    Malecot c.
    Malecot reentry c.
    nasopancreatic c.
    Nélaton c.
    olive-tip c.
    oral suction c.
    Pezzer c.
    pigtail c.
    prostatic c.
    self-retaining c.
    solid-state esophageal man-
     ometry c.
    Tenckhoff c.
    Tenckhoff peritoneal c.
    two-way c.
    ureteral c.
    urethral c.
    whistle-tip c.
    winged c.

catheterization
    cystic duct c.
    hepatic vein c.
    retrourethral c.
    Seldinger cystic duct c.
    transpapillary c.
    umbilical vein c.

catheterize

cauda *pl.* caudae
    c. epididymidis
    c. equina

cauda *(continued)*
    c. equina lesion
    c. pancreatis

caudal
    c. artery
    c. pancreaticojejunostomy
    c. peduncle of thalamus
    c. tubercle of liver

caudate
    c. eminence of liver
    c. lobe
    c. lobe of liver
    c. process

caustic
    c. acid
    c. alkali
    c. colitis
    c. esophagitis

cautery
    blind c.

caveolated cells

cavern
    c's of corpora cavernosa of
        penis
    c's of corpus spongiosum

caverna *pl.* cavernae
    cavernae corporis spon-
        giosi
    cavernae corporum caver-
        nosorum penis

cavernitis
    fibrous c.

cavernosal abscess

cavernositis

cavernosography
    dynamic infusion c.

cavernosometry
    dynamic infusion c.

cavernous
    c. fibrosis
    c. hemangioma

cavitas *pl.* cavitates
    c. abdominalis

cavitas *(continued)*
    c. abdominis
    c. pelvica
    c. pelvina
    c. pelvis
    c. peritonealis

cavity
    abdominal c.
    abdominopelvic c.
    anterior mediastinal c.
    greater peritoneal c.
    intraperitoneal c.
    lesser peritoneal c.
    middle mediastinal c.
    peritoneal c.
    posterior mediastinal c.
    retroperitoneal c.
    Retzius c.
    superior mediastinal c.
    visceral c.

CDD
    common bile duct
        CBD 2 choledocho-
            scope
        CBD stone

CBDE
    common bile duct explora-
        tion

C bile

CCK
    cholecystokinin

CDAI
    Crohn disease activity in-
        dex

CDCA
    chenodeoxycholic acid

cDNA
    complementary deoxyribo-
        nucleic acid

CEA
    carcinoembryonic antigen

ceca

cecal
    c. appendage

cecal *(continued)*
    c. appendix
    c. bascule
    c. colonoscopy
    c. fissure
    c. folds
    c. hernia
    c. imbrication procedure
    c. mucosal nodule
    c. serosa
    c. ulcer
    c. vascular ectasia
    c. volvulus

cecectomy

Cecil operation

cecitis

Ceclor

cecocele

cecocolic
    c. intussusception

cecocolon

cecocolopexy

cecocolostomy

cecofixation

cecoileostomy

cecopexy

cecoplication

cecorrhaphy

cecosigmoidostomy

cecostomy

cecotomy

cecum
    antimesocolic side of the c.
    coned c.
    cone-shaped c.
    high c.
    mobile c.
    c. mobile
    watermelon c.

cefaclor

Celestin
    C. endoprosthesis
    C. esophageal tube
    C. graduated dilator

celiac
    c. angiogram
    c. angiography
    c. axis
    c. disease
    c. flux
    c. infantilism
    c. lymph node
    c. plexus reflex
    c. rickets
    c. sprue
    c. syndrome
    c. tumor

celiectomy

celiocentesis

celioenterotomy

celiogastrotomy

celiomyomotomy

celioparacentesis

celioscope

celioscopy

celiotomy
    exploratory c.
    c. incision
    ventral c.

cell
    absorptive c.
    acid c's
    acinar c.
    acinar c. carcinoma
    acinic c.
    acinous c.
    algoid c's
    antral D-c.
    antral EC-c.
    antral gastric c.
    Armanni-Ebstein c's
    atypical ductular c.
    autologous liver c.

cell *(continued)*
   B c.
   bile duct epithelial c.
   border c's
   caveolated c's
   central c.
   centroacinar c's
   chief c's
   clear c.
   clear c. carcinoma
   clear c. hepatocellular carcinoma
   clear c. nonpapillary carcinoma
   Davidoff (Davidov) c's
   Dukes A, B, C signet c.
   fat c's
   fat-storing c's of liver
   flow c.
   follicular dendritic c's (FDC)
   foot c's
   G c's
   gastrin c.
   gastrin c. function
   gastrin-secreting c.
   Gaucher c.
   germ c's
   germ c. carcinoma
   germ c. mutation
   germ c. tumor
   germinal c.
   giant c.
   Gley c's
   glial c.
   glitter c's
   Goormaghtigh c's
   ground-glass c.
   HBV-specific T c.
   Heidenhain c's
   hematopoietic c.
   hepatic c's
   initial c's
   intercalated c's
   intercapillary c's
   interstitial c's
   interstitial c's of Cajal
   interstitial c's of Leydig
   intestinal absorptive c.

cell *(continued)*
   islet c. carcinoma
   islet c. of Langerhans
   Ito c's
   juxtaglomerular c's
   Kulchitsky c.
   Kulchitsky-c. carcinoma
   Kupffer c's
   lacis c's
   Langerhans c.
   Langhans c.
   Leydig c's
   lipid-laden clear c.
   littoral c.
   liver c's
   liver-deprived epithelial clonic c.
   mast c.
   mesangial c's
   mononuclear c.
   mucous neck c's
   mucus-secreting c.
   myenteric ganglion c.
   myoepithelioid c's
   c. necrosis
   neuroendocrine c.
   non-alpha, non-beta pancreatic islet c.
   non-antigen-expressing target c.
   noncleaved B c.
   nuclear-tagged c.
   nurse c's
   nursing c's
   oat c.
   OK c.
   osteoclast-like giant c.
   owl eye c's
   oxyntic c's
   P c.
   pancreatic acinar c.
   pancreatic islet c.
   Paneth c's
   parenchymal hepatic c's
   parenchymal liver c's
   parietal c's
   peptic c's
   peripheral blood mononuclear c.

cell *(continued)*
  peripheral T c.
  phagocytic stellate c.
  Pick c.
  PMN c.
  pocket c.
  polymorphonuclear c.
  postreceptor signaling of
    parietal c.
  PP-immunoreactive c.
  primed c.
  principal c's
  proliferating c.
  c. proliferation
  ptyocrinous c.
  pulpar c.
  Q c.
  rectal epithelial c.
  renal c. carcinoma
  C. Saver
  Schwann c.
  schwannian spindle c.
  seminal c's
  senescent c.
  c. separation technique
  serotonin c.
  Sertoli c's
  Sertoli-Leydig c.
  sex c's
  sexual c's
  signet-ring c.
  sinusoid-lining c.
  C. Soft System
  somatostatin c.
  sperm c.
  spermatogenic c.
  spermatogonial c.
  spillage of tumor c's
  spindle c.
  squamous c.
  stellate c.
  suppressor T c.
  c. surface area
  c. surface receptor
  c. swelling
  T c.
  target c.
  T effector c.
  thymus-derived c.

cell *(continued)*
  trans-blotting c.
  transitional c.
  trypan blue–stained c.
  tubular epithelial c.
  tumor c.
  undifferentiated c.
  vascular permeation of tu-
    mor c.
  vascular smooth muscle c.
  von Hansemann c's
  von Kupffer c's
  xanthoma c.
  zymogenic c's

cell–cell
  c. adhesion
  c. contact
  c. interaction

Cellcept

cell-mediated
  c.-m. hepatic injury
  c.-m. immunity
  c.-m. immunohistological
    response
  c.-m. mechanism
  c.-m. suppression

cellobiose/mannitol sugar test

cell-positive margin

cell-substratum

Cell-Track

cellular
  c. atypia
  c. differentiation
  c. enzyme
  c. immune response
  c. immunity
  c. infiltration
  c. peptide
  c. proliferation

cellules

cellulitis
  candidal c.
  periurethral c.
  vaginal cuff c.

cellulose
   c. acetate

celoscope

celoscopy

celotomy

Celsius thermometer

center
   anospinal c.
   dark zone germinal c.
   germinal c.
   light zone germinal c.
   vomiting c.

centesis

centigrade thermometer

central
   c. adrenergic agent
   c. arteries of spleen
   c. cell
   c. echogenicity
   c. hyperalimentation
   c. necrosis
   c. peduncle of thalamus
   c. vein of suprarenal gland
   c. veins of hepatic lobules
   c. venous alimentation
   c. venous pressure

centrifugation
   Ficoll-Hypaque gradient c.

centrilobar
   c. pancreatitis

centrilobular
   c. cholestasis
   c. region of liver

centroacinar
   c. cells

cerebral
   c. gigantism

cerebrohepatorenal syndrome

cerumen obstruction

cervical
   c. intraepithelial neoplasia

cervical *(continued)*
   c. motion tenderness
   c. polyp
   c. wart

cervix *pl.* cervices
   c. glandis
   c. vesicae

CESD
   cholesteryl ester storage
     disease

Cestoda
   C. tapeworm

Cetacaine topical anesthetic

Ceylon sore mouth

CF-HM endoscope

CGM
   coffee-ground material

CH-40 activated charcoal

Chagas
   C. disease
   C.-Cruz disease

chagasic megaesophagus

chain
   gamma c.
   gamma heavy c's
   gamma heavy c's of immu-
     noglobulins

challenge
   c. diet
   food c.
   gluten c.
   rectal gluten c.
   solid bolus c.

chancre

chancroid

change
   Armanni-Ebstein c.
   degenerative c.
   enzyme c.
   erosive prepyloric c.
   fibrocystic c.

change *(continued)*
   fractional weight c.
   mesenchymal c.
   orthostatic c.
   pancreatic ductal morphol-
      ogical c.
   phlegmonous c.
   postsurgical c.
   segmental c.
   sensorium c.
   spatial c.
   trophic c.
   ultrastructural basket-
      weave c.

channel
   biopsy c.
   common c.
   8-c. cross-sectional anal
      sphincter probe
   gastric c.
   ligand-gated c.
   lymph c.
   Mitrofanoff catheteriza-
      tion c.
   pancreaticobiliary com-
      mon c.
   pyloric c.
   stoma-like c.
   treatment c.
   voltage-gated c.

Charcoaid

charcoal
   activated c.
   CH-40 activated c.
   c. filter
   c. hemoperfusion
   hemoperfusion with c.
   C. Plus
   c. suspension

CharcoCaps

Charcodote

Charcot
   C. cirrhosis
   C. fever
   C. intermittent fever
   C. syndrome
   C. triad

Charcot *(continued)*
   C. triangle
   C.-Böttcher crystalloids

chaude-pisse

cheesy nephritis

chemical
   c. anoxia
   c. cholecystitis
   c. colitis
   cystogenic c.
   c. gastritis
   c. litholysis
   c. peritonitis
   c. prostatitis

chemical-induced esophagitis

chemoembolization

chemolysis
   infrarenal c.

chemoprophylaxis

chemoradiation therapy

chemoradiotherapy

chemoreceptor
   c. trigger zone

chemosensitivity

chemosis

chemotactic
   c. factor
   c. peptide

chemotherapeutic agent
   c. a. hepatotoxicity

chemotherapy
   adjuvant c.
   continuous infusion c.
   cytotoxic c.
   c.-induced vomiting
   intraperitoneal c.
   intrathecal c.
   intravesical c.

chenodeoxycholate

chenodeoxycholic acid (CDCA)

chenodeoxycholylglycine

chenodeoxycholyltaurine

cherry angioma

Chevalier Jackson
    C. J. esophagoscope
    C. J. gastroscope

chevron incision

chew-and-spit test

CHF
    congenital hepatic fibrosis

Chiari
    C. malformation
    C. syndrome

Chiba
    C. needle
    C. percutaneous cholangio-
        gram

chief cells

Chilaiditi syndrome

Child
    C. class A
    C. class B
    C. class C
    C. classification
    C. classification of liver dis-
        ease
    C. C-minus patient
    C. criteria
    C. esophageal varices clas-
        sification
    C. hepatic dysfunction clas-
        sification
    C. liver criterion
    C. liver disease classifica-
        tion
    C. pancreaticoduodenos-
        tomy
    C.-Phillips bowel plication
    C.-Pugh classification
    C.-Turcotte classification

child
    c. esophagoscope

chili bean pseudopolyp

chill
    urethral c.

Chiron
    C. RIBA HCV test

chittem bark

chlorhydria

chloride balance

chloridorrhea
    familial c.

chloro-azotemic nephritis

chloroma
    gastric c.

chlorpromazine
    c.-induced cholestasis

chloruresis

chloruria

choana pl. choanae

Cho/Dyonics two-portal endo-
    scope

cholagogic

cholagogue

cholaic acid

cholaneresis

cholangeitis

cholangiectasis

cholangioadenoma

cholangiocarcinoma
    hilar c.
    metastatic c.
    peripheral c.

cholangiocath catheter

cholangiocatheter
    cystic duct c.
    saline-filled c.

cholangiocellular
    c. carcinoma

cholangiocholecystocholedo-
  chectomy

cholangiodrainage

cholangiodysplastic pseudocirrhosis

cholangioenterostomy

cholangiofibroma

cholangiofibromatosis

cholangiogastrostomy

cholangiogram
  balloon c.
  Chiba percutaneous c.
  common duct c.
  contrast selective c.
  cystic duct c.
  endoscopic retrograde c.
  fine-needle percutaneous c.
  fine-needle transhepatic c.
  intravenous c.
  operative c.
  percutaneous transhepa-
    tic c.
  pernasal c.
  serial c.
  thin-needle percutaneous c.
  transgastric c.
  transhepatic c.
  T-tube c.

cholangiographic
  c. catheter
  c. finding

cholangiography
  balloon occlusion c.
  direct c.
  drip infusion c.
  endoscopic c.
  endoscopic retrograde c.
  fine-needle transhepatic c.
  intravenous c.
  percutaneous c.
  percutaneous transhepat-
    ic c.
  retrograde c.
  transhepatic c.

cholangiohepatitis
  Oriental c.
  recurrent pyogenic c.

cholangiohepatoma

cholangiojejunostomy
  intrahepatic c.

cholangiolar

cholangiole

cholangiolitic
  c. cirrhosis
  c. hepatitis

cholangiolitis

cholangioma

cholangiopancreatography
  endoscopic retrograde c.
    (ERCP)

cholangiopathy
  eosinophilic c.

cholangioscopy
  peroral c.

cholangiostomy

cholangiotomy

cholangiovenous
  c. communication
  c. reflux

cholangitic
  c. abscess
  c. biliary cirrhosis
  c. hepatitis

cholangitis
  acute obstructive c.
  acute obstructive suppura-
    tive c. (AOSC)
  acute suppurative c.
  ascending c.
  bacterial c.
  c. carcinoma
  chronic nonsuppurative
    destructive c.
  fibrous obliterative c.

cholangitis *(continued)*
  granulomatous c.
  idiopathic autoimmune c.
  intrahepatic sclerosing c.
  c. lenta
  lymphoid c.
  nonsuppurative destructive c.
  Oriental c.
  pleomorphic destructive c.
  postendoscopic c.
  primary sclerosing c.
  progressive nonsuppurative c.
  progressive suppurative c.
  pyogenic c.
  recurrent pyogenic c.
  sclerosing c.
  secondary c.
  septic c.
  suppurative c.
  transient c.
  viral c.

cholanopoiesis

cholanopoietic

cholate

cholebilirubin

Cholebrine
  C. contrast medium

cholechromopoiesis

cholecyanin

cholecyst

cholecystagogic

cholecystagogue

cholecystalgia

cholecystatony

cholecystectasia

cholecystectomy
  laparoscopic c.
  laparoscopy-guided subhepatic c.
  minilaparoscopic c.

cholecystectomy *(continued)*
  prophylactic c.
  transpapillary endoscopic c. (TEC)

cholecystenteric
  c. fistula

cholecystenteroanastomosis

cholecystenterorrhaphy

cholecystenterostomy

cholecystenterotomy

cholecystic

cholecystis

cholecystitis
  acalculous c.
  acute c.
  acute acalculous c.
  calculous c.
  chemical c.
  c. with cholelithiasis
  chronic c.
  c. emphysematosa
  emphysematous c.
  erythromycin-induced c.
  follicular c.
  gangrenous c.
  gaseous c.
  c. glandularis proliferans
  perforated c.
  c. treatment
  xanthogranulomatous c.

cholecystocholangiography

cholecystocholedochal fistula

cholecystocolonic
  c. fistula

cholecystocolostomy

cholecystocolotomy

cholecystoduodenal
  c. fistula
  c. ligament

cholecystoduodenocolic
  c. fistula

cholecystoduodenocolic *(continued)*
  c. fold

cholecystoduodenostomy
  Jenckel c.

cholecystoendoprosthesis
  endoscopic retrograde c.

cholecystoenterostomy

cholecystogastric

cholecystogastrostomy

cholecystogogic

cholecystogram
  oral c.

cholecystography

cholecystoileostomy

cholecystointestinal

cholecystojejunostomy

cholecystokinetic
  c. food

cholecystokinin (CCK)

cholecystolithiasis

cholecystolithotripsy

cholecystonephrostomy

cholecystopathy

cholecystopexy

cholecystoptosis

cholecystopyelostomy

cholecystorrhaphy

cholecystosis
  hyperplastic c.

cholecystotomy

choledochal
  c. basal pressure
  c. cyst
  c. region
  c. sphincter

choledochectomy

choledochendysis

choledochitis

choledochocele

choledochocholedochostomy

choledochocolonic fistula

choledochoduodenal
  c. fistulotomy
  c. junctional stenosis

choledochoduodenostomy

choledochoenteric fistula

choledochoenterostomy

choledochogastrostomy

choledochohepatostomy

choledochoileostomy

choledochojejunostomy
  loop c.
  retrocolic end-to-side c.
  Roux-en-Y c.

choledocholith

choledocholithiasis

choledocholithotomy

choledocholithotripsy

choledochopancreatic ductal
  junction

choledochoplasty

choledochorrhaphy

choledochoscope
  Berci-Shore c.
  CBD 2 c.
  flexible fiberoptic c.
  Hopkins rod-lens system
    for rigid c.
  Machida c.
  Olympus CHF-P-series c.
  URF-P2 c.

choledochoscopic guidance

choledochoscopy
  operative c.

choledochostomy

choledochotomy
  c. incision
  longitudinal c.

choledochous
  c. duct

choledochus
  c. cyst

choleglobin

choleic

choleic acid

cholelith

cholelithiasis
  cholecystitis with c.
  intrahepatic c.
  c. prevalence

cholelithic
  c. dyspepsia

cholelithotomy

cholelithotripsy

cholelithotrity

cholemesis

cholemia
  familial c.
  Gilbert c.

cholemic
  c. nephrosis

choleperitoneum

choleperitonitis

cholepoiesis

cholepoietic

choleprasin

cholera
  Asiatic c.
  c. morbus

cholera *(continued)*
  pancreatic c.
  c. sicca
  summer c.
  c. toxin
  c. toxin–induced diarrhea

choleraic
  c. diarrhea

choleresis

choleretic
  c. effect

choleriform
  c. enteritis

cholerigenic

cholerigenous

choleroid

cholerrhagia

cholescintigram

cholescintigraphy

cholestasia

cholestasis
  acute drug-induced c.
  benign recurrent intrahe-
    patic c.
  canalicular c.
  centrilobular c.
  chlorpromazine-induced c.
  drug-induced c.
  estrogen-induced c.
  extrahepatic c.
  familial c.
  hepatocanalicular c.
  hepatocellular c.
  high-grade c.
  intrahepatic c.
  methyltestosterone-in-
    duced c.
  neonatal c.
  tolbutamide-induced c.

cholestatic
  chronic c. liver disease
  c. hepatitis
  c. hypersensitivity

cholestatic *(continued)*
  c. jaundice
  c. liver disease
  c. reaction
  c. syndrome
  c. viral hepatitis

cholesterol
  biliary c. secretion
  c. calculus
  c.-containing gallstone
  c. crystal embolization
  c. embolism
  c. gallstone
  high-density lipoprotein c. (HDL-C)
  low-density lipoprotein c.
  c. polyps

cholesteroleresis

cholesterolopoiesis

cholesterolosis
  c. of gallbladder
  c. of mucosal surface

cholesteryl
  c. ester storage disease (CESD)

choletherapy

choleverdin

cholic acid (CA)

cholochrome

cholocyanin

chologenetic

Cholografin contrast medium

cholohemothorax

cholelith

chololithiasis

chololithic

cholopoiesis

cholorrhea

choloscopy

cholothorax

cholylglycine

cholyltaurine

chorda *pl.* chordae
  c. spermatica

chordee

chorditis

Christie gallbladder retractor

Christmas
  C. tree appearance of pancreas
  C. tree sign

chromargentaffin

chromatography
  gas c.
  gel filtration c.

chromatopectic

chromatopexis

chromatoscopy

chromaturia

chromic gut

chromocystoscopy

chromopectic

chromopexic

chromopexy

chromoscopy time

chromosomal abnormality

chromospermism

chromoureteroscopy

chromourinography

chronic
  c. active gastritis
  c. active hepatitis
  c. active liver disease
  c. active viral hepatitis

chronic *(continued)*
    c. active viral hepatitis, non-A, non-B
    c. active viral hepatitis, type B
    c. aggressive hepatitis
    c. alcoholic cirrhosis
    c. alcoholic pancreatitis
    c. ambulatory peritoneal dialysis
    c. anoplasty treatment
    c. appendicitis
    c. atrophic duodenitis
    c. atrophic gastritis
    c. autoimmune hepatitis
    c. bacterial enteropathy
    c. calcifying pancreatitis
    c. cholecystitis
    c. cholestatic liver disease
    c. cicatrizing enteritis
    c. circumscribed plasmocytic balanoposthitis
    c. cystic gastritis
    c. diarrhea
    c. diverticulitis
    c. erosion
    c. erosive gastritis
    c. fibrosing hepatitis
    c. follicular gastritis
    c. functional constipation
    c. functional symptomatology
    c. gastritis
    c. glomerulonephritis
    c. graft-versus-host disease
    c. hepatitis
    c. hypocomplementemic glomerulonephritis
    c. idiopathic constipation
    c. idiopathic intestinal pseudo-obstruction
    c. idiopathic jaundice
    c. inflammatory disease
    c. interstitial cystitis
    c. interstitial hepatitis
    c. intestinal dysmotility
    c. intestinal ischemic syndrome
    c. lead poisoning

chronic *(continued)*
    c. liver disease
    c. lobar hepatitis
    c. metabolic acidosis
    c. nephritis
    c. nephrosis
    c. nonsuppurative destructive cholangitis
    c. pancreatitis
    c. parenchymatous nephritis
    c. peptic esophagitis
    c. persistent hepatitis
    c. persisting hepatitis
    c. progressive hepatitis
    c. pyelonephritis
    c. regurgitation
    c. relapsing pancreatitis
    c. renal failure
    c. sclerosing hyaline fibrosis
    c. superficial gastritis
    c. suppurative nephritis
    c. transplant rejection
    c. ulcerative colitis (CUC)
    c. ulcerative proctitis
    c. urate nephropathy
    c. uric acid nephropathy
    c. viral hepatitis

chronically
    c. inflamed gallbladder

chylangioma

chyle
    c. cyst
    c. spaces

chyliform ascites

chylomediastinum

chyloperitoneum

chylous
    c. ascites
    c. ascitic fluid
    c. hydrocele
    c. leukemia

chyluria

chylus

chyme

chymification

chymorrhea

cicatricial
    c. kidney
    c. stricture
    c. tissue

cigarette drain

ciguatera

ciliary
    c. dysentery

ciliate
    c. dysentery

Cimino shunt

cine-esophagogram

cinefluorographic study

cinegastroscopy

cineradiographic analysis

circadian
    c. gastric acidity

circuit
    short c.

circular
    c. enterorrhaphy
    c. folds
    c. folds of Kerckring
    c. layer of muscular coat of
        colon
    c. layer of muscular coat of
        rectum
    c. layer of muscular coat of
        small intestine
    c. layer of muscular coat of
        stomach

circulation
    enterohepatic c.
    hepatic c.
    portal c.
    portoumbilical c.

circumanal
    c. glands

circumcaval
    c. ureter

circumcise

circumcision

circumintestinal

circumrenal

circumscribed
    chronic c. plasmocytic bal-
        anoposthitis
    c. peritonitis

Circumstraint

circumumbilical incision

cirrhosis
    acholangic biliary c.
    acute juvenile c.
    alcoholic c.
    atrophic c.
    autoimmune c.
    bacterial c.
    biliary c.
    Budd c.
    calculous c.
    calculus c.
    capsular c. of liver
    cardiac c.
    Charcot c.
    cholangiolitic c.
    cholangitic biliary c.
    chronic alcoholic c.
    compensated c.
    congestive c.
    CPH-CAH c.
    Cruveilhier-Baumgarten c.
    cryptogenic c.
    decompensated c.
    decompensated alcohol-
        ic c.
    drug-induced c.
    end-stage c.
    fatty c.
    fatty micromedionodular c.
    focal biliary c.

cirrhosis *(continued)*
    frank c.
    glabrous c.
    Glisson c.
    Hanot c.
    hemochromatotic c.
    hepatic c.
    histologic c.
    hypertrophic c.
    hypochlorhydric c.
    incomplete c.
    juvenile c.
    Laënnec c.
    liver c.
    c. of liver
    macronodular c.
    malarial c.
    medionodular c.
    metabolic c.
    micronodular c.
    mixed c.
    multilobular c.
    necrotic c.
    nonazotemic c.
    nutritional c.
    obstructive biliary c.
    periportal c.
    pigment c.
    pigmentary c.
    pipestem c.
    portal c.
    posthepatitic c.
    postnecrotic c.
    primary biliary c.
    progressive familial c.
    secondary biliary c.
    stasis c.
    c. of stomach
    syndrome of primary biliary c.
    syphilitic c.
    Todd c.
    toxic c.
    type C c.
    unilobular c.
    vascular c.

cirrhotic
    c. ascites
    c. gastritis

cirrhotic *(continued)*
    c. hydrothorax
    c. liver
    c. nodule
    c. patient

cirsocele

citrate
    lead c.
    c. of magnesia
    piperazine c.
    potassium c.
    sodium c.
    c. synthase
    c. test

Citrotein liquid feeding

Claggett Barrett
    C. B. esophagogastroscopy
    C. B. esophagogastrostomy

clam
    c. enterocystoplasty
    c. ileocystoplasty

clamp
    Adson c.
    Allis c.
    Bainbridge intestinal c.
    Best right-angle colon c.
    Buie c.
    Buie pile c.
    Cope c.
    Crile appendix c.
    Crile hemostatic c.
    DeMartel appendix c.
    DeMartel-Wolfson anastomosis c.
    Dennis c.
    Doyen c.
    Doyen intestinal c.
    Earle hemorrhoid c.
    Foss intestinal c.
    Furniss anastomosis c.
    Furniss-Clute c.
    Gant c.
    Goldblatt c.
    Haberer intestinal c.
    Heaney c.
    Hirschmann pile c.
    intestinal c.

clamp *(continued)*
>Jarvis hemorrhoid c.
>Jarvis pile c.
>McLean pile c.
>Martel c.
>Masters intestinal c.
>Masters-Schwartz liver c.
>Mayo abdominal c.
>Mayo-Robson c.
>Mayo-Robson intestinal c.
>Mikulicz c.
>Moynihan c.
>noncrushing bowel c.
>Nussbaum intestinal c.
>occlusive c.
>O'Hanlon intestinal c.
>Payr c.
>Rankin c.
>Redo intestinal c.
>Yellen c.

clamp applier
>Stone c. a.

class
>Child c. A
>Child c. B
>Child c. C

classic
>c. achalasia
>c. seminoma

classification
>Anderson c.
>Ann Arbor cancer staging
>bismuth benign bile duct
>   stricture c.
>Borrmann gastric cancer c.
>Child c.
>Child esophageal varices c.
>Child hepatic dysfunction c.
>Child c. of liver disease
>Child liver disease c.
>Child-Pugh c.
>Child-Turcotte c.
>Dagradi esophageal vari-
>   ces c.
>Dukes c. of carcinoma
>Hara c. of gallbladder in-
>   flammation

classification *(continued)*
>Japanese c. of cancer
>Kasugai c.
>Lauren gastric carcinoma c.
>McNeer c.
>Marseille pancreatitis c.
>Ming gastric carcinoma c.
>Nyhus c.
>Ranson acute pancreatitis c.
>Sydney system gastritis c.
>TNM c. of carcinoma
>UICC tumor c.
>Visick dysphagia c.
>WHO gastric carcinoma c.

clay-colored stool

cleansing hypertonic phos-
>phate enema

clear
>c. discharge
>enemas until c.
>c. liquid diet

clearance
>blood-urea c.
>hepatic c.
>renal c.
>urea c.

clear cell
>c. c. adenocarcinoma
>c. c. carcinoma
>c. c. hepatocellular carci-
>   noma
>lipid-laden c. c.
>c. c. nonpapillary carci-
>   noma
>c. c. sarcoma of kidney

clearing
>esophageal c.

cleft palate

Clinifeed Iso enteral feeding

Clinitest
>C.-negative stool
>C.-positive stool
>C. stool test

clip
  absorbable c.
  endoscope c.

clip applier
  AcuClip endoscopic multi-
    ple c. a.

clitoric epispadias

cloacal
  c. exstrophy
  c. malformation
  c. remnant

cloacogenic
  c. anal carcinoma

CLO biopsy

clonic contraction

clonorchiasis
  biliary c.

clonorchiosis

clonus
  left-sided c.

C-loop
  duodenal C-l.

Cloquet
  C. hernia
  C. ligament

closed
  c. afferent loop
  c. drainage
  c. efferent loop
  c.-end ostomy pouch
  c. esophagus
  c. hemorrhoidectomy
  c. hydronephrosis
  c.-loop intestinal obstruc-
    tion

closing pressure

Clostridium difficile–associated
  diarrhea

closure
  ileostomy c.

closure *(continued)*
  secondary c.

clot
  adherent c.
  blood c.
  intraluminal c.
  sentinel c.

CLOtest

clotted blood

clotting abnormality

cloudy
  c. ascites
  c. bile

cloxacillin
  c.-induced cholestatic jaun-
    dice

clump kidney

clysma *pl.* clysmata

clyster

c-mount adapter

CMV
  cytomegalovirus
    CMV-associated ulcer-
      ation
    CMV esophagitis
    CMV-induced esopha-
      geal ulceration
    CMV infection

coagulation
  heater probe c.
  c. necrosis

coagulopathy
  iatrogenic c.
  c. pancreatitis

coarse nodularity

coat
  dartos c.
  external c. of esophagus
  external c. of ureter
  fibrous c. of corpus caver-
    nosum of penis

coat *(continued)*
>   fibrous c. of testis
>   vaginal c. of testis
>   vascular c. of stomach
>   villous c. of small intestine

cobalophilin

cobblestone
>   c.-like appearance
>   c. pattern
>   c. pattern of hepatocyte

Cobelli glands

cocaine hepatotoxicity

coccygeal fistula

Cochin China diarrhea

cocktail
>   GI c.
>   lytic c.

coefficient
>   ultrafiltration c.

coeliac

coffee-ground
>   c.-g. emesis
>   c.-g. material (CGM)
>   c.-g. vomit

Coffey ureterointestinal anastomosis

Cohen
>   C. antireflux procedure

Colace

cold
>   c. biopsy
>   c. cup biopsy
>   c. forceps ablation
>   c. snare ablation

colectomy
>   abdominal c.
>   laparoscopic c.
>   left c.
>   right c.
>   sigmoid c.
>   subtotal c.

colectomy *(continued)*
>   total abdominal c.
>   transverse c.

coles

colic
>   accessory superior c. artery
>   appendicular c.
>   c. artery
>   biliary c.
>   bilious c.
>   copper c.
>   Devonshire c.
>   endemic c.
>   episodic c.
>   esophageal c.
>   flatulent c.
>   gallstone c.
>   gastric c.
>   hepatic c.
>   c. impression of liver
>   infantile c.
>   inferior right c. artery
>   intermediate c. vein
>   intestinal c.
>   lead c.
>   left c. artery
>   left c. vein
>   middle c. artery
>   middle c. vein
>   multiple recurrent renal c.
>   nephric c.
>   c. omentum
>   painter's c.
>   pancreatic c.
>   c. part of omentum
>   c. patch
>   c. patch esophagoplasty
>   pseudoesophageal c.
>   renal c.
>   right c. artery
>   right c. vein
>   saturnine c.
>   stercoral c.
>   ureteral c.
>   uterine c.
>   vermicular c.
>   verminous c.

colic *(continued)*
  worm c.
  zinc c.

colicky
  c. abdominal pain

colicystitis

colicystopyelitis

coliform bacteria

coliplication

colipuncture

colitis *pl.* colitides
  acute infectious c.
  acute self-limited c. (ASLC)
  adenovirus c.
  allergic c.
  amebic c.
  antibiotic-associated c.
  bacterial c.
  balantidial c.
  Behçet c.
  cathartic c.
  caustic c.
  chemical c.
  chronic ulcerative c. (CUC)
  collagenous c.
  Crohn c.
  c. cystica profunda
  c. cystica superficialis
  cytomegalovirus c.
  diabetic c.
  diversion c.
  familial ulcerative c.
  focal c.
  fulminant c.
  fulminating ulcerative c.
  gangrenous ischemic c.
  granulomatous c.
  granulomatous transmural c.
  c. gravis
  hemorrhagic c.
  iatrogenic c.
  idiopathic c.
  infectious c.
  inflammatory c.
  intractable ulcerative c.

colitis *(continued)*
  irradiation c.
  ischemic c.
  left-sided c.
  lymphocytic c.
  microscopic c.
  milk-sensitive c.
  mucosal ulcerative c.
  mucous c.
  myxomembranous c.
  necrotic hemorrhagic c.
  necrotizing amebic c.
  nonantibiotic c.
  nonspecific c.
  pantothenic acid deficiency–induced c.
  c. perineal complication
  c. polyposa
  progesterone-associated c.
  pseudomembranous c.
  radiation c.
  radiation induced c.
  regional c.
  salmonella c.
  segmental c.
  segmental ischemic c.
  soap c.
  toxic c.
  transmural c.
  c. ulcerativa
  ulcerative c. (UC)
  uremic c.
  viral c.

collagen
  alpha$_2$-beta$_1$ integrin cell-surface c.

collagenous
  c. colitis
  c. sprue

colla *(plural of* collum)

collapsing glomerulopathy

collar
  Spanish c.

collar-button
  c.-b. appearance in colon
  c.-b. ulceration

collateral fibers of Winslow

collecting
    c. duct
    c. tubes
    c. tubule

collection
    American Type Culture C.
      (ATCC)
    duodenal fluid c.
    fluid c.
    pus c.
    quantitative stool c.

Colles
    C. fascia
    triangular ligament of C.

colliculectomy

colliculitis

colliculus *pl.* colliculi
    bulbar c.
    cervical c. of female ure-
      thra (of Barkow)
    c. seminalis

colliquative diarrhea

Collis
    C. antireflux operation
    C. gastroplasty
    C. repair

colloidal aluminum hydroxide

colloid-producing adenocarcinoma

collum *pl.* colla
    c. glandis penis
    c. vesicae biliaris
    c. vesicae felleae

colocecostomy

colocentesis

colocholecystostomy

coloclysis

coloclyster

colocolic
    c. intussusception

colocolonic
    c. anastomosis

colocolostomy

colocutaneous
    c. fistula

colodyspepsia

colofixation

coloenteritis

cologastrocutaneous fistula

Cologel

colohepatopexy

coloileal
    c. fistula

cololysis

colometrometer

colon
    c. ascendens
    ascending c.
    c. cancer screening
    c. carcinoma
    collar-button appearance
      in c.
    c. conduit
    c. consciousness
    c. cutoff sign
    c. descendens
    descending c.
    distal c.
    c. dyspepsia
    giant c.
    iliac c.
    c. incarceration
    irritable c.
    lead-pipe c.
    left c.
    loops of redundant c.
    midsigmoid c.
    pelvic c.
    perforation of c.
    rectosigmoid c.

colon *(continued)*
c. resection
right c.
saccular c.
c. sigmoideum
spastic c.
toxic dilation of c.
transverse c.
c. transversum

colonalgia

colonic
c. adenocarcinoma
c. adenoma
c. arterial spider
c. bacteria
c. dilatation
c. dilation
c. distention
c. diverticula
c. diverticulosis
c. diverticulum
c. explosion
c. fistula
c. foreign body
c. gas
c. hemorrhage
c. hyperalgesia
c. ileus
c. inertia
c. infiltration
c. interposition
c. ischemia
c. J-pouch
c. lavage
c. lavage solution
c. lesion
c. lipoma
c. loop
c. lymphoid nodule
c. mass
c. metastasis
c. motility
c. mucosal line
c. mucosal pattern
c. necrosis
c. neoplasia
c. obstruction
c. patch

colonic *(continued)*
c. perforation
c. pitting
c. polyp
c. pseudo-obstruction
c. transabdominal sonography (CTAS)
c. transit
c. transit study
c. transit test
c. transit time
c. tuberculosis
c. ulcer
c. urticaria
c. varix
c. vascular lesion
c. villus
c. volvulus
c. wall

Colonlite
C. bowel prep

colonopathy

colonorrhagia

colonoscope
ACMI fiberoptic c.
fiberoptic c.
forward-viewing video c.
video c.

colonoscopic
c. appendectomy
c. biopsy
c. decompression
c. diagnosis
c. disimpaction
c. polypectomy
c. removal
c. tattoo

colonoscopy
cecal c.
c. complication
diagnostic c.
emergency c.
high-magnification c.
pediatric c.
c. screening
screening c.

colonoscopy *(continued)*
    splenic flexure c.
    tandem c.
    therapeutic c.
    total c.
    upper endoscopy and c.

colony-stimulating factor (CSF)

colopathy

colopexia

colopexotomy

colopexy

Coloplast
    C. Flange pouch
    C. mini pouch
    C. ostomy irrigation set

coloplication

coloproctectomy

coloproctitis

coloproctostomy

coloptosis

colopuncture

color
    stool c.

colorectal
    c. adenocarcinoma
    c. biopsy
    c. bleeding
    c. cancer
    c. carcinogenesis
    c. carcinoma
    c. disease
    c. endometriosis
    hereditary nonpolyposis c.
        carcinoma
    c. lymphoma
    c. mucosa
    mutated c. carcinoma
    c. neoplasm
    c. physiologic dysfunction
    c. physiologic study
    c. polyp
    c. snare

colorectal *(continued)*
    c. stricture
    c. surgery
    c. trauma
    c. ulcer
    c. villous adenoma

colorectitis

colorectostomy

colorectum

colorrhaphy

colorrhea

coloscope

coloscopy

Coloscreen Self-test

colosigmoidostomy

colosigmoid resection

colostomy
    c. bag
    c. bridge
    continent c.
    ConvaTec c. pouch
    decompression c.
    descending loop c.
    Devine c.
    diverting c.
    diverting loop c.
    divided-stoma c.
    double-barrel c.
    dry c.
    end c.
    end-loop c.
    end-sigmoid c.
    exteriorization c.
    Hartmann c.
    ileosigmoid c.
    ileotransverse c.
    irrigation c.
    juxta-anal c.
    loop transverse c.
    Mikulicz c.
    permanent end c.
    c. pyloric autotransplanta-
        tion
    c. rod

colostomy *(continued)*
    sigmoid-end c.
    sigmoid-loop rod c.
    c. soiling
    c. takedown
    takedown of c.
    temp end c.
    temporary end c.
    terminal c.
    transverse-loop rod c.
    Turnbull c.
    wet c.

colotomy

colovaginal
    c. fistula

colovesical
    c. fistula

colpocystoureterocystotomy

colpopoiesis

colporectopexy

colpoureterocystotomy

colpoureterotomy

column
    anal c's
    c's of Bertin
    c's of Morgagni
    rectal c's
    renal c's of Bertin
    c. of Sertoli

columna *pl.* columnae
    columnae anales
    columnae ani
    columnae bertini
    columnae rectales [Morgagnii]
    columnae renales
    columnae renales [Bertini]

columnar
    c.-lined esophagus
    c. metaplasia

colypeptic

coma
    acute hepatic c.

coma *(continued)*
    c. cast
    hepatic c.

combination calculus

combined hemorrhoid

Comfeel skin adhesive

common
    c. bile duct
    c. bile duct exploration
    c. bile duct obstruction
    c. bile duct stent
    c. bile duct stone
    c. bile duct varices
    c. buckthorn
    c. cavity phenomenon
    c. channel
    c. duct cholangiogram
    c. duct exploration
    c. duct sound
    c. duct stone
    c. hepatic artery
    c. hepatic duct
    c. iliac artery
    pancreaticobiliary c. channel
    c. sheath of testis and spermatic cord

communicating hydrocele

communication
    cholangiovenous c.
    anomalous pancreaticobiliary c.

Companion feeding pump

Compat feeding pump

compensated cirrhosis

competent
    c. ileocecal valve

Compleat-B liquid feeding

complement
    c. activation
    c. hemolytic activity

complementary deoxyribonucleic acid (cDNA)

complete
  c. bowel obstruction
  c. epispadias
  c. surgical exploration

complex
  AIDS-related c. (ARC)
  immune c.
  juvenile nephronophthisis–
    medullary cystic dis-
    ease c.
  juxtaglomerular c.
  Meyenburg c's
  ureterotrigonal c.
  urobilin c.

compliance
  dynamic c.
  rectal c.
  static c.

complication
  benign pneumatic colonos-
    copy c.
  bowel preparation c.
  colitis perineal c.
  colonoscopy c.
  endoscopy c.
  extraintestinal c.
  feeding c.
  gastrointestinal c.
  hematologic c.
  infectious c.
  opportunistic c.

compound
  bismuth c.

compression
  c. button gastrojejunos-
    tomy
  duodenal c.
  esophageal c.
  extrinsic c.
  gastric c.
  c. syndrome

compressor
  c. muscle of urethra
  c. urethrae
  c. vaginae

concealed
  c. hemorrhage
  c. umbilical stoma
  c. vomiting

concentrate
  lactulose c.

concentration
  amylase c.
  limiting isorrheic c.
  maximum urinary c.
  minimal isorrheic c.

concretion
  bile c.
  fecal c.
  preputial c.
  prostatic c's

concussion
  hydraulic abdominal c.

condition
  acid-peptic c.

conduit
  antirefluxing colonic c.
  colon c.
  cutaneous appendiceal c.
  ileal c.
  Mitrofanoff c.

condyloma *pl.* condylomas,
  condylomata
    c. acuminatum
    anal c.
    esophageal c. acuminatum

cone
  Haller c's
  c. pedicle

coned cecum

cone-shaped cecum

configuration
  germ line c.
  germline c.

congenital
  c. adrenal hyperplasia
    (CAH)

congenital *(continued)*
  c. aganglionosis
  c. chloride diarrhea
  c. diaphragm
  c. diverticulosis
  c. familial nonhemolytic jaundice
  c. hepatic fibrosis (CHF)
  c. hydrocele
  c. hyperbilirubinemia
  c. hypertrophic pyloric stenosis
  c. lactic acidosis
  c. megacolon
  c. megaloureter
  c. mesoblastic nephroma
  c. nonhemolytic jaundice
  c. portacaval shunt
  c. pyloric stenosis
  c. splenomegaly
  c. stenosis

congenitally altered anatomy

congested kidney

congestion
  active c.

congestive
  c. cirrhosis
  c. gastropathy
  c. hepatomegaly
  c. hypertensive gastropathy
  c. splenomegaly

conic bougie

conical catheter

conjugated
  c. bile acid
  c. bilirubin
  c. hyperbilirubinemia

connecting
  c. canal
  c. tubule

connective tissue

Connell suture

Conradi line

consciousness
  colon c.

consumption
  alcohol c.

constipated

constipation
  antepartum c.
  atonic c.
  chronic functional c.
  chronic idiopathic c.
  drug-induced c.
  functional c.
  gastrojejunal c.
  geriatric c.
  idiopathic c.
  intractable c.
  outlet obstruction c.
  postpartum c.
  c.-predominant irritable bowel syndrome
  proctogenous c.
  psychogenic c.
  slow transit c.
  spastic c.

constitutional
  c. hepatic dysfunction
  c. hyperbilirubinemia

constricting pain

constriction
  duodenopyloric c.
  hourglass c. of gallbladder

constrictor
  c. urethrae
  c. vaginae

contact
  cell–cell c.
  c. laxative

contamination
  fecal c.

contents
  abdominal c.
  bowel c.
  gastric c.

contents *(continued)*
 intestinal c.

contiguous loop

continence
 fecal c.
 urinary c.

continent
 c. colostomy
 c. cutaneous appendicocystostomy
 c. cutaneous diversion
 c. ileal pouch
 c. ileal reservoir
 c. ileostomy
 c. of stool
 c. urinary diversion

continuous
 c. ambulatory peritoneal
 dialysis
 c. arteriovenous hemofiltration
 c. cycling peritoneal dialysis
 c. drip feeding
 c. infusion chemotherapy
 c. suction drainage
 c. venovenous hemofiltration

continuity
 bowel c.

contour
 c. ERCP cannula
 isodose c.
 sawtooth irregularity of
 bowel c.

contracted kidney

contractile
 c. ring dysphagia
 c. stricture

contractility
 detrusor c.

contraction
 anal sphincter c.
 clonic c.

contraction *(continued)*
 fat-induced gallbladder c.
 gallbladder c.
 isotonic c.
 paradoxical c.
 peristaltic c.
 secondary c.
 segmentation c.
 tertiary c.
 tonic c.

contralateral
 c. reflux

contrast
 c. agent
 c.-associated renal failure
 c. selective cholangiogram

contrast medium
 Baricon c. m.
 Baroflave c. m.
 Barosperse c. m.
 Biligrafin c. m.
 Biliscopin c. m.
 Bilivist c. m.
 Bilopaque c. m.
 Biloptin c. m.
 Cholebrine c. m.
 Cholografin c. m.
 extravasation of c. m.
 Gastrografin c. m.
 Gastrovist c. m.
 Hypaque c. m.
 Oragrafin c. m.

control
 bleeding c.
 feedback c.
 hemorrhage c.
 pain c.

controlled drain

conus *pl.* coni
 coni epididymidis
 coni vasculosi

ConvaTec
 C. Active Life stoma cap
 C. colostomy pouch
 C. Durahesive Water os-
 tomy

ConvaTec *(continued)*
    C. Little One Sur-Fit pouch
    C. Sur-Fit two-piece pouch

conversion

convex margin of testis

convoluted
    distal c. tubule
    first c. tubule
    proximal c. tubule
    second c. tubule
    c. seminiferous tubules
    c. tubule

Cook
    C. plastic Luer lock adapter
    C. speculum

Cooper
    C. fascia
    C. hernia
    C. herniotome
    C. irritable testis
    C. ligament operation
    C. ligament repair

Cope
    C. clamp
    C. sign

copper colic

copracrasia

copremesis

coprolith

coproma

coprostasis

coral calculus

Corbus disease

cord
    c. bladder
    common sheath of testis
        and spermatic c.
    hepatic c's
    c. hydrocele
    palpable c.
    spermatic c.

corditis

core needle biopsy

corkscrew esophagus

corona *pl.* coronas, coronae
    c. glandis penis

coronal
    c. adhesion
    c. planes

coronavirus gastroenteritis

corporal biopsy

corporeal fibrosis

corpus *pl.* corpora
    c. adiposum pararenale
    c. cavernosum penis
    c. cavernosum urethrae vi-
        rilis
    c. epididymidis
    c. gastricum
    c. glandulae bulboure-
        thralis
    c. glandulare prostatae
    c. Highmori
    c. highmorianum
    c. pancreatis
    c. penis
    c. spongiosum penis
    c. ventriculare
    c. ventriculi
    c. vesicae biliaris
    c. vesicae felleae
    c. vesicae urinariae

corpuscle
    Jaworski c's
    malpighian c's of kidney
    renal c's
    Weber c.

corpusculum *pl.* corpuscula
    corpuscula renis

Correctol

corrosive
    c. esophageal stricture
    c. esophagitis

corrosive *(continued)*
  c. gastritis

Cortenema
  C. retention enema

cortex *pl.* cortices
  adrenal c.
  c. of kidney
  renal c.
  c. renalis
  c. renis

cortical
  c. adenomas
  c. collecting duct
  c. collecting tubule
  c. labyrinth
  c. lobules of kidney
  c. substance of kidney

cortices *plural of* cortex

corticoadenoma

corticotropin
  c.-releasing factor (CRF)
    CRF action
    CRF regulation

cortisone acetate

costive

costiveness

costochondral tenderness

costocolic
  c. fold
  c. ligament

costophrenic blunting

costovertebral angle tenderness

cottonseed oil

coulombic force

count
  Addis c.

counterbalance
  renal c.

countercurrent
  c. mechanism

Courvoisier
  C. gallbladder
  C. gastroenterostomy
  C. law
  C. sign
  C.-Terrier syndrome

Couvelaire ileourethral anastomosis

cover
  Foxy Pouch c.
  laparotomy pad c.
  pad c.
  Sur-Fit Pouch c.

Cowper gland

cowperian duct

cowperitis

cow's milk allergy

coxsackievirus
  c. infection

CPA
  cyproterone acetate

CPH-CAH cirrhosis

cramping pain

crampy abdominal pain

cream
  rectal c.
  c. of tartar

crease
  inguinal c.
  midline abdominal c.
  skin c.

creatorrhea

Credé method

creeping mesenteric fat

cremaster
  c. muscle

cremasteric
  c. artery
  c. fascia

cremasteric *(continued)*
    c. fiber

Creon
    C. 10
    C. 20

crepitus

crescent
    epithelial c.
    c. gastric cardia
    glomerular c.

crescentic glomerulonephritis

crest
    seminal c.
    female urethral c.
    male urethral c.

cribriform area of renal papilla

cricoesophageal tendon

cricopharyngeal
    c. achalasia
    c. bar
    c. diverticulum
    c. muscle
    c. myotomy
    c. spasm
    c. sphincter

cricopharyngeus
    c. muscle

Crigler
    C.-Najjar disease
    C.-Najjar jaundice
    C.-Najjar syndrome

Crile
    C. angle retractor
    C. appendix clamp
    C. bile duct forceps
    C. hemostat
    C. hemostatic clamp
    C. nerve hook

crisis *pl.* crises
    Dietl c.
    hepatic c.

crista *pl.* cristae
    c. urethralis
    c. urethralis muliebris
    c. urethralis virilis

criterion *pl.* criteria
    Child criteria
    Child liver c.
    Ranson criteria

Criticare HN elemental liquid
    feeding

Crohn
    C. colitis
    C. and Colitis Foundation
        of America
    C. disease
    C. disease activity index
        (CDAI)
    C. disease of colon
    C. Disease Endoscopic In-
        dex of Severity
    C. duodenal ulcer
    familial C. disease
    gastroduodenal C. disease
    C. ileitis
    C. ileocolitis
    C. regional enteritis
    C. small intestine

Cronkhite-Canada syndrome

Crosby capsule

crossbar deformity

crossed renal ectopia

crossmatched blood

croupous cystitis

cruciate incision

crural
    deep c. arch
    c. fold
    c. fossa
    c. fovea
    c. hernia
    c. ring

crus *pl.* crura
    anterior c. of anterior ingui-
        nal ring
    c. of diaphragm
    external c. of anterior in-
        guinal ring
    c. inferius anuli inguinalis
        subcutanei
    internal c. of anterior ingui-
        nal ring
    lateral c. of superficial in-
        guinal ring
    c. laterale anuli inguinalis
        superficialis
    medial c. of superficial in-
        guinal ring
    c. mediale anuli inguinalis
        superficialis
    posterior c. of anterior in-
        guinal ring

crush
    c. kidney
    c. syndrome

Cruveilhier
    C. fascia
    C. ulcer
    C.-Baumgarten cirrhosis
    C.-Baumgarten syndrome

Cruz
    Chagas-C. disease

cryobank

cryogenic ablation

cryosurgical ablation

cryotherapy for hemorrhoids

crypt
    c. abscess
    anal c's
    c's of Haller
    ileal c.
    c's of Lieberkühn
    c's of Littre
    Luschka c's
    c. of Morgagni

crypt *(continued)*
    mucous c's of duodenum
    odoriferous c's of prepuce
    c's of Tyson

crypta *pl.* cryptae
    cryptae mucosae duodeni
    cryptae odoriferae
    cryptae praeputiales
    cryptae urethrae muliebris

cryptitis
    anal c.

cryptogenic cirrhosis

cryptoglandular

cryptorchid

cryptorchidectomy

cryptorchidism

cryptorchidopexy

cryptorchidy

cryptorchism

cryptosporidial
    c. infection

cryptosporidium *pl.* crypto-
sporidia
    c.-induced diarrhea

crystal
    Lubarsch c's
    oxalate c.
    c's of Reinke

crystalloid
    c. body
    Charcot-Böttcher c's
    c's of Reinke

crystalluria

CT
    computed tomography
        CT-guided fine-needle
            aspiration
        CT-guided liver biopsy
        CT-guided needle-aspi-
            ration biopsy

CT *(continued)*
    CT-guided pseudocyst
        drainage
    helical CT

CTAS
    colonic transabdominal so-
        nography

CUC
    chronic ulcerative colitis

cuff abscess

cuffed
    c. endotracheal tube
    c. esophageal endopros-
        thesis

cul-de-sac
    c.-de-s. of Douglas
    c.-de-s. fluid
    c.-de-s. mass

culdocentesis

Cullen sign

Culp-DeWeerd ureteropelvio-
    plasty

culposuspension
    Burch c.

culture
    aerobic c.
    American Type C. Collec-
        tion (ATCC)
    anaerobic c.
    blood c.
    stool c.
    tissue c.

culture-negative neutrocytic as-
    cites

cuprophane

curative resection

curling

currant jelly stool

curvatura *pl.* curvaturae
    c. gastrica major
    c. gastrica minor

curvatura *(continued)*
    c. major gastris
    c. minor gastris
    c. ventricularis major
    c. ventricularis minor

curvature
    greater gastric c.
    lesser gastric c.
    greater c. of stomach
    lesser c. of stomach

curve
    gallbladder emptying-refill-
        ing c.

curved end-to-end anastomosis

CUSA

Cushing
    C. suture
    C. ulcer
    C.-Rokitansky ulcers

cushingoid facies

cushion
    hemorrhoidal c.

cutaneous
    c. appendiceal conduit
    c. fissure
    c. fungus
    c. lesion
    c. metastasis
    c. opening of male urethra
    c. ureterostomy
    c. vesicostomy

cutback anoplasty

cut surface of liver

cyanosis
    autotoxic c.
    enterogenous c.

cyanotic
    c. induration
    c. kidney

cycle
    biliary c.
    gastric c.
    Schiff biliary c.

cyclic vomiting

cylinder
 Bence Jones c's
 Külz c.
 urinary c.

cylindrical bougie

cylindroid

cylindruria

cyproterone acetate (CPA)

cyst
 adventitious c.
 biliary c.
 choledochal c.
 choledochus c.
 chyle c.
 endoscopic transpapillary
  c. drainage
 enteric c.
 enterogenous c.
 esophageal duplication c.
 false c.
 hepatic c.
 ileal duplication c.
 intraepithelial c's
 intraluminal c's
 liver c.
 macroscopic liver c.
 mesenteric c.
 morgagnian c.
 noncommunicating bili-
  ary c.
 nonparasitic c. of liver
 omental c's
 ovarian dermoid c.
 pancreatic c.
 paranephric c.
 parapyelitic c's
 pyelogenic renal c.
 retention c.
 seminal c.

cystadenocarcinoma
 pancreatic mucinous c.
 papillary serous c.

cystadenoma
 bile duct c.

cystadenoma *(continued)*
 ductal c.
 ductectatic mucinous c.
 glycogen-rich c.
 mucinous c.

cystalgia

cystatrophia

cystauchenitis

cystauchenotomy

cystectasia

cystectasy

cystectomy
 radical c.

cystelcosis

cysterethism

cysthypersarcosis

cystic
 acquired c. disease of kidney
 c. artery
 c. bile
 chronic c. gastritis
 c. cystitis
 c. fibrosis
 c. hamartoma
 c. kidney
 c. renal dysplasia
 Seldinger c. duct catheterization
 c. vein

cystic duct
 c. d. angiogram
 c. d. catheterization
 c. d. cholangiocatheter
 c. d. cholangiogram
 c. d. leakage

cysticoduodenal
 c. ligament

cysticolithectomy

cysticolithotripsy

cysticorrhaphy

cysticotomy

cystides (*plural of* cystis)

cystine
    c. calculus

cystinuria

cystinuric

cystirrhagia

cystirrhea

cystis *pl.* cystides
    c. fellea

cystistaxis

cystitis
    acute catarrhal c.
    allergic c.
    bacterial c.
    chronic interstitial c.
    c. colli
    croupous c.
    cystic c.
    c. cystica
    diphtheritic c.
    c. emphysematosa
    eosinophilic c.
    exfoliative c.
    follicular c.
    c. follicularis
    c. glandularis
    hemorrhagic c.
    incrusted c.
    interstitial c.
    mechanical c.
    panmural c.
    c. papillomatosa
    c. senilis feminarum
    submucous c.

cystocele

cystochromoscopy

cystocolostomy

cystodiaphanoscopy

cystoduodenostomy

cystodynia

cystoelytroplasty

cystoenterocele

cystoepiplocele

cystogastric fistula

cystogastrostomy

cystogenic
    c. chemical

cystohepatic
    c. triangle

cystojejunostomy

cystolith

cystolithectomy

cystolithiasis

cystolithic

cystolithotomy

cystometer

cystometrogram
    filling c.

cystometrography

cystometry

cystonephrosis

cystoneuralgia

cystoparalysis

cystoparesis

cystopexy

cystophotography

cystophthisis

cystoplasty
    augmentation c.
    sigmoid c.

cystoplegia

cystoproctostomy

cystoprostatectomy
    radical c.

cystoptosis

cystopyelitis

cystopyelonephritis

cystorectostomy

cystorrhagia

cystorrhaphy

cystorrhea

cystoschisis

cystoscope
   French c.

cystoscopic

cystoscopy

cystospasm

cystospermitis

cystostaxis

cystostomy
   suprapubic c.
   tubeless c.

cystotome

cystotomy
   suprapubic c.

cystotrachelotomy

cystoureteritis

cystoureteropyelitis

cystoureteropyelonephritis

cystourethritis

cystourethrocele

cystourethroscope

cytogenetic analysis

cytokine antagonist

cytologic biopsy

cytology
   exfoliative c.
   fine-needle aspiration c.
   gastric brush c.

cytolytic action

cytomegalovirus (CMV)
   c. colitis
   c. esophagitis
   c. infection

cytometer
   flow c.

cytometry
   flow c.
   flow cell c.

cytoprotectant

cytoprotection

cytoprotective
   c. effect

cytotoxic
   c. agent
   c. chemotherapy

cytotoxicity
   antibody-dependent cell-
      mediated c. (ADCC)

Czerny
   C. suture
   C.-Lembert suture

Dacron
    D. graft
    D. interposition graft
    D. mesh

DAG
    diffuse antral gastritis

Dagradi esophageal varices
    classification

DAEC
    diffusely adherent *Esche-
    richia coli*

Dairy-Ease chewable tablet

damage
    drug-induced d.
    gastric mucosal d.
    Graham scale for drug-in-
        duced gastric d.
    histologic d.
    oropharyngeal d.

Dansac
    D. Karaya Seal one-piece
        drainage pouch
    D. ostomy irrigation set

dark stool

darting incision

dartoic

dartoid

dartos
    d. coat
    d. fascia
    d. fascia of scrotum
    d. muscle
    d. muscle of scrotum
    d. pouch procedure

Davidoff (*spelled also* Davidov)
    D. cells

Davidov (*variant of* Davidoff)

dead
    d. bowel
    d. space

dearterialization

death
    hepatocellular d.
    liver d.

debris
    purulent d.

decapsulation
    renal d.

decay
    d.-accelerating factor (DAF)

decidual umbilicus

declining glucose tolerance

decompensated
    d. alcoholic cirrhosis
    d. cirrhosis

decompression
    balloon d.
    biliary d.
    colonoscopic d.
    d. colostomy
    ductal d.
    endoscopic d.
    endoscopic biliary d.
    gastric d.
    intestinal d.
    nasogastric d.
    operative d.
    PEG-assisted d.
    percutaneous transhepa-
        tic d.
    transduodenal endoscop-
        ic d.
    tube d.
    d. tube
    variceal d.

decortication

decreased peristalsis

decubitus calculus

deep
    d. abdominal ring
    d. crural arch

deep *(continued)*
 d. external pudendal artery
 d. fascia of perineum
 d. inguinal ring
 d. interloop abscess
 d. layer of triangular ligament
 d. pain
 d. perineal fascia
 d. postanal anorectal space
 d.-seated fungal infection

de-epithelialized flap

defecation
 balloon d.
 fragmentary d.
 infrequent d.
 obstructed d.
 painful d.
 d. reflex
 d. syncope

defecatory
 d. difficulty
 d. dyschezia
 d. straining
 d. urgency

defecogram

defecography

defecometry

defect
 acidemia d.
 fascial d.
 filling d.
 frondlike filling d.
 intraluminal filling d.

deferent duct

deferentectomy

deferential

deferentitis

deficiency
 acquired lactose d.
 d. anemia
 nutritional d.

defloration pyelitis

deformity
 bulb d.
 crossbar d.
 duodenal bulb d.
 hourglass d.
 keyhole d.
 limb d.

degeneration
 acute hepatocellular d.
 Armanni-Ebstein d.
 ballooning d. of hepatocytes

degenerative
 d. change
 d. nephritis

deglutible

deglutition
 d. disorder
 d. mechanism

deglutitive

deglutitory

degraded liver

dehiscence
 abdominal incision d.
 staple line d.
 d. of stump
 suture line d.
 wound d.

dehydration
 absolute d.
 d. fever
 hypernatremic d.
 relative d.
 voluntary d.

dehydrobilirubin

dehydrocholaneresis

dehydrogenase
 lactate d. (LDH)

delayed
 d. gastric emptying
 d. hyperacute transplant rejection

delayed *(continued)*
 d. nephrogram
 d. primary intention
 d. primary intention healing

del Castillo syndrome

deletion
 functional d.

Delorme rectal prolapse operation

delta hepatitis

DeMartel
 D. appendix clamp
 D. appendix forceps
 D.-Wolfson anastomosis
  clamp

dementia
 dialysis d.

demeclocycline
 d.-induced ascites

demucosalized augmentation
 with gastric segment

Denck esophagoscope

denervated bladder

dengue
 d. fever
 hemorrhagic d.
 d. hemorrhagic fever
 d. hemorrhagic fever infection
 d. virus

Denis Browne
 D. B. abdominal retractor
 D. B. operation

Dennis
 D. clamp
 D. forceps
 D. intestinal forceps
 D. intestinal tube
 D. tube
 D.-Brooke ileostomy

Dennis *(continued)*
 D.-Varco pancreaticoduo-
  denostomy

Denonvilliers
 D. aponeurosis
 D. fascia

de novo
 d. n. liver cancer
 d. n. malignancy

dense
 d. adhesion
 d. deposit disease

dentate
 d. line
 d. margin

Dent disease

Denver
 D. peritoneovenous shunt
 D. shunt

deoxycholaneresis

deoxycholate

deoxycholic acid

deoxycholylglycine

deoxycholyltaurine

deoxyribonucleic acid (DNA)
 complementary d. a.
  (cDNA)

Depage-Janeway gastrostomy

dependent rubor

depepsinized

de Pezzer catheter

depletion
 mucous d.

depletional hyponatremia

deposit
 hemosiderin d.

depression
 orbital d.

depressed adenoma

dermatitis herpetiformis

DeRoyal Surgical grab bag

descending
    d. aorta
    d. colon
    d. diaphragm
    d. duodenum
    d. limb
    d. loop colostomy

desexualize

Desferal
    D. challenge for hemochromatosis

Desjardins
    D. gallbladder forceps
    D. gallbladder probe
    D. gallbladder scoop
    D. gallstone forceps
    D. gallstone probe
    D. point

Desmarres paracentesis knife

destructive
    chronic nonsuppurative d. cholangitis
    nonsuppurative d. cholangitis
    pleomorphic d. cholangitis

detection
    anti–liver microsomal antibody d.

de Toni-Fanconi syndrome

detorsion

Detrol

detrusor
    d. contractility
    d. hyperreflexia
    d. instability
    d.-sphincter dyssynergia
    d. urinae

detubularized right colon reservoir

devascularization
    paraesophagogastric d.

developer
    Hemoccult Sensa d.

deviation
    axis d.
    tongue d.

device
    ACMI ulcer measuring d.
    angled delivery d. (ADD)
    bioartificial liver support d.
    feeding d.
    flexible delivery d.
    Gastro-Port II feeding d.
    GIA autosuture d.
    OraSure salivary collection d.

Devine colostomy

devisceration

devolvulization

Devonshire colic

DEXA
    dual-energy x-ray absorption

Dexon polyglycolic acid mesh

dexpanthenol

dextrinizing time

dextrogastria

diabetes
    adult-onset d. mellitus
    alimentary d.
    brittle d.
    bronze d.
    bronzed d.
    fibrocalculous pancreatic d.
    gestational d.
    d. home screening test
    d. insipidus
    insulin-dependent d.
    insulin-dependent d. mellitus (IDDM)

diabetes *(continued)*
    juvenile d. mellitus
    juvenile-onset d. mellitus
    ketosis-prone d. mellitus
    ketosis-resistant d. mellitus
    malnutrition-related d. mellitus (MRDM)
    d. mellitus (DM) (types 1 and 2)
    nephrogenic d. insipidus
    non–insulin-dependent d. mellitus (NIDDM)
    renal d.

diabetic
    d. colitis
    d. diet
    d. enteropathy
    d. gastroparesis
    d. gastropathy
    d. glomerulopathy
    d. glomerulosclerosis
    d. impotence
    d. ketoacidosis
    d. nephropathy
    d. neuropathy
    d. patient

diabeticorum
    gastroparesis d.

Diabinese

diabrosis

diachorema

diachoresis

diagnosis
    colonoscopic d.
    histologic d.

diagnostic
    d. angiography
    d. colonoscopy
    d. paracentesis

dialysance

dialysate

dialysis
    d. amyloidosis

dialysis *(continued)*
    chronic ambulatory peritoneal d.
    continuous ambulatory peritoneal d.
    continuous cycling peritoneal d.
    d. dementia
    d. dysequilibrium
    d. dysequilibrium syndrome
    d. encephalopathy
    intermittent peritoneal d.
    d.-related ascites
    peritoneal d.

dialyzable

dialyzed

dialyzer

diaphragm
    accessory d.
    antral d.
    congenital d.
    crus of d.
    descending d.
    duodenal d.
    mucosal ileal d.
    pelvic d.
    pyloric d.
    secondary d.
    urogenital d.

diaphragma *pl.* diaphragmata
    d. urogenitale

diaphragmatic
    d. abscess
    d. breathing
    d. hernia
    d. hiatus
    d. peritonitis
    d. surface of liver

diaphragmlike stricture

diarrhea
    acute infectious d.
    Aeromonas d.
    antibiotic-associated d.
    antibiotic-induced d.

diarrhea *(continued)*
    anxiety-related d.
    beta-lactam–associated d.
    bile salt d.
    bilious d.
    bloody d.
    cachectic d.
    choleraic d.
    cholera toxin–induced d.
    chronic d.
    d. chylosa
    Clostridium difficile–asso-
      ciated d.
    Cochin China d.
    colliquative d.
    congenital chloride d.
    cryptosporidium-indu-
      ced d.
    dientameba d.
    dysenteric d.
    enteral d.
    enterotoxin d.
    explosive d.
    familial chloride d.
    fatty d.
    fermental d.
    fermentative d.
    flagellate d.
    functional d.
    gastrogenic d.
    gluten-sensitive d.
    hemorrhagic d.
    hill d.
    ileostomy d.
    infantile d.
    infectious d.
    inflammatory d.
    intermittent d.
    intractable d.
    irritative d.
    lactose-associated d.
    lienteric d.
    liquid d.
    malabsorptive d.
    maldigestive d.
    mechanical d.
    morning d.
    mucous d.
    nocturnal d.

diarrhea *(continued)*
    osmotic d.
    d. pancreatica
    pancreatogenous fatty d.
    paradoxical d.
    parenteral d.
    putrefactive d.
    postvagotomy d.
    rotavirus d.
    secretory d.
    serous d.
    stercoral d.
    d. stool
    summer d.
    toxic d.
    toxigenic d.
    traveler's d.
    tropical d.
    unrelenting d.
    viral d.
    virulent d.
    virus d.
    watery d.
    white d.

diarrheal

diarrheic

diarrheogenic
    d. syndrome

diastasis
    d. recti abdominis
    palpable rib d.
    rectus d.

diastatic serosal tear

diathermic fistulotomy

dibasic sodium phosphate

dibucaine

didymalgia

didymitis

didymodynia

didymus

dientameba diarrhea

diet
    absolute d.
    acid-ash d.
    ADA (American Diabetes
        Association) d.
    advance to regular d.
    alkaline-ash d.
    balanced d.
    basal d.
    bland d.
    blenderized d.
    BRAT d.
    BRATT d.
    CAPS-free d.
    challenge d.
    clear liquid d.
    diabetic d.
    elimination d.
    fasting d.
    fiber-deficient d.
    fractionated d.
    full liquid d.
    gluten-free d.
    high bulk, low fat d.
    high calorie d.
    high carbohydrate d.
    high fat d.
    high protein d.
    high roughage d.
    lactose-free d.
    low calorie d.
    low fat d.
    low fiber d.
    low residue d.
    low roughage d.
    low sodium d.
    modified liver d.
    Portagen d.
    progressive d.
    regular d.
    Sippy d.
    smooth d.
    soft d.
    soft bland d.
    vegetarian d.
    Weight Watchers d.
dietary
    d. fat

dietary (continued)
    d. fiber
    d. habits

dietetic regimen

diethylenetriamine pentaacetic
    acid (DTPA)

Dietl crisis

Dieulafoy
    D. cirsoid aneurysm
    D. disease
    D. gastric erosion
    D. lesion
    D. triad
    D. ulcer
    D. vascular malformation

differentiation
    cellular d.
    osteogenic d.

difficulty
    defecatory d.

diffuse
    d. angiodysplasia
    d. antral gastritis (DAG)
    d. corporal atrophic gastri-
        tis
    d. esophageal spasm
    d. glomerulonephritis
    d. lobular fibrosis
    d. metastasis
    d. pain
    d. pancreatitis
    d. peritonitis
    d. tenderness

diffused hydrocele

diffusely
    d. adherent *Escherichia coli*
    d. tender abdomen

diffusion
    fluid phase d.
    pericapillary d.

digastric
    d. impression
    d. triangle

Di-Gel

digestion
  solid food d.

digestive
  d. apparatus
  d. canal
  d. fever
  d. gastrosuccorrhea
  d. organs
  d. system
  d. tract
  d. tube

digital
  d. rectal examination
  d. rectal evacuation
  d. subtraction angiography

digitally guided biopsy

dihydroxyaluminum
  d. aminoacetate
  d. sodium carbonate

diisopropyl iminodiacetic acid
  (DISIDA)

dilatation
  anal d.
  aneurysmal d.
  biliary d.
  bowel d.
  colonic d.
  esophageal d.
  d. of esophagus
  gastric d.
  prognathic d.
  prognathion d.
  pyloric d.
  rectal d.
  d. of the stomach

dilate

dilated
  d. bile duct
  d. gallbladder
  d. loops of bowel

dilating bougie

dilation
  achalasia balloon d.

dilation *(continued)*
  anal d.
  balloon d.
  balloon d. of the papilla
  biliary d.
  bowel d.
  colonic d.
  ductal d.
  Eder-Puestow d.
  endoscopic d.
  endoscopic papillary bal-
    loon d.
  esophageal d.
  d. of esophagus
  extrahepatic biliary cys-
    tic d.
  gastric d.
  d. of hemorrhoids
  hepatic web d.
  inadequate d.
  intrahepatic biliary cys-
    tic d.
  intrahepatic ductal d.
  percutaneous balloon d.
  peroral esophageal d.
  pneumatic esophageal d.
  pyloric d.
  rectal d.
  through-the-scope d.
  toxic d. of colon

dilator
  achalasia d.
  Achiever balloon d.
  American Dilation Sys-
    tem d.
  American Endoscopy d.
  anal d.
  Bakes common duct d.
  balloon d.
  biliary balloon d.
  biliary d. catheter
  bougie d.
  Celestin graduated d.
  d. placement failure
  Einhorn d.
  Eliminator PET biliary bal-
    loon d.
  ERCP d.
  esophageal d.

dilator *(continued)*
 esophageal balloon d.
 Ferris biliary duct d.
 French d.
 Hegar rectal d.
 Kollmann d.
 Kron bile duct d.
 Kron gall duct d.
 Murphy common duct d.
 pneumatic d.
 rectal d.
 Rigiflex achalasia d.
 Sippy esophageal d.
 Starck d.

dilution
 agar d.

dilutional hyponatremia

diminished
 d. bowel sounds
 d. branching abnormality
 d. gag reflex

diminutive
 d. adenomatous polyp
 d. colonic polyp
 d. hyperplastic polyp

dimpling
 focal d.
 postanal d.
 skin d.

diphtheritic
 d. cystitis
 d. enteritis

direct
 d. bilirubin
 d. cholangiography
 d. hernia
 d. inguinal hernia
 d. laryngoscopy
 d. vision liver biopsy

discharge
 anal d.
 bloody d.
 clear d.
 nasal d.

discharge *(continued)*
 purulent d.

discoloration

discomfort
 epigastric d.

discrete mass

disease
 α_1-antitrypsin d.
 acalculous gallbladder d.
 acid-peptic d.
 acquired cystic d. of kidney
 acquired cystic kidney d.
  (ACKD)
 acute abdominal vascular d.
 acute graft-versus-host d.
 acute idiopathic inflammatory bowel d.
 acute polycystic d.
 Addison d.
 adrenal d.
 adult celiac d.
 adult familial hyaline membrane d.
 adult polycystic d.
 adult polycystic kidney d.
 adult polycystic liver d.
  (APLD)
 alcoholic liver d.
 alpha-chain d.
 alpha heavy-chain d.
 Alström d.
 Anderson d.
 anemia of chronic d.
 anorectal d.
 anti-GBM antibody d.
 anti–glomerular basement membrane antibody d.
 atheroembolic renal d.
  (AER)
 atypical gallbladder d.
 autoimmune d.
 Barrett d.
 Behçet d.
 benign anorectal d. (BAD)

disease *(continued)*
    Berger d.
    biliary tract d.
    black liver d.
    bleeding acid-peptic d.
    Bouchard d.
    Bradley d.
    Bright d.
    Brinton d.
    Budd d.
    Cacchi-Ricci d.
    calculous gallbladder d.
    calculus d.
    Caroli d.
    celiac d.
    Chagas d.
    Chagas-Cruz d.
    Child classification of liver d.
    cholestatic liver d.
    cholesteryl ester storage d. (CESD)
    chronic active liver d.
    chronic cholestatic liver d.
    chronic graft-versus-host d.
    chronic inflammatory d.
    chronic liver d.
    colorectal d.
    Corbus d.
    Crigler-Najjar d.
    Crohn d.
    Crohn d. activity index (CDAI)
    Crohn d. of colon
    Crohn D. Endoscopic Index of Severity
    dense deposit d.
    Dent d.
    Dieulafoy d.
    diverticular d.
    early-onset graft-versus-host d.
    Ebstein d.
    end-stage d.
    end-stage renal d. (ESRD)
    Fabry d.
    Fahr-Volhard d.
    familial Crohn d.

disease *(continued)*
    fatty liver d.
    febrile d.
    Fenwick d.
    fibrocystic d. of the pancreas
    foot process d.
    Fournier d.
    fourth venereal d.
    fulminant Crohn d.
    fungal d.
    gallbladder d.
    gamma heavy chain d.
    gastric mucosal d.
    gastritis-associated peptic ulcer d.
    gastroduodenal Crohn d.
    gastroesophageal reflux d. (GERD)
    gastrointestinal d.
    Gaucher d.
    Gee d.
    Gee-Herter d.
    Gee-Herter-Heubner d.
    Gee-Thaysen d.
    Gilbert d.
    graft-versus-host d.
    granulomatous d.
    Gross d.
    hepatic Hodgkin d.
    hepatic metastatic d.
    hepatic veno-occlusive d.
    hepatobiliary d.
    hepatocellular d.
    Herter d.
    Herter-Heubner d.
    Heubner-Herter d.
    Hirschsprung d.
    idiopathic inflammatory bowel d.
    ileocolic d.
    ileocolonic Crohn d.
    immunoproliferative small intestine d.
    infantile celiac d.
    inflammatory bowel d. (IBD)
    intramural atheromatous d.

disease *(continued)*
    ischemic bowel d.
    Klebs d.
    Laënnec d.
    Lane d.
    Leyden d.
    liver d.
    malabsorption d.
    Malassez d.
    Marion d.
    medullary cystic d.
    medullary cystic kidney d.
    Ménétrier d.
    metastatic d.
    minimal change d.
    monoclonal immunoglobu-
      lin deposition d.
    neoplastic d.
    nil d.
    nonobstructive hepatic
      parenchymal d.
    obstructive gastroduodenal
      Crohn d.
    oral d.
    Ormond d.
    Osler-Weber-Rendu d.
    ovarian d.
    Paget d.
    Paget extramammary d.
    Paget perianal d.
    Paget d. of perianal area
    pancreatic d.
    pancreaticobiliary d.
    parenchymal liver d.
    Patella d.
    Payr d.
    peptic ulcer d. (PUD)
    Peyronie d.
    polycystic kidney d.
    polycystic d. of kidneys
    polycystic liver d.
    polycystic d. of liver
    polycystic renal d.
    radiation-induced d.
    reflux d.
    Rokitansky d.
    Rossbach d.
    Ruysch d.
    schistosomal liver d.

disease *(continued)*
    scleroderma bowel d.
    sigmoid d.
    Spencer d.
    steroid-dependent Crohn d.
    Thaysen d.
    transfusion-related chronic
      liver d.
    ulceroerosive d.
    uremic bone d.
    van Buren d.
    van den Bergh d.
    venereal d.
    veno-occlusive d. of the
      liver
    Whipple d.
    white spot d.

DISIDA
    diisopropyl iminodiacetic
      acid

disimpaction
    colonoscopic d.

disk
    anal d.
    d. kidney

dismembered reimplanted ap-
    pendicocystostomy

disorder
    autoimmune connective tis-
      sue d.
    deglutition d.
    esophageal motility d.
    evacuation d.
    feeding d.
    functional bowel d. (FBD)
    functional d. of the stom-
      ach
    gastric motility d.
    intestinal motility d.
    motility d.
    nonspecific esophageal mo-
      tility d. (NEMD)

displacement
    bowel d.
    fish-hook d.
    gallbladder d.

disruption
    pancreatic duct d.

dissecting
    d. abdominal aneurysm
    d. balloon

dissection
    aortic d.
    blunt d.
    blunt and sharp d.
    en bloc d.
    sharp d.

Disse
    spaces of D.

dissector
    water-jet d.

disseminated
    d. CMV infection
    d. histoplasmosis

dissemination
    metastatic d.

dissolution of gallstone

distal
    d. bile duct
    d. blind stomach
    d. colon
    d. convoluted tubule
    d. duodenum
    d. esophageal ring
    d. esophageal stenosis
    d. esophageal stricture
    d. esophagus
    d. gastrectomy
    d. ileitis
    d. pancreatectomy
    d. renal tubular acidosis
        (dRTA)
    d. splenorenal shunt
    d. straight tubule

distended
    d. abdomen

distensibility

distension (*variant of* disten-
    tion)

distention
    abdominal d.
    colonic d.
    esophageal balloon d.
    gaseous d.
    gastric d.
    postprandial d.
    rectal d.
    visible abdominal d.

distress
    epigastric d.
    functional bowel d. (FBD)
    moderate d.

disturbance
    acid-base d.

Dittel operation

diurese

diuresis *pl.* diureses
    osmotic d.
    postobstructive d.

diuretic
    loop d.
    osmotic d.
    d. salt

diuria

diversion
    biliopancreatic d.
    Bricker urinary d.
    Camey enterocystoplasty
        urinary d.
    d. colitis
    continent cutaneous d.
    continent urinary d.
    fecal d.
    ileocolic urinary d.
    ileocolonic pouch urinary d.
    d. proctitis

diversionary ileostomy

diversity
    germ line d.
    germline d.

diverticula *plural of* diverticu-
    lum

diverticular
  d. bleeding
  d. disease
  d. hemorrhage
  d. hernia

diverticulectomy
  Harrington esophageal d.
  pharyngoesophageal d.

diverticulitis
  acute d.
  chronic d.
  duodenal d.
  d. evaluation
  Meckel d.
  sigmoid d.

diverticulopexy

diverticulosis
  acquired d.
  colonic d.
  congenital d.
  gastric d.

diverticulum *pl.* diverticula
  d. of Åkerlund
  diverticula ampullae ductus deferentis
  biliary d.
  caliceal d.
  calyceal d.
  cervical d.
  diverticula of colon
  colonic diverticula
  cricopharyngeal d.
  duodenal d.
  esophageal d.
  false d.
  Ganser d.
  giant d.
  Graser d.
  hepatic d.
  Hutch d.
  hypopharyngeal d.
  d. ilei verum
  intestinal d.
  intraluminal duodenal d.
  intramural d.

diverticulum *(continued)*
  inverted sigmoid d.
  juxtapapillary duodenal d.
  Kirchner d.
  Meckel d.
  midesophageal d.
  mucosal d.
  noncommunicating d.
  Nuck d.
  pancreatic d.
  perforated d.
  periampullary duodenal d.
  pharyngeal d.
  pharyngoesophageal d.
  pressure d.
  pulsion d.
  Rokitansky d.
  ruptured sigmoid d.
  sigmoid d.
  supradiaphragmatic d.
  traction d.
  urachal d.
  vesical d.
  Zenker d.

diverting
  d. colostomy
  d. loop colostomy
  d. loop ileostomy
  d. stoma

divided-stoma colostomy

divisum
  pancreas d.

divulsor

DNA
  deoxyribonucleic acid
    DNA fragmentation

Dobbhoff
  D. feeding tube
  D. gastric decompression tube
  D. PEG tube

docusate
  d. calcium
  d. potassium
  d. sodium

dog-ear
    d.-e. anastomosis

Dohlman esophagoscope

dolichocolon

dome of liver

donation
    organ d.

Donnatal

donor
    d. hepatectomy
    living nonrelated d.
    living related d.
    living unrelated d.

dopamine agonist

Doppler
    Accuson-128 color flow D.
        machine
    D. ultrasound
    D. ultrasound intestinal
        blood flow measurement

dorsal
    d. pancreatic artery
    d. point

dorsum *pl.* dorsa
    d. penis
    d. of penis
    d. of testis

double
    d. bladder
    d. gallbladder
    d. J-shaped reservoir
    d. penis
    d. pyloroplasty
    d. urethra

double-barrel
    d.-b. colostomy
    d.-b. ileostomy
    d.-b. reservoir

double-bubble duodenal sign

double-channel
    d.-c. endoscope

double-channel *(continued)*
    d.-c. fistulotomy
    d.-c. videoendoscope

double-contrast
    d.-c. air barium enema
    d.-c. barium enema

double-current catheter

double-lumen
    d.-l. catheter
    d.-l. endoprosthesis

double-pigtail endoprosthesis

double-stapled ileal reservoir

doubly ligated

doughnut kidney

doughy abdomen

Douglas
    D. abscess
    cul-de-sac of D.
    D. fold
    D. pouch
    D. rectal snare

Doyen
    D. abdominal retractor
    D. abdominal scissors
    D. clamp
    D. forceps
    D. gallbladder forceps
    D. intestinal clamp
    D. intestinal forceps
    D. retractor
    D. rib elevator

DPEG
    dual percutaneous endo-
        scopic gastrostomy

drain
    cigarette d.
    controlled d.
    Jackson-Pratt d.
    Mikulicz d.
    nasobiliary d.
    Penrose d.
    Penrose sump d.
    stab wound d.

drain *(continued)*
    sump d.
    sump-Penrose d.
    Teflon nasobiliary d.

drainage
    biliary d.
    button d.
    capillary d.
    closed d.
    continuous suction d.
    CT-guided pseudocyst d.
    endoscopic d.
    endoscopic biliary d.
    endoscopic nasobiliary
      catheter d.
    endoscopic pancreatic d.
    endoscopic transpapillary
      cyst d.
    endosonography-guided d.
      of pancreatic pseudocyst
    external d.
    gravity-dependent d.
    incision and d.
    J-Vac closed wound d.
    nasobiliary d.
    nasogastric d.
    nasopancreatic d.
    open d.
    percutaneous d.
    percutaneous abscess d.
    percutaneous antegrade
      biliary d.
    percutaneous biliary d.
    percutaneous transhepa-
      tic d.
    percutaneous transhepatic
      biliary d.
    postoperative irrigation-
      suction d.
    serosanguineous d.
    suction d.
    through d.
    tidal d.
    transduodenal d.
    transgastric d.
    transhepatic biliary d.
    transmural d.
    transpapillary d.
    T-tube d.

drainage *(continued)*
    d. tube
    Wangensteen d.
    wound d.

drastic

dressing
    Adaptic d.
    adhesive d.
    bio-occlusive d.
    bolus d.
    occlusive d.
    occlusive collodion d.
    Op-Site d.
    pressure d.
    sterile d.
    Tegaderm d.
    Telfa d.

dried aluminum hydroxide gel

drinking habit

drip
    alkaline milk d.
    d. feeding
    d. infusion cholangiogra-
      phy
    Murphy d.

dromedary hump

droperidol

dropsical nephritis

dropsy
    abdominal d.
    nutritional d.

dRTA
    distal renal tubular acido-
      sis

drug
    anorectic d.
    anticholinergic d.
    antiemetic d.
    antilipemic d.
    antimotility d.
    antispasmodic d.
    d. hepatotoxicity
    H_2 receptor–blocking d.
    hydrochloretic d.

drug *(continued)*
  lipid-lowering d.
  d. metabolism
  nonnephrotoxic d.
  nonsteroidal antiinflamma-
    tory d.
  prokinetic d.
  d. reaction
  recreational d.
  d. resistance
  d. therapy

drug-induced
  d.-i. acute hepatic injury
  d.-i. cholestasis
  d.-i. cirrhosis
  d.-i. constipation
  d.-i. damage
  d.-i. esophagitis
  d.-i. gastritis
  d.-i. hepatitis
  d.-i. pain
  d.-i. pancreatitis
  d.-i. renal failure
  d.-i. steatosis
  d.-i. ulcer

drug-related liver disease

drum belly

dry
  d. colostomy
  d. heaves
  d. skin
  d. swallow
  d. vomiting

DTPA
  diethylenetriamine pentaa-
    cetic acid

dual
  d.-energy x-ray absorptiom-
    etry
  d.-energy x-ray absorption
    (DEXA)
  d. percutaneous endo-
    scopic gastrostomy
    (DPEG)
  d.-photon absorptiometry

Dubin
  D.-Johnson syndrome

Dubin *(continued)*
  D.-Sprinz syndrome

duct
  accessory d. of Luschka
  accessory pancreatic d.
  accessory d. of Santorini
  anomalous pancreaticobi-
    liary d. (APBD)
  beaded hepatic d.
  Bellini d.
  Bernard d.
  bile d.
  biliary d.
  choledochous d.
  collecting d.
  common bile d.
  common hepatic d.
  cortical collecting d.
  cowperian d.
  cystic d.
  deferent d.
  ejaculatory d.
  d. of epididymis
  excretory d. of seminal
    gland
  excretory d. of seminal ves-
    icle
  excretory d. of testis
  gall d.
  gall d. spoon
  d. of gallbladder
  Guérin d's
  Haller aberrant d.
  hepaticopancreatic d.
  hepatic d.
  hepatocystic d.
  impacted cystic d.
  interlobular bile d's
  left hepatic d.
  Luschka d's
  medullary collecting d.
  metanephric d.
  minor pancreatic d.
  nephric d.
  nontransected pancrea-
    tic d.
  normal caliber d.
  pancreatic d.
  papillary d.

duct *(continued)*
   paraurethral d's of female urethra
   paraurethral d's of male urethra
   persistent müllerian d.
   d's of prostate gland
   prostatic d's
   renal d.
   right hepatic d.
   Rokitansky-Aschoff d's
   d. of Santorini
   Schüller d's
   seminal d's
   d. of seminal gland
   d. of seminal vesicle
   Skene d's
   spermatic d.
   testicular d.
   upstream pancreatic d.
   d. of Wirsung

ductal
   d. adenocarcinoma of the prostate
   d. carcinoma of the prostate
   d. cystadenoma
   d. decompression
   d. dilation
   d. epithelial hyperplasia
   d. hypertension
   d. stricture
   d. system
   d. system perforation

ductectatic mucinous cystadenoma

ductopenia

ductule
   bile d's
   biliary d's
   efferent d's of testis
   inferior aberrant d.
   interlobular d's
   d's of prostate
   superior aberrant d.

ductulus *pl.* ductuli
   ductuli aberrantes

ductulus *(continued)*
   d. aberrans inferior
   d. aberrans superior
   ductuli biliferi
   ductuli efferentes testis
   ductuli interlobulares
   ductuli prostatici

ductus *pl.* ductus
   d. aberrans
   d. aberrans halleri
   d. biliaris
   d. biliferi
   d. choledochus
   d. cysticus
   d. deferens
   d. ejaculatorius
   d. epididymidis
   d. excretorius glandulae seminalis
   d. excretorius glandulae vesiculosae
   d. excretorius vesiculae seminalis
   d. glandulae bulbourethralis
   d. hepaticus communis
   d. hepaticus dexter
   d. hepaticus sinister
   d. interlobulares
   d. lobi caudati dexter
   d. lobi caudati sinister
   d. pancreaticus
   d. pancreaticus accessorius
   d. papillaris
   d. paraurethrales urethrae femininae
   d. paraurethrales urethrae masculinae
   d. prostatici
   d. spermaticus

Duecollement
   D. hemicolectomy
   D. maneuver

Duhamel
   D. colon operation
   D. operation
   D. pull-through

Duhamel *(continued)*
    Lester Martin modification
      of D. operation

Dukes
    D. A, B, C signet cell
    D. classification of carci-
      noma
    D. staging system

Dulcolax
    D. bowel prep

dull
    d. pain
    d. to percussion abdomen

dullness
    hepatic d.
    liver d.
    d. to percussion
    shifting d.
    splenic d.
    tympanitic d.

dumping
    d. stomach
    d. syndrome

duodenal
    d. adenocarcinoma
    d. adenoma
    d. ampulla
    d. atresia
    d. bleeding
    d. bulb
    d. bulb deformity
    d. cancer
    d. cap
    d. carcinoid
    d. C-loop
    d. compression
    d. diaphragm
    d. diverticulitis
    d. diverticulum
    d. effect
    d. erosion
    d. fistula
    d. fluid collection
    d. foreign body
    d. glands
    d. hemangiomatosis

duodenal *(continued)*
    d. hematoma
    d. impression of liver
    inferior d. fossa
    d. injury
    d. loop
    d. lumen
    d. lymphoma
    d. mass
    d. metastasis
    d. mucosa
    d. neurofibroma
    d. obstruction
    d. opening of stomach
    d. orifice of stomach
    d. papilla
    d. perforation
    d. polyp
    d. reflux
    d. stenosis
    d. stump
    superior d. fossa
    d. sweep
    d. telangiectasia
    d. terminus
    d. trauma
    d. tuberculosis
    d. tumor
    d. ulcer
    d. ulceration
    d. varix
    d. villus
    d. wall hamartoma
    d. web

duodenectomy

duodenitis
    chronic atrophic d.
    erosive d.

duodenobiliary
    d. pressure gradient
    d. reflux

duodenocaval fistula

duodenocholangeitis

duodenocholecystostomy

duodenocholedochotomy

duodenocolic
d. fistula

duodenocystostomy

duodenoduodenostomy

duodenoenterostomy

duodenogastric
d. reflux

duodenogastroesophageal
d. reflux

duodenohepatic
d. ligament

duodenoileal
d. bypass

duodenoileostomy

duodenojejunal
d. flexure
d. fold
d. fossa
d. hernia
d. junction

duodenojejunostomy

duodenolysis

duodenomesocolic
d. fold

duodenopancreatectomy

duodenopancreatic reflux

duodenopancreaticocholedo-
chal rupture

duodenopyloric
d. constriction

duodenorenal
d. ligament

duodenorrhaphy

duodenoscope
video d.

duodenoscopy

duodenostomy
Witzel d.

duodenotomy
transverse d.

duodenum
descending d.
distal d.

Duphalac

Duplay operation

duplex ileum

duplication
alimentary tract d.
esophageal d. cyst
gastric d.

Dupuytren
D. hydrocele
D. suture

dusky stoma

Duval pancreaticojejunostomy

Duverney
D. foramen
D. gland

dwarf
renal d.

dwarfism
renal d.

dye
fluorescent d.
d. workers' cancer

dynamic
d. closure pressure
d. compliance
d. fluorescein angiography
d. ileus
d. infusion cavernosogra-
phy
d. infusion cavernosometry

dyschesia (*variant of* dyschezia)

dyschezia
defecatory d.

dyscholia

dysenteric
  d. algid malaria
  d. diarrhea

dysenteriform

dysentery
  amebic d.
  bacillary d.
  balantidial d.
  bilharzial d.
  catarrhal d.
  ciliary d.
  ciliate d.
  epidemic d.
  flagellate d.
  Flexner d.
  fulminant d.
  fulminating d.
  helminthic d.
  institutional d.
  Japanese d.
  malarial d.
  malignant d.
  protozoal d.
  schistosomal d.
  scorbutic d.
  Sonne d.
  spirillar d.
  sporadic d.
  viral d.

dysequilibrium
  dialysis d.

dysfunction
  anal sphincter d.
  anorectal sensorimotor d.
  Child hepatic d. classification
  colorectal physiologic d.
  constitutional hepatic d.
  erectile d.
  esophageal body motor d.
  gastric d.
  graft d.
  late graft d.
  outlet d.
  postgastrectomy d.
  posttransplant renal d.

dysfunction *(continued)*
  sphincter d.

dysfunctional bleeding

dysgenesis
  anorectal d.

dysgenetic fibrous band

dyshepatia

dyskinesia
  bile duct d.
  biliary d.

dyslipidemia

dysmotility
  chronic intestinal d.
  esophageal d.
  gallbladder d.

dyspareunia

dyspepsia
  acid d.
  adhesion d.
  appendicular d.
  appendix d.
  atonic d.
  biliary d.
  catarrhal d.
  cholelithic d.
  colon d.
  fermentative d.
  flatulent d.
  functional d.
  gastric d.
  gastroduodenal d.
  intestinal d.
  nervous d.
  nonorganic d.
  nonulcer d.
  postcholecystectomy flatulent d.
  reflex d.
  ulcerlike d.

dyspeptic

dysperistalsis

dysphagia
  d. aortica

dysphagia *(continued)*
  Atkinson scoring system
    for d.
  contractile ring d.
  esophageal d.
  d. inflammatoria
  liquid food d.
  d. lusoria
  d. nervosa
  oropharyngeal d.
  d. paralytica
  postvagotomy d.
  progressive d.
  sideropenic d.
  soft food d.
  solid food d.
  d. spastica
  vallecular d.
  Visick d. classification

dysphagy

dysplasia
  Barrett d.
  cystic renal d.
  epithelial d.
  fibrous d.
  high-grade d.
  low-grade d.
  malignant d.
  mucosal d.
  multicystic renal d.
  neuronal colonic d.
  neuronal intestinal d.
  nonulcer d.
  polypoid d.
  renal d.
  renal-retinal d.
  ureteral neuromuscular d.

dysplasia-associated lesion or
  mass

dysplasia-to-carcinoma sequence

dysplastic
  d. focus
  d. nodule

dyspnea
  renal d.

dyspragia
  d. intermittens angiosclero-
    tica intestinalis

dysraphism
  occult spinal d.

dysrhythmia
  esophageal d.

dysspermia

dyssynergia
  biliary d.
  detrusor–external sphinc-
    ter d.
  detrusor-sphincter d.
  detrusor–striated sphinc-
    ter d.
  rectoanal d.
  vesico-sphincter d.

dystonia

dystrophic calcification

dystrypsia

dysuresia

dysuria
  spastic d.

dysuriac

dysuric

dyszoospermia

EAEC
  enteroadherent *Escherichia coli*

EAggEC
  enteroaggregative *Escherichia coli*

Eagle-Barrett syndrome

ear
  dog-e.

Earle
  E. hemorrhoid clamp
  E. rectal probe

early
  e. B-cell factor (EBF)
  e. satiety

early-onset graft-versus-host disease

Easi-Lav lavage

easily reducible hernia

eater
  liver e.

eating habits

EBA
  extrahepatic biliary atresia

Ebner reticulum

Ebstein
  E. disease
  E. lesion

echinococcal
  e. abscess
  e. liver abscess

echinococcosis
  biliary e.

Echinococcus

echoendoscopy

echogastroscope

echogenic
  e. liver

echogenicity
  central e.

echo pattern

Eck fistula

Eckhout vertical gastroplasty

ecstrophy

ectacolia

ectasia
  antral vascular e.
  cecal vascular e.
  gastric antral vascular e.
  tortuous venous e.
  tubular e.
  vascular e.

ectatic
  e. vascular lesion

ectocolon

ectoperitoneal

ectoperitonitis

ectopia
  e. cloacae
  crossed renal e.
  gastric mucosal e. in rectum
  renal e.
  e. renis
  e. testis
  e. vesicae

ectopic
  e. anus
  e. gastric mucosa
  e. gestation
  e. kidney
  e. pancreas
  e. pregnancy
  e. testis
  e. ureter
  e. ureterocele
  e. varices

ectopy
  acquired gastric e.

ectopy *(continued)*
    gastric mucosal e.

ectoscopy

edema
    angioneurotic e.
    antral e.
    e. bullosum vesicae
    bullous e.
    focal e.
    idiopathic e.
    laryngeal e.
    nephrotic e.
    pedal e.
    perianal e.
    pericholecystic e.
    peripheral e.
    pitting e.
    pulmonary e.
    renal e.
    sacral e.

edematous
    e. gallbladder
    e. pancreatitis
    e. tag

edentulous

Eder
    E. gastroscope
    E.-Bernstein gastroscope
    E.-Chamberlin gastroscope
    E.-Hufford gastroscope
    E.-Hufford rigid esophago-
        scope
    E.-Palmer semiflexible fiber-
        optic endoscope
    E.-Palmer semiflexible gas-
        troscope
    E.-Puestow dilation
    E.-Puestow guidewire
    E.-Puestow olive

edge
    heaped-up e's
    hepatic e.
    liver e.
    ulcer with heaped-up e's

Edmondson grading system for
    hepatocellular carcinoma

EEA
    EEA AutoSure stapler
    EEA stapler

effect
    choleretic e.
    cytoprotective e.
    duodenal e.
    esophageal e.
    gastric e.
    halo e.
    irradiation e.
    metabolic e.
    octreotide e.
    physiological trophic e.
    placebo e.
    prokinetic e.
    systemic e.
    tubulotoxic e.

effective
    e. renal blood flow
    e. renal plasma flow

effector T cell
    e. T c. function

efferent
    e. artery of glomerulus
    e. ductules of testis
    e. glomerular arteriole
    e. limb
    e. loop
    e. vessel of glomerulus

effluent
    anal e.
    ileostomy e.
    transverse colostomy e.

egagropilus

EGD
    esophagogastroduodenos-
        copy
        Sand-Eze EGD pillow

EGE
    eosinophilic gastroenteritis

egesta

egestion

egophony

Egyptian splenomegaly

EHEC
    enterohemorrhagic *Escherichia coli*

EHM
    extrahepatic metastasis

EIEC
    enteroinvasive *Escherichia coli*

Einhorn
    E. dilator
    E. string test

ejaculate

ejaculatio
    e. deficiens
    e. praecox

ejaculation
    premature e.
    retrograde e.

ejaculator
    e. seminis

ejaculatory
    e. duct

ejaculum

ejecta

ejection
    e. fraction
    gallbladder e. fraction
    gallbladder e. rate
    e. rate

elastance

elastic
    e. band ligation
    e. bougie
    e. ligature
    e. recoil

elbowed
    e. bougie
    e. catheter

electrocoagulation necrosis

electrocystography

electrode
    abdominal patch e.

electrodialyzer

electroejaculation

electrogastrogram

electrogastrograph

electrogastrography

electrolyte
    e. abnormality
    e. balance
    balanced e. solution
    e. flush solution

electromyography
    ureteral e.

electrophoresis
    agarose gel e.
    e. immunoblot analysis

electrostatic force

electrosurgical fulguration

electroureterogram

electroureterography

elevator
    Doyen rib e.

eleventh rib flank incision

elimination diet

Eliminator
    E. biliary stent
    E. nasal biliary catheter set
    E. pancreatic stent
    E. PET biliary balloon dilator

eliminator
    fecal odor e.

Elliot position

Elliott gallbladder forceps

elliptical incision

Ellsner gastroscope

elusive
    e. polyp
    e. ulcer

emasculate

emasculation

embolic agent

embolism
    arterial e.
    bile pulmonary e.
    cholesterol e.
    mesenteric arterial e.
    pulmonary e.

embolization
    angiographic e.
    angiographic variceal e.
    arterial e.
    bilateral pudendal artery e.
    cholesterol crystal e.
    splenic arterial e.
    transcatheter arterial e.
    transcatheter hepatic arter-
        ial e.
    transcatheter splenic arter-
        ial e.
    transcatheter variceal e.
    transhepatic e.

embolus *pl.* emboli
    metallic e.
    pulmonary e.
    talc e.

embryoma
    e. of kidney

embryonal
    e. adenoma
    e. adenomyosarcoma
    e. carcinoma
    e. carcinosarcoma
    infantile e. carcinoma
    juvenile e. carcinoma
    e. nephroma
    e. sarcoma

embryonic testicular regression
    syndrome

emergency
    e. appendectomy
    e. colonoscopy
    e. laparotomy

emergent
    e. appendectomy

emesia

emesis
    bilious e.
    coffee-ground e.

emetatrophia

emetic

emetocathartic

emetogenic

Emetrol

eminence
    caudate e. of liver
    omental e. of body of pan-
        creas

emission
    gamma e.

EMLA anesthetic

emodin

emphysema
    endoscopy-related e.
    intestinal e.

emphysematous
    e. cholecystitis
    e. gastritis
    e. pyelonephritis

empty intestine

emptying
    delayed gastric e.
    gastric e.
    gastric e. time
    neorectal e.
    rectal e.
    solid e.
    e. time

empyema
  e. of gallbladder

empyocele

Emulsoil
  E. bowel prep

enalapril

en bloc
  e. b. dissection
  e. b. distal pancreatectomy
  e. b. resection

encelialgia

enceliitis

encelitis

encephaloid gastric carcinoma

encephalopathy
  bilirubin e.
  dialysis e.
  hepatic e.
  portal-systemic e.
  uremic e.
  Wernicke e.

encirclement
  anal e.

encopresis

encrusted pyelitis

encysted
  e. calculus
  e. hernia
  e. hydrocele
  e. peritonitis

end
  e. colostomy
  e. ileostomy
  e. stoma

endemic
  e. colic
  e. funiculitis
  e. nonbacterial infantile
    gastroenteritis

end-expiratory intragastric
  pressure

end-fire transrectal probe

end-hole catheter

end-loop
  e.-l. colostomy
  e.-l. ileocolostomy
  e.-l. ileostomy
  e.-l. stoma

endoabdominal
  e. fascia

endoanal mucosectomy

endoappendicitis

endobronchial fistula

endocervical
  e. gland

Endoclip

EndoCoil biliary stent

endocolitis

endocrine
  e. gland

endocrinologic impotence

endocystitis

endodermal sinus tumor

endoenteritis

endoesophagitis

endogastric

endogastritis

endogenous
  e. obesity
  e. opioid

endoherniorrhaphy

Endolav
  E. lavage pump

EndoMate grab bag

endometrioma
  ovarian e.

endometriosis
  colorectal e.

endopelvic

endoperitoneal

endoperitonitis

endophlebitis
  e. hepatica obliterans

endoprosthesis
  biliary e.
  Celestin e.
  cuffed esophageal e.
  double-lumen e.
  double-pigtail e.
  esophageal e.
  expandable biliary e.
  large-bore biliary e.
  pancreatic e.
  peroral e.
  pigtail e.

endoradiosonde

endorectal
  e. ileal pouch
  e. ileal pull-through
  e. pull-through
  e. pull-through procedure
  e. ultrasound

endoscope
  AccuSharp e.
  ACMI e.
  battery-powered e.
  CF-HM e.
  Cho/Dyonics two-portal e.
  e. clip
  double-channel e.
  Eder-Palmer semiflexible fi-
    beroptic e.
  end-viewing e.
  FCS two-channel ultra-high-
    magnification e.
  FG-series two-channel e.
  FGS-ML-series two-chan-
    nel e.
  FGS-series two-channel e.
  fiberoptic e.

endoscope *(continued)*
  flexible e.
  flexible fiberoptic e.
  forward-viewing e.
  Fujinon EG-FP series e.
  Fujinon EVE series e.
  Fujinon EVG-CT series e.
  Fujinon EVGFP series e.
  Fujinon EVG-F series e.
  Fujinon FP series e.
  Fujinon UGI-FP series vid-
    eo e.
  Hirschowitz e.
  e. impaction
  JFB III e.
  J-shaped e.
  Karl Storz e.
  Kussmaul e.
  LoPresti e.
  magnifying e.
  Messerklinger e.
  mother/daughter e.
  oblique-viewing e.
  Olympus Aloka Gf-EU-se-
    ries e.
  Olympus CV-series e.
  Olympus DES-series e.
  Olympus EUS-series e.
  Olympus EVIS series e.
  Olympus GF-UM-series e.
  Olympus GIF-HM-series e.
  Olympus GIF-J-series e.
  Olympus GIF-Q-series e.
  Olympus GIF-T-series e.
  Olympus GIF-XP-series e.
  Olympus JF-T-series e.
  Olympus JF-TV-series e.
  Olympus JF-V-series e.
  Olympus PFJ-series pediat-
    ric e.
  Olympus P-series e.
  Olympus TJF-series e.
  Olympus UM-series e.
  Olympus V-series e.
  Olympus XCV-XK-series e.
  Olympus XP-series e.
  Olympus XQ-series e.
  pediatric e.
  Pentax EC-series video e.

endoscope *(continued)*
  Pentax EG-series video e.
  Pentax FD-series video e.
  Pentax FG-series video e.
  rigid e.
  semiflexible e.
  semirigid e.
  side-viewing e.
  Toshiba video e.
  two-channel e.
  UGI e.
  upper GI e.
  video e.
  Welch Allyn video e.

endoscopic
  e. assessment
  e. atrophic gastritis
  e. band ligation
  e. biliary decompression
  e. biliary drainage
  e. biopsy
  e. cholangiography
  e. color Doppler assessment
  e. decompression
  e. dilation
  e. drainage
  e. enterogastric reflux gastritis
  e. esophagitis
  e. extirpation cicatricial obliteration
  e. finding
  e. fistulotomy
  e. fulguration
  e. gastritis
  e. gastrostomy
  e. hemorrhagic gastritis
  e. hemostasis
  e. incision
  e. manometry
  e. nasobiliary catheter drainage
  e. pancreatic drainage
  e. pancreatic stenting
  e. papillary balloon dilation
  e. raised erosive gastritis
  e. removal
  e. retrograde cannulation

endoscopic *(continued)*
  e. retrograde cholangiogram
  e. retrograde cholangiography
  e. retrograde cholangiopancreatography (ERCP)
  e. retrograde cholecystoendoprosthesis
  e. retrograde pancreatography
  e. retrograde parenchymography of pancreas (ERPP)
  e. rugal hyperplastic gastritis
  e. sclerosis
  e. small bowel biopsy
  e. sphincterotomy-induced pancreatitis
  e. stenting
  e. tattoo
  e. transpapillary cannulation
  e. transpapillary catheterization of the gallbladder
  e. transpapillary cyst drainage
  e. variceal ligation

endoscopist

endoscopy
  advanced therapeutic e.
  anal e.
  e. complication
  fiberoptic e.
  flexible e.
  gastrointestinal e.
  high-magnification e.
  intestinal e.
  intraoperative e.
  intraoperative biliary e.
  outpatient e.
  pancreaticobiliary e.
  pediatric e.
  peripartum e.
  peroral e.
  postsurgical e.
  primary diagnostic e.

endoscopy *(continued)*
    e. procedure
    e.-related emphysema
    e. suite
    therapeutic e.
    therapeutic upper e.
    transcolonic e.
    transesophageal e.
    transnasal e.
    upper alimentary e.
    upper e. and colonoscopy
    upper gastrointestinal e.
    video e.

Endoshears

endosnare

endosonography
    e.-guided drainage of pancreatic pseudocyst

Endostapler

endothelium
    gastrointestinal e.

Endotorque
    Greenen E.

endotoxin
    bacterial e.
    e.-induced fever

endotracheal
    e. intubation
    e. tube

endourethral

endourology

end-sigmoid colostomy

end-stage
    e.-s. cirrhosis
    e.-s. disease
    e.-s. renal disease (ESRD)
    e.-s. renal failure

end-to-end
    e.-t.-e. anastomosis
    e.-t.-e. reanastomosis

end-to-side
    e.-t.-s. anastomosis

end-to-side *(continued)*
    e.-t.-s. portacaval shunt
    e.-t.-s. reimplantation
    right-angled e.-t.-s. anastomosis

end-viewing
    e.-v. endoscope
    e.-v. gastroscope

enema
    air contrast barium e. (ACBE)
    analeptic e.
    antegrade e.
    antegrade continuous e. procedure
    5-ASA e.
    barium e. (BE)
    barium e. with air contrast
    barium e. reduction
    blind e.
    cleansing hypertonic phosphate e.
    Cortenema retention e.
    double-contrast air barium e.
    double-contrast barium e.
    flatus e.
    Fleet e.
    Fleet Baby e.
    Fleet Babylax e.
    flexible barium e.
    full-column barium e.
    Gastrografin e.
    high e.
    hydrocortisone e.
    hydrogen peroxide e.
    Kayexalate e.
    lactulose e.
    mesalamine e.
    methylene blue e.
    NuLYTELY e.
    nutrient e.
    oil retention e.
    Phospho-Soda e.
    prednisolone e.
    retention e.
    retrograde flow on barium e.

enema *(continued)*
 Rowasa e.
 saline cleansing e.
 single-contrast barium e.
 small-bowel e.
 soapsuds e.
 sodium phosphates e.
 sodium phosphate and bi-
  phosphate e.
 tap water e.
 theophylline olamine e.
 e's until clear
 water soluble contrast e.

enemator

engorgement
 liver e.

engraftment

enlargement
 ovarian e.

Enrich feeding

Ensure
 E. Plus
 E. Plus feeding

Entamoeba histolytica
 Entamoeba histolytica abscess

enteraden

enteradenitis

enteral
 e. absorption
 e. alimentation
 e. diarrhea
 e. feeding
 e. nutrition

enteralgia

enterectasis

enterectomy

enterepiplocele

enteric
 e. adenovirus
 e. cyst

enteric *(continued)*
 e. fever
 e. fistula
 e. hyperoxaluria
 e. infection

enteric-coated
 e.-c. aspirin

enterically transmitted non-A,
 non-B hepatitis

enteritis
 Campylobacter e.
 choleriform e.
 chronic cicatrizing e.
 Crohn regional e.
 e. cystica chronica
 diphtheritic e.
 eosinophilic e.
 granulomatous e.
 e. gravis
 idiopathic diffuse ulcerative nongranulomatous e.
 leishmanial e.
 mucomembranous e.
 mucous e.
 e. necroticans
 e. nodularis
 phlegmonous e.
 e. polyposa
 protozoan e.
 pseudomembranous e.
 radiation e.
 regional e.
 segmental e.
 streptococcus e.
 terminal e.
 tuberculous e.
 ulcerative e.
 viral e.

enteroadherent
 e. *Escherichia coli*

enteroaggregative
 e. *Escherichia coli*

enteroanastomosis

Enterobacter aerogenes

enterobiliary

enterocele
  partial e.

enterocentesis

enterocholecystostomy

enterocholecystotomy

enterocinesia

enterocinetic

enterocleisis
  omental e.

enteroclysis

enterocolectomy

enterocolitis
  Aeromonas-associated e.
  antibiotic-associated e.
  antibiotic-induced e.
  bacterial e.
  gangrenous ischemic e.
  granulomatous e.
  hemorrhagic e.
  Hirschsprung-associated e.
  necrotizing e.
  pseudomembranous e.
  radiation e.
  regional e.
  Salmonella typhimurium e.

enterocolostomy

enterocutaneous
  e. fistula

enterocyst

enterocystocele

enterocystoma

enterocystoplasty
  Camey e.
  Camey e. urinary diversion
  clam e.
  sigmoid e.

enterocyte

enterodynia

enteroenteral fistula

enteroenteric fistula

enteroenterostomy
  Parker-Kerr e.
  two-layer e.

enteroepiplocele

enterogastric
  e. reflex

enterogastritis

enterogenous
  e. cyanosis
  e. cyst

enterogram

enterograph

enterography

enterohemorrhagic
  e. *Escherichia coli* (EHEC)

enterohepatic
  e. circulation

enterohepatitis

enterohydrocele

enterointestinal

enteroinvasive
  e. *Escherichia coli*

enterokinesia

enterokinetic

enterolith
  calcified e.

enterolithiasis

enterology

enterolysis

enteromegalia

enteromegaly

enteromerocele

enteromesenteric
  e. occlusion

enteromycodermitis

enteromycosis
   e. bacteriacea

enteromyiasis

enteron

enteroneuritis

enteronitis

enteroparesis

enteropathic
   e. arthritis

enteropathogen

enteropathogenesis

enteropathogenic

enteropathy
   allergic e.
   bile salt–losing e.
   chronic bacterial e.
   diabetic e.
   food-sensitive e.
   gluten e.
   gluten-sensitive e.
   idiopathic e.
   protein-losing e.
   radiation e.
   soya-induced e.

enteroperitoneal
   e. abscess

enteropexy

enteroplasty

enteroplegia

enteroplication

enterorrhagia

enterorrhaphy
   circular e.

enterorrhea

enterorrhexis

enteroscope

enteroscopy
   Roux-en-Y limb e.
   transgastrostomic e.
   video small bowel e.

enterosepsis

enterospasm

enterostasis

enterostaxis

enterostenosis

enterostomal

enterostomy
   gun-barrel e.

enterotome

enterotomy
   antimesenteric e.
   longitudinal e.

enterotoxin
   e. diarrhea

enterotropic

enterourethral fistula

enterovaginal fistula

enterovenous

enterovesical
   e. fistula

enteruria

entrapment of bowel

Entrition Entri-Pak feeding

enuresis

enuretic

environment
   bactericidal stomach e.

enzyme
   angiotensin-converting e.
   (ACE)
   cellular e.
   e. change
   liver e.

enzyme *(continued)*
    pancreatic e.

eosin
    hematoxylin and e. (H&E)
    hematoxylin and e. stain

eosinophil
    e. chemotactic factor of an-
      aphylaxis

eosinophilic
    e. ascites
    e. ballooning
    e. cholangiopathy
    e. cystitis
    e. enteritis
    e. esophagitis
    e. gastritis
    e. gastroenteritis (EGE)
    e. gastroenteropathy
    e. granuloma
    e. ileal perforation
    e. prostatitis

EPEC
    enteropathogenic *Esche-*
      richia coli

epicardia

epicardial

epicritic pain

epicystitis

epicystotomy

epidemic
    e. dysentery
    e. gangrenous proctitis
    e. gastritis
    e. gastroenteritis
    e. hemorrhagic fever
    e. hepatitis
    e. jaundice
    e. nausea
    e. nephropathy
    e. nonbacterial gastroenter-
      itis
    e. vomiting

epidemica
    nausea e.

epididymal

epididymectomy

epididymis *pl.* epididymides

epididymitis
    spermatogenic e.

epididymodeferentectomy

epididymodeferential

epididymo-orchitis

epididymotomy

epididymovasectomy

epididymovasostomy

epigastralgia

epigastric
    e. angle
    e. discomfort
    e. distress
    e. fold
    e. hernia
    e. incision
    inferior e. artery
    inferior e. vein
    e. pain
    e. spot
    superficial e. artery
    superficial e. vein
    superior e. artery
    superior e. veins

epigastrium

epigastrocele

epiorchium

epiplocele

epiploectomy

epiploenterocele

epiploic
    e. abscess
    e. appendages
    e. appendagitis
    e. appendix
    e. foramen

epiploic *(continued)*
  left e. vein
  e. orifice
  right e. vein
  e. sac

epiploitis

epiplomerocele

epiplomphalocele

epiploon
  great e.
  lesser e.

epiplopexy

epiploplasty

epiplorrhaphy

epiploscheocele

episodic
  e. colic
  e. vomiting

epispadia

epispadiac

epispadial

epispadias
  balanic e.
  balanitic e.
  clitoric e.
  complete e.
  glandular e.
  incomplete e.
  penile e.
  penopubic e.
  subsymphyseal e.

epistaxis
  Gull renal e.

epithalaxia

epithelial
  bile duct e. cell
  e. cast
  e. cell
  e. crescent
  e. dysplasia
  e. inclusion body

epithelial *(continued)*
  rectal e. cell
  tubular e. cell

epithelioid
  e. granuloma
  e. leiomyoma

epithelium *pl.* epithelia
  airway e.
  Barrett e.
  capsular e.
  gastric e.
  glomerular e.
  seminiferous e.
  villous e.

epityphlitis

epityphlon

epsilon-aminocaproic acid

Epstein
  E.-Barr viral infection
  E. nephrosis
  E. syndrome

equal fluid balance

equilibrium
  acid-base e.

equivalent

equivocal

ERCP
  endoscopic retrograde
    cholangiopancreatogra-
    phy
      Bilisystem ERCP can-
        nula
      ERCP cannulation
      contour ERCP cannula
      ERCP dilator
      Fluoro Tip ERCP can-
        nula
      ERCP-guided biopsy
      ERCP manometry
      post-ERCP induced
        pancreatitis
      postsphincterotomy
        ERCP cannulation
      Teflon ERCP cannula

erectile dysfunction

erection

eroded polyp

erosion
    cancerous e.
    chronic e.
    Dieulafoy gastric e.
    duodenal e.
    gastric antral e.
    gastric mucosal e.
    idiopathic chronic e.
    linear e.
    salt-and-pepper duodenal e.
    stress e.

erosive
    e. balanitis
    chronic e. gastritis
    e. duodenitis
    e. esophagitis
    e. gastritis
    e. gastropathy
    e. prepyloric change

erosive/hemorrhagic gastritis

erotic vomiting

eructation

erythema
    e. multiforme

erythematopultaceous
    e. stomatitis

erythematous
    e. gastropathy

erythrocyte aggregation

erythrocytosis
    absolute e.

erythromycin
    e.-induced cholecystitis

erythroplasia
    Zoon e.

Escherichia coli
    enterohemorrhagic *E. coli*
    (EHEC)

escutcheon
    female e.
    male e.

esogastritis

EsophaCoil esophageal stent

esophagalgia

esophageal
    e. achalasia
    e. acid infusion test
    e. adenocarcinoma
    e. A ring
    e. atresia
    e. balloon dilator
    e. balloon distention
    e. balloon tamponade
    e. banding
    e. biopsy
    e. body motor dysfunction
    e. B ring
    e. cancer
    e. candidiasis
    e. carcinoma
    Child e. varices classifica-
      tion
    e. clearing
    e. colic
    e. compression
    e. condyloma acuminatum
    e. condyloma virus
    e. contractile ring
    e. dilatation
    e. dilation
    e. dilator
    e. diverticulum
    e. duplication cyst
    e. dysmotility
    e. dysphagia
    e. effect
    e. endoprosthesis
    e. fistula
    e. foreign body
    e. function test
    e. fungal infection
    e. glands
    e. groove
    e. hematoma

esophageal *(continued)*
- e. hiatus
- e. hyperkeratosis
- e. impression of liver
- e. infection
- e. inlet
- e. intramural hematoma
- e. intubation
- e. Lewy body
- lower e. sphincter
- e. lumen
- e. malignancy
- e. manometric sequence
- e. manometry
- e. mass
- e. motility
- e. motility disorder
- e. mucosa
- e. mucosal ring
- e. muscular ring
- e. myotomy
- e. obstruction
- e. osteophyte
- e. perforation
- e. perfusate
- e. peristalsis
- e. peristaltic pressure
- e. pH monitoring
- e. photodynamic therapy
- e. plexus
- e. polyp
- e. prosthesis
- e. reflux
- e. resection
- e. ring
- e. rupture
- e. scleroderma
- e. shunt
- e. sound
- e. spasm
- e. sphincter
- e. sphincter relaxation
- e. squamous cell carcinoma
- e. squamous papilloma
- e. stenosis
- e. stricture
- e. stricture repair
- superficial e. carcinoma

esophageal *(continued)*
- e. tear
- e. transection
- e. transit time
- transthoracic resection of e. carcinoma
- e. trauma
- e. tube
- e. tuberculosis
- e. tumor
- e. ulcer
- e. ulceration
- upper e. sphincter
- e. variceal bleeding
- e. variceal sclerosis
- e. variceal sclerotherapy
- e. varix
- e. wall
- e. wall thickness
- e. web

esophagectasia

esophagectasis

esophagectomy
- Ivor Lewis two-stage subtotal e.
- e. with thoracotomy
- transhiatal e.
- transthoracic e.

esophagism

esophagismus

esophagitis
- acid-pepsin reflux e.
- acid-peptic e.
- alkaline reflux e.
- aspergillosis e.
- bacterial e.
- Barrett e.
- *Candida* e.
- candidal e.
- caustic e.
- chemical-induced e.
- chronic peptic e.
- CMV (cytomegalovirus) e.
- corrosive e.
- cytomegalovirus e.
- e. dissecans superficialis

esophagitis *(continued)*
  drug-induced e.
  endoscopic e.
  eosinophilic e.
  erosive e.
  fungal e.
  herpes simplex e.
  herpetic e.
  herpetiform e.
  histologic e.
  infectious e.
  Leishmania e.
  monilial e.
  nonreflux e.
  nonspecific e.
  peptic e.
  pill e.
  polycystic chronic e.
  radiation e.
  reflux e.
  refractory e.
  retention e.
  severe erosive e.
  severe reflux e.
  stasis e.
  streptococcal e.
  tuberculous e.
  tuberculous infectious e.
  ulcerative e.
  viral e.

esophagobronchial
  e. fistula

esophagocardiomyotomy

esophagocele

esophagocolic
  e. anastomosis

esophagocologastrostomy

esophagocoloplasty

esophagoduodenostomy

esophagodynia

esophagoenterostomy

esophagoesophagostomy

esophagofundopexy

esophagogastrectomy

esophagogastric
  e. fat pad
  e. junction
  e. tamponade
  e. variceal bleeding

esophagogastroanastomosis

esophagogastroduodenal

esophagogastroduodenoscopy
  (EGD)

esophagogastromyotomy

esophagogastroplasty

esophagogastroscopy
  Abbott e.
  Claggett Barrett e.
  intrathoracic e.
  Johnson e.
  Thal e.
  Woodward e.

esophagogastrostomy
  Abbott e.
  Claggett Barrett e.

esophagogram
  barium e.

esophagojejunogastrostomosis

esophagojejunogastrostomy

esophagojejunoplasty

esophagojejunostomy
  loop e.
  Roux-en-Y e.

esophagology

esophagomalacia

esophagomediastinal fistula

esophagomycosis

esophagomyotomy
  Heller e.

esophagoplasty
  colic patch e.

esophagoplication

esophagoproximal gastrectomy

esophagoptosis

esophagopulmonary fistula

esophagorespiratory fistula

esophagosalivary
    e. reflex

esophagoscope
    ACMI fiberoptic e.
    balloon e.
    Blom-Singer e.
    Bruening e.
    Chevalier Jackson e.
    child e.
    Denck e.
    Dohlman e.
    Eder-Hufford rigid e.
    fiberoptic e.
    Foregger rigid e.
    Foroblique fiberoptic e.
    full-lumen e.
    Haslinger e.
    Holinger e.
    Hufford e.
    infant e.
    Jackson e.
    Jasbee e.
    Jesberg e.
    J-scope e.
    Kalk e.
    large-bore rigid e.
    LoPresti fiberoptic e.
    Moersch e.
    Mosher e.
    Olympus EF-series e.
    optical e.
    oval e.
    oval-open e.
    Roberts e.
    Roberts-Jesberg e.
    Sam Roberts e.
    Schindler e.
    Storz e.
    Tesberg e.
    Universal e.
    Yankauer e.

esophagoscopy

esophagospasm

esophagostenosis

esophagostoma

esophagostomy

esophagotome

esophagotomy

esophagus *pl.* esophagi
    abdominal e.
    achalasialike e.
    aperistaltic e.
    atonic e.
    Barrett e.
    cervical e.
    closed e.
    columnar-lined e.
    corkscrew e.
    dilatation of e.
    dilation of e.
    distal e.
    nutcracker e.
    scleroderma of e.
    spastic e.
    strictured e.
    thoracic e.
    tortuous e.
    variceal sclerotherapy in e.

ESRD
    end-stage renal disease

essential
    e. amino acid
    e. fatty acid
    e. hematuria

esterified fecal acid

estrogen-induced cholestasis

état
    é. mammelonné

ETEC
    enterotoxigenic *Escherichia coli.*

ethacrynic acid

ethanol (ETOH)
   e. abuse
   e.-induced tumor necrosis

ethyl alcohol

ET-NANB
   enterically transmitted
     non-A, non-B hepatitis

ETOH
   ethanol
     ETOH abuse

euchlorhydria

eucholia

euchylia

Eulexin

eunuchoid
   e. gigantism

eupancreatism

eupepsia

eupepsy

eupeptic

euperistalsis

euvolemic

Evac-Q-Kit bowel prep

Evac-Q-Kwik bowel prep

evacuation
   digital rectal e.
   e. disorder
   rectal e.
   stool e.

evacuator

evaluation
   diverticulitis e.
   followup e.

evanescent

eventration

evisceration
   total abdominal e.

Ewald
   E. breakfast
   E. gastroscope
   E. test meal
   E. tube

Ewing sarcoma

exacerbation of pain

examination
   digital rectal e.
   followup e.
   microscopic urine e.
   rectal e.

exania

excavated gastric carcinoma

excavatio *pl.* excavationes
   e. rectovesicalis

excavation
   rectovesical e.

excavatum
   pectus e.

excess
   base e.
   e. mucus

excessive bleeding

exchange resin
   anion e. r.

excision
   abdominoperineal e.
   laser hemorrhoid e.

excoriation

excrement

excrementitious

excretion
   basal renal e.
   biliary e.

excretory
   e. duct of seminal gland
   e. duct of seminal vesicle
   e. duct of testis

excretory *(continued)*
    e. function

exenteration
    anterior e.
    anterior pelvic e.
    pelvic e.
    posterior pelvic e.
    supralevator pelvic e.
    total pelvic e.

exenterative

exenteritis

exercise
    e.-associated acute renal
      failure
    Kegel e's
    thallium e. stress test

exfoliative
    e. cystitis
    e. cytology
    e. gastritis

exit site infection

Ex-Lax

Exna

exocolitis

exocrine
    e. gland
    e. pancreas
    e. part of pancreas

exogastric

exogastritis

exogenous obesity

exophytic
    e. adenocarcinoma
    e. mass
    e. wart

expandable
    e. biliary endoprosthesis
    e. olive

expanding retroperitoneal hematoma

expansile abdominal mass

exploration
    common bile duct e.
      (CBDE)
    common duct e.
    complete surgical e.

exploratory
    e. biopsy
    e. celiotomy
    e. laparotomy

explosion
    colonic e.

explosive diarrhea

exposure
    occupational toxin e.

exquisite
    e. pain
    e. tenderness

exquisitely tender abdomen

exsanguinating hemorrhage

exstrophy
    e. of the bladder
    e. of cloaca
    cloacal e.

extension fiber

exteriorization colostomy

external
    e. abdominal ring
    e. anal sphincter
    aponeurosis of e. oblique
    e. appliance
    e. beam radiation
    e. beam radiation therapy
    e. biliary fistula
    e. biliary lavage
    e. coat of esophagus
    e. coat of ureter
    e. cooling appliance
    e. crus of anterior inguinal
      ring
    e. drainage
    e. fistula
    e. genital organs
    e. hemorrhoid

external *(continued)*
    e. hernia
    e. iliac artery
    e. inguinal ring
    e. ligament
    e. margin of testis
    e. oblique
    e. oblique aponeurosis
    e. oblique fascia
    e. oblique muscle of abdomen
    e. orifice of urethra
    e. proctotomy
    e. rectal sphincter
    e. ring
    e. rotation
    e. shock wave lithotripsy
    e. skin tag
    e. spermatic fascia
    e. sphincter muscle of anus
    e. sphincterotomy
    e. stimulus
    e. swelling
    e. trauma
    e. urethral orifice
    e. urethrotomy

extirpation
    surgical e.

extract
    belladonna e.

extractor
    basket e.

extracystic

extraglomerular
    e. mesangium

extrahepatic
    e. bile duct
    e. bile duct cancer
    e. bile duct carcinoma
    e. bile duct obstruction
    e. biliary atresia
    e. biliary cystic dilation
    e. biliary obstruction
    e. biliary stricture

extrahepatic *(continued)*
    e. cancer
    e. cholestasis
    e. metastasis
    e. obstruction
    e. shunt

extraintestinal
    e. complication

extralymphatic metastasis

extramucosal
    e. mass

extramural lesion

extrapancreatic

extraparotid lymph gland

extraperitoneal
    e. fascia
    e. space
    e. tissue

extraprostatic

extraprostatitis

extrarenal
    e. azotemia
    e. pelvis

extrasaccular
    e. hernia

extrasphincteric anal fistula

extravasated
    e. contrast material

extravasation
    e. of contrast medium
    peripelvic e.
    urinary e.

extravascular
    e. space

extravesical anastomosis

extremitas *pl.* extremitates
    e. inferior renis
    e. inferior testis
    e. superior renis

extremitas *(continued)*
  e. superior testis

extrinsic
  e. compression
  e. mass

extrophia

extrude

extubate

exudate
  pharyngeal e.

exudate-transudate concept

exudative
  e. ascites
  e. nephritis
  e. peritonitis
  e. pharyngitis

ex vivo

Fabry disease

faceted gallstone

facies *pl.* facies
  f. abdominalis
  f. anterior corporis pancreatis
  f. anterior prostatae
  f. anterior renis
  f. anteroinferior corporis pancreatis
  f. anterosuperior corporis pancreatis
  cushingoid f.
  f. diaphragmatica hepatis
  f. hepatica
  f. inferior hepatis
  f. inferior pancreatis
  f. inferolateralis prostatae
  f. lateralis testis
  f. medialis testis
  moon f.
  f. posterior corporis pancreatis
  f. posterior hepatis
  f. posterior prostatae
  f. posterior renis
  Potter f.
  f. superior hepatis
  f. urethralis penis
  f. visceralis hepatis

facilitator neuron

FACS
  fluorescence-activated cell sorter
  fluorescence-activated cell sorting

factitial proctitis

factor
  alcoholic prognostic f.
  Am f.
  antinucleoprotein f.
  atrial natriuretic f.
  f. B
  B cell growth f.

factor *(continued)*
  Castle intrinsic f.
  chemotactic f.
  colony-stimulating f. (CSF)
  corticotropin-releasing f. (CRF)
  f. D
  decay-accelerating f. (DAF)
  early B-cell f. (EBF)
  eosinophil chemotactic f. of anaphylaxis
  gamma-activated f. (GAV)
  granulocyte colony-stimulating f. (G-CSF)
  granulocyte-macrophage colony-stimulating f. (GM-CSF)
  growth hormone–releasing f. (GHRF)
  f. H
  hepatocyte growth f. (HGF)
  homologous restriction f.
  f. I
  inhibiting f.
  intrinsic f. (IF)
  leukemia inhibitory f.
  leukotactic f.
  macrophage migration inhibitory f.
  migration inhibitory f.
  mitogenic f.
  nucleocapsid core f.
  f. P (properdin)
  releasing f.
  rheumatoid f.
  spreading f.
  T cell growth f.
  transcription-activating f.
  transfer f.
  tumor necrosis f.

FAG
  fundic atrophic gastritis

Fahey test

Fahrenheit thermometer

Fahr-Volhard disease

failure
  acute hepatic f.
  acute intrinsic renal f.
  acute renal f.
  anemia of chronic renal f.
  chronic renal f.
  contrast-associated renal f.
  dilator placement f.
  drug-induced renal f.
  end-stage renal f.
  exercise-associated acute
    renal f.
  fulminant hepatic f. (FHF)
  fulminant hepatocellular f.
  fulminant liver f.
  intubation f.
  irradiation f.
  kidney f.
  late-onset hepatic f.
  liver f.
  multiorgan system f.
  multiple organ f.
  nephrotoxic acute renal f.
  nonoliguric acute renal f.
  oliguric renal f.
  parenchymatous acute
    renal f.
  postischemic acute renal f.
  radiocontrast-induced
    acute renal f.
  renal f.
  subfulminant liver f.
  f. to thrive
  treatment f.
  vascular access f.

falciform ligament of liver

falciparum malaria

fallopian
  f. tube
  f. valve

false
  f. cast
  "f. channel" formation
  f. colonic obstruction
  f. cyst
  f. diverticulum

false (continued)
  f. hematuria
  f.-negative
  f.-positive
  f. spermatic vesicle
  f. straight arterioles of kid-
    ney
  f. tympanites

familial
  f. adenomatous polyposis
  f. aggregation
  f. amyloidosis
  f. chloride diarrhea
  f. chloridorrhea
  f. cholemia
  f. cholestasis
  f. chronic idiopathic jaun-
    dice
  f. colonic varices
  f. colorectal polyposis
  f. Crohn disease
  f. dysalbuminemic hyper-
    thyroxinemia
  f. fat-induced hyperlipid-
    emia
  f. gastrointestinal polyposis
  f. hamartomatous polypo-
    sis
  f. hepatitis
  f. hypercholesterolemia
  f. hypercholesterolemia
    with hyperlipidemia
  f. hyperchylomicronemia
  f. hyperchylomicronemia
    with hyperprebetalipo-
    proteinemia
  f. hyperlipoproteinemia
  f. hyperprebetalipoprotei-
    nemia
  f. hypertriglyceridemia
  f. intestinal polyposis
  f. intestinal pseudo-ob-
    struction
  f. isolated hyperthyroxine-
    mia
  f. juvenile nephrolithiasis
  f. juvenile nephronophthi-
    sis

familial *(continued)*
   f. juvenile nephrophthisis
   f. juvenile polyposis
   f. Mediterranean fever
   f. medullary thyroid carcinoma-pheochromocytoma syndrome
   f. nephritis serum
   f. nephrosis
   f. nonhemolytic jaundice
   f. pancreatitis
   f. pheochromocytoma
   f. polyposis
   f. polyposis coli
   f. polyposis syndrome
   progressive f. cirrhosis
   f. recurrent polyserositis
   f. ulcerative colitis

family screening

Fanconi syndrome

Ian-type laparoscopic retractor

farmer's lung

Farr technique

Farre tubercles

Fas (CD95)
   F. ligand
   F. protein

fascia *pl.* fasciae
   anal f.
   anoscrotal f.
   anterior rectus f.
   anterior renal f.
   Buck f.
   f. of Camper
   Colles f.
   fasciae of colon
   Cooper f.
   cremasteric f.
   f. cremasterica
   Cruveilhier f.
   dartos f.
   dartos f. of scrotum
   deep penile f.

fascia *(continued)*
   deep perineal f.
   deep f. of perineum
   Denonvilliers f.
   f. diaphragmatis pelvis inferior
   f. diaphragmatis pelvis superior
   f. diaphragmatis urogenitalis inferior
   f. diaphragmatis urogenitalis superior
   endoabdominal f.
   external oblique f.
   external spermatic f.
   extraperitoneal f.
   f. extraperitonealis
   fusion f.
   Gerota f.
   f. of Gerota
   f. inferior diaphragmatis pelvis
   inferior f. of urogenital diaphragm
   infundibuliform f.
   intercolumnar f.
   internal abdominal f.
   internal oblique f.
   internal spermatic f.
   ischiorectal f.
   middle perineal f.
   pelviprostatic f.
   f. pelvis visceralis
   f. penis profunda
   f. penis superficialis
   perineal f., superficial
   f. perinei superficialis
   peritoneoperineal f.
   f. peritoneoperinealis
   f. propria cooperi
   f. prostatae
   f. of prostate
   rectal f.
   rectovesical f.
   renal f.
   f. renalis
   Scarpa f.
   f. spermatica externa
   f. spermatica interna

fascia *(continued)*
  subperitoneal f.
  f. subperitonealis
  superficial penile f.
  superficial f. of perineum
  f. superficialis perinei
  f. superior diaphragmatis pelvis
  superior f. of urogenital diaphragm
  f. transversalis
  transverse f.
  Tyrrell f.
  f. of urogenital trigone
  visceral pelvic f.
  visceral f. of pelvis

fascial
  f. defect
  f. layer
  f. sheath of prostate
  f. sling
  f. sling approach

fascicular

fasciculated
  f. bladder

fasciculation

fasciculus *pl.* fasciculi
  longitudinal fasciculi of colon

fasciitis
  necrotizing f.
  perirenal f.

Fasciola

fashion
  helical f.
  retrograde f.

fasting
  f. blood sugar (FBS)
  f. diet
  f. plasma glucose (FPG)

fat
  abdominal f.
  abdominal f. pad

fat *(continued)*
  f. cell
  creeping mesenteric f.
  dietary f.
  esophageal f. pad
  f. hernia
  herniated preperitoneal f.
  high bulk, low f. diet
  high f. diet
  ileocecal f. pad
  f. indigestion
  f.-induced gallbladder contraction
  low f. diet
  f. pad
  paranephric f.
  pararenal f.
  pericolonic f.
  perinephric f.
  perirenal f.
  perivesical f.
  preperitoneal f.
  properitoneal f.
  protruding f.
  f.-soluble
  f.-soluble bilirubin
  f.-storing cells of liver
  f.-storing liver cells
  subcutaneous f.

fatty
  f. acid
  f. ascites
  f. capsule of kidney
  f. cirrhosis
  f. diarrhea
  f. food
  f. food intolerance
  f. infiltration of liver
  f. kidney
  f. liver
  f. liver disease
  f. liver hepatitis
  f. liver of pregnancy
  f. meal
  f. micromedionodular cirrhosis
  f. necrosis
  f. omental apron

fatty *(continued)*
    f. stool
    f. tissue

FBD
    functional bowel disorder
    functional bowel distress

FBS
    fasting blood sugar

FCS two-channel ultra-high-magnification endoscope

FDH
    familial dysalbuminemic hyperthyroxinemia

Fe
    Slow F.

febrile
    f. agglutinins
    f. disease
    f. pleomorphic anemia

fecal
    f. abscess
    f. analysis
    f. bile acid
    f. concretion
    f. contamination
    f. continence
    f. diversion
    f. fat test
    f. fistula
    f. flora
    f. fluid
    f. impaction
    f. incontinence
    f. leukocyte
    f. marker
    f. material
    f. obstruction
    f. occult blood test
    f. odor eliminator
    f.-oral route
    f.-oral transmission
    f. peritonitis
    f. reservoir
    f. residue
    f. spillage
    f. stasis

fecal *(continued)*
    f. tumor
    f. vomiting

fecalith

fecaloma

fecaluria

Fecatest

feces
    impacted f.
    inspissated f.
    retained f.

feculence

feculent
    f. vomitus

fecundity

Federici sign

feedback
    antibody f.
    f. control

feeding
    Amin-Aid powdered f.
    bolus f.
    Build Up enteral f.
    Citrotein liquid f.
    Clinifeed Iso enteral f.
    Compleat-B liquid f.
    f. complication
    continuous drip f.
    Criticare HN elemental liquid f.
    f. device
    f. disorder
    drip f.
    Enrich f.
    Ensure Plus f.
    enteral f.
    Entrition Entri-Pak f.
    Finkelstein f.
    Flexical enteral f.
    forced f.
    forcible f.
    Fortison enteral f.
    gastric f.
    gastrostomy f.

feeding *(continued)*
  f. gastrostomy
  gavage f.
  half-strength f.
  Hepatic-Aid powdered f.
  HN f.
  hyperosmotic f.
  intermittent drip f.
  intravenous f.
  Isocal HCN liquid f.
  Isotein HN f.
  isotonic f.
  jejunostomy elemental
    diet f.
  jejunostomy tube f.
  lactose-free f.
  Lonalac f.
  low residue f.
  Magnacal liquid f.
  Meritene liquid f.
  nasal f.
  nasojejunal f.
  Osmolite HN enteral f.
  parenteral f.
  Portagen f.
  Precision Isotonic pow-
    dered f.
  Renu enteral f.
  Resource enteral f.
  sham f.
  Stresstein liquid f.
  Sustacal HC liquid f.
  Sustagen liquid f.
  Trauma-Aid HBC enteral f.
  TraumaCal enteral f.
  Travasorb HN powdered f.
  Travasorb MCT liquid f.
  Travasorb STD liquid f.
  tube f.
  f. tube
  Vital f.
  Vitaneed f.
  Vivonex HN powdered f.
  Vivonex TEN f.
feeding pump
  Companion f. p.
  Compat f. p.
  Frenta Mat f. p.
  Frenta System II f. p.

feeding pump *(continued)*
  Nutromat Pad S f. p.

feeding tube
  Bard gastrostomy f. t.
  Compat f. t.
  Dobbhoff f. t.
  Keofeed f. t.
  nasoduodenal f. t.
  nasoenteric f. t.
  nasogastric f. t.
  postpyloric f. t.

Feen-A-Mint

female
  f. catheter
  f. escutcheon
  f. hypospadias

feminization
  male f.
  testicular f.

femoral
  f. fossa
  f. fovea
  f. hernia
  f. ring

femorocele

femur

Fenger gallbladder probe

Fenwick
  F. disease
  F.-Hunner ulcer

Feosol

Ferguson gallstone scoop

fermental diarrhea

fermentative
  f. diarrhea
  f. dyspepsia

Ferrein
  pyramid of F.
  F. tubes
  F. tubules

Ferris biliary duct dilator

ferritin
　　anionic f.
　　f. conjugated antibody
　　serum f.

ferrous
　　f. sulfate

fertile

fertility

fetoprotein
　　alpha f. (AFP)

fetor
　　f. hepaticus

fetus
　　allogeneic f.

fever
　　Aden f.
　　bilious remittent f.
　　breakbone f.
　　cachectic f.
　　Charcot f.
　　dehydration f.
　　dengue f.
　　dengue hemorrhagic f.
　　digestive f.
　　endotoxin-induced f.
　　enteric f.
　　epidemic hemorrhagic f.
　　familial Mediterranean f.
　　glandular f.
　　hemorrhagic f.
　　hepatic f.
　　hormonal f.
　　inanition f.
　　f. index
　　intermittent hepatic f.
　　low-grade f.
　　spiking f.
　　thirst f.
　　typhoid f.
　　urethral f.
　　urinary f.
　　urticarial f.
　　viral hemorrhagic f.
　　Yangtze Valley f.

fever (continued)
　　yellow f.

FG-series two-channel endo-
　　scope

FGS-ML-series two-channel en-
　　doscope

FGS-series two-channel endo-
　　scope

FHF
　　fulminant hepatic failure

F1 hybrid

fiber
　　afferent f.
　　archiform f's
　　f. bundle
　　collateral f's of Winslow
　　cremasteric f.
　　f.-deficient diet
　　dietary f.
　　extension f.
　　intercolumnar f's
　　intercrural f's
　　low f. diet
　　oblique f's of stomach
　　viscoelastic collagen f.

Fiberall

fibercolonoscope

FiberCon

fiberduodenoscope

fiberendoscope

fibergastroscope

fiberoptic
　　f. bundle
　　f. catheter
　　f. colonoscope
　　f. endoscope
　　f. endoscopy
　　f. esophagoscope
　　flexible f. choledochoscope
　　flexible f. endoscope
　　f. gastroscope
　　f. injection sclerotherapy

fiberoptic *(continued)*
    f. instrument technique
    f. panendoscopy
    f. sigmoidoscope
    f. sigmoidoscopy

FiberOptic
    F. sensor

fiberoptics

fiberscope
    Hirschowitz gastroduodenal f.

fibra *pl.* fibrae
    fibrae intercrurales
    fibrae obliquae gastricae
    fibrae obliquae ventriculi

fibrillary glomerulonephritis

fibrin
    f. calculus
    f. tissue adhesive

fibrinogen

fibrinoid
    f. necrosis

fibrinolytic activity

fibrinous
    f. cast

fibroadenomatosis
    biliary f.

fibroadipose
    f. tissue

fibroblast
    f. growth factor
    f. interferon

fibrocalculous pancreatic diabetes

fibrocaseous
    f. peritonitis

fibrocystic
    f. change
    f. disease of the pancreas

fibrodysplasia

fibrodysplastic

fibroelastic
    f. connective tissue
    f. tissue

fibrofatty adventitia

fibrogenesis
    f. imperfecta ossium

fibroid
    f. polyp
    uterine f.

fibrolamellar
    f. carcinoma
    f. hepatoma

fibrolipomatous
    f. nephritis

fibroma
    ovarian f.

fibromatosis
    f. ventriculi

fibromyoma

fibromyomata

fibrosing
    chronic f. hepatitis
    f. piecemeal necrosis

fibrosis
    alcoholic f.
    arachnoid f.
    cavernous f.
    chronic sclerosing hyaline f.
    congenital hepatic f.
    corporeal f.
    cystic f.
    diffuse lobular f.
    hepatic f.
    idiopathic retroperitoneal f.
    interstitial f.
    noncirrhotic portal f.
    pancreatic f.
    panmural f. of the bladder
    paravariceal f.

fibrosis *(continued)*
    periductal f.
    perilobular f.
    peripancreatic f.
    periportal f.
    periureteric f.
    pipestem f.
    portal-to-portal f.
    portal tract f.
    retroperitoneal f.
    secondary biliary f.
    sinusoidal f.
    Symmers f.
    transmural f.
    vesical f.

fibrous
    f. appendage of liver
    f. capsule of corpora caver-
        nosa of penis
    f. capsule of kidney
    f. capsule of liver
    f. capsule of testis
    f. cavernitis
    f. coat of corpus caver-
        nosum of penis
    f. coat of testis
    f. dysplasia
    f. nephritis
    f. obliterative cholangitis
    f. tissue
    f. tunic of liver

Ficoll
    F. gradient
    F.-Hypaque gradient cen-
        trifugation

field
    high-power f. (hpf)

filament
    actin f.

filarial
    f. funiculitis
    f. hydrocele

filiform
    f. bougie
    f. polyp

filiform *(continued)*
    f. polyposis
    f. stricture
    f. tip
    f.-tipped catheter

filling
    f. cystometrogram
    f. defect

filmy adhesion

filter
    Baermann stool f.
    charcoal f.

filtrate
    glomerular f.

filtration
    f. barrier
    f. fraction
    reverse f.
    f. slits

fimbria

fimbriae

finasteride

finding
    cholangiographic f.
    endoscopic f.
    focal f.
    manometric f.
    sensory f.
    spinal fluid f.
    ultrasonographic f.

fine
    f. gastric mucosal pattern
    f. needle
    f. tissue forceps
    f.-toothed forceps

finely fatty foamy liver

fine-needle
    f.-n. aspiration
    f.-n. aspiration biopsy
    f.-n. aspiration cytology
    f.-n. biopsy
    CT-guided f.-n. aspiration

fine-needle *(continued)*
  f.-n. percutaneous cholangiogram
  f.-n. transhepatic cholangiogram
  f.-n. transhepatic cholangiography

fingerlike villus

fingertip lesion

Finkelstein feeding

Finney
  F. gastroenterostomy
  F. operation
  F. pyloroplasty

Finochietto retractor

first
  f. convoluted tubule
  f. set

fish
  f.-hook displacement
  f.-mouth incision
  f.-mouth meatus
  f.-scale gallbladder
  f. tapeworm

Fishberg concentration test

fissura *pl.* fissurae
  f. in ano
  f. ligamenti teretis
  f. ligamenti venosi

fissural

fissure
  anal f.
  f. in ano
  cecal f.
  cutaneous f.
  f. for ligamentum teres
  f. for ligamentum venosum
  longitudinal f.
  portal f.
  f. of round ligament
  sagittal f. of liver
  transverse f.
  umbilical f.

fissured tongue

fistula *pl.* fistulae, fistulas
  abdominal f.
  anal f.
  f. in ano
  anorectal f.
  antecubital arteriovenous f.
  aortoduodenal f.
  aortoenteric f.
  aortoesophageal f.
  aortogastric f.
  aortograft duodenal f.
  aortosigmoid f.
  arterial-enteric f.
  AV f.
  benign duodenocolic f.
  biliary f.
  biliary-bronchial f.
  biliary-cutaneous f.
  biliary-duodenal f.
  biliary-enteric f.
  bilioenteric f.
  f. bimucosa
  Blom-Singer tracheoesophageal f.
  brachiocephalic f.
  brachiosubclavian bridge graft f.
  Brescia-Cimino f.
  bronchoesophageal f.
  calyceal f.
  cholecystenteric f.
  cholecystocholedochal f.
  cholecystocolonic f.
  cholecystoduodenal f.
  cholecystoduodenocolic f.
  choledochocolonic f.
  choledochoduodenal f.
  choledochoenteric f.
  coccygeal f.
  colocutaneous f.
  cologastrocutaneous f.
  coloileal f.
  colonic f.
  colovaginal f.

fistula *(continued)*
colovesical f.
cystogastric f.
duodenal f.
duodenocaval f.
duodenocolic f.
Eck f.
endobronchial f.
enteric f.
enterocutaneous f.
enteroenteral f.
enteroenteric f.
enterourethral f.
enterovaginal f.
enterovesical f.
esophageal f.
esophagobronchial f.
esophagomediastinal f.
esophagopulmonary f.
esophagorespiratory f.
external f.
external biliary f
extrasphincteric anal f.
fecal f.
forearm graft arteriove-
nous f.
gastric f.
gastrocolic f.
gastrocutaneous f.
gastroduodenal f.
gastroenteric f.
gastrointestinal f.
gastrojejunocolic f.
genitourinary f.
graft-enteric f.
hepatic f.
hepatopleural f.
horseshoe f.
ileosigmoid f.
ileovesical f.
intersphincteric anal f.
intestinal f.
intrahepatic AV f.
intrahepatic spontaneous
arterioportal f.
jejunocolic f.
mesenteric f.
mesenteric arteriovenous f.
mucous f.

fistula *(continued)*
pancreatic f.
pancreatic cutaneous f.
pararectal f.
parietal f.
perianal f.
pleurobiliary f.
perineal f.
postbiopsy f.
postoperative f.
posttraumatic pancreatic-
cutaneous f.
f. probe
pseudocystobiliary f.
radiocephalic f.
rectal f.
rectolabial f.
rectourethral f.
rectourinary f.
rectovaginal f.
rectovesical f.
rectovestibular f.
rectovulvar f.
renogastric f.
retroperitoneal f.
saphenous loop f.
spermatic f.
splenic AV f.
stercoral f.
sylvian f.
thigh graft arteriovenous f.
thoracic f.
tracheoesophageal f.
transsphincteric anal f.
ulcerogenic f.
umbilical f.
urachal f.
ureterocolic f.
urethrovaginal f.
urinary f.
urinary umbilical f.
urogenital f.
vaginal f.
vesical f.
vesicocolic f.
vesicocutaneous f.
vesicovaginal f.
vestibular f.

fistulatome

fistulectomy

fistulization

fistuloenterostomy

fistulogram

fistulotomy
    anal f.
    choledochoduodenal f.
    diathermic f.
    double-channel f.
    endoscopic f.
    needle-knife f.
    Parks method of anal f.

fistulous
    f. orifice
    f. tract

Fitz-Hugh–Curtis syndrome

fixation
    intestinal f.
    Zamboni f.

fixed segment of bowel

FK506 (tacrolimus)

flabby abdomen

flagellate
    f. diarrhea
    f. dysentery

flagellin

flagellum

Flagyl

flank
    bulging f.
    f. incision
    f. mass

flap
    abdominal fasciocuta-
      neous f.
    advancement of rectal f.
    Boari f.
    de-epithelialized f.
    island pedicle f.
    liver f.

flap *(continued)*
    myocutaneous f.
    surgical f.
    tubularized cecal f.
    f.-valve mechanism

flask ulcer

flat
    f. abdomen
    f. adenoma
    f. depressed lesion
    f. elevated lesion
    f. plate of abdomen

flatulence

flatulent
    f. colic
    f. dyspepsia

Flatulex

flatus
    f. enema
    f. tube insertion

flea-bitten kidney

fleckmilz

Fleet
    F. Baby enema
    F. Babylax enema
    F. enema
    F. Phospho-Soda

flexible
    f. aspiration needle
    f. barium enema
    f. delivery device
    f. endoscope
    f. endoscopy
    f. fiberoptic choledocho-
      scope
    f. fiberoptic endoscope
    f. forward-viewing panen-
      doscope
    f. gastroscope
    f. laparoscopy
    f. sigmoidoscope

Flexical enteral feeding

Flexner dysentery

flexura *pl.* flexurae
  f. anorectalis recti
  f. coli dextra
  f. coli hepatica
  f. coli sinistra
  f. coli splenica
  f. duodeni inferior
  f. duodeni superior
  f. duodenojejunalis
  f. hepatica coli
  f. lienalis coli
  f. perinealis recti
  f. sacralis recti

flexure
  anorectal f. of rectum
  duodenojejunal f.
  hepatic f. of colon
  inferior f. of duodenum
  left f. of colon
  left colonic f.
  perineal f. of rectum
  right f. of colon
  right colonic f.
  sacral f. of rectum
  sigmoid f.
  splenic f.
  splenic f. carcinoma
  splenic f. of colon
  splenic f. colonoscopy
  superior f. of duodenum

floating
  f. gallbladder
  f. gallstone
  f. kidney
  f. liver
  f. stool

flocculation
  f. test

floor
  inguinal f.
  f. of inguinal canal
  f. of pelvis

floppy type of Nissen fundoplication

flora
  bacterial f.
  fecal f.
  gastrointestinal tract f.
  GI tract f.
  intestinal f.
  normal f.
  vaginal f.

florid duct lesion

flow
  f. cell
  f. cell cytometry
  f. cytometer
  f. cytometry
  effective renal blood f.
  effective renal plasma f.
  obstruction of bile f.
  renal plasma f.

fluctuant
  f. mass

fluctuation

fluid
  f. analysis
  ascitic f.
  bile-stained f.
  bloody peritoneal f.
  chylous ascitic f.
  f. collection
  cul-de-sac f.
  fecal f.
  f.-filled sac
  f.-filled small bowel
  follicular f.
  f. phase diffusion
  seminal f.
  sequestration of f.
  f. shift
  straw-colored f.
  turbid peritoneal f.

fluidextract
  aromatic cascara f.
  cascara sagrada f.
  senna f.

fluke
  liver f.

flulike syndrome

fluorescein
  f.-labeled antihuman globulin

fluorescence
  f.-activated cell sorter
  (FACS)
  f.-activated cell sorting
  (FACS)
  f. angiography

fluorescent
  f. antibody
  f. antibody (FA) assay
  f. antigen assay
  f. dye
  f. labels
  f. microscope
  f. microscopy
  f. treponemal antibody absorption test (FTA-ABS)

fluoride

fluorochrome

fluoroscopic guidance

Fluoro Tip ERCP cannula

fluphenazine
  f. hydrochloride

flush
  f.-tank sign

flushing

flutamide

flux
  celiac f.
  proton f.

FNH
  focal nodular hyperplasia

foamy
  f. liver
  f. stool

focal
  f. biliary cirrhosis

focal *(continued)*
  f. colitis
  f. colonic mucosal ulcer
  f. dimpling
  f. edema
  f. embolic glomerulonephritis
  f. fatty infiltration of liver
  f. finding
  f. glomerular sclerosis
  f. glomerulonephritis
  f. glomerulosclerosis
  f. ileus
  f. nodular hyperplasia
  f. nonfatty infiltration of
  liver
  f. pancreatitis
  f. sclerosis
  f. segmental glomerulosclerosis
  f. tenderness
  f. tumor

focus *pl.* foci
  dysplastic f.
  f. formation

folate
  f. anemia
  f. malabsorption

fold
  aryepiglottic f.
  cecal f's
  cholecystoduodenocolic f.
  circular f's
  circular f's of Kerckring
  costocolic f.
  crural f.
  Douglas f.
  duodenojejunal f.
  duodenomesocolic f.
  epigastric f.
  gastric f's
  gastropancreatic f.
  Guérin f.
  haustral f.
  Heister f.
  Hensing f.
  hepatopancreatic f.
  horizontal f's of rectum

fold *(continued)*
  ileocecal f.
  ileocolic f.
  inferior duodenal f.
  inguinal f.
  interureteric f.
  Kerckring (Kerkring) f's *(of small intestine)*
  Kohlrausch f's
  f's of large intestine
  left gastropancreatic f.
  left pancreaticogastric f.
  longitudinal f. of duodenum
  mucous f's of rectum
  Nélaton f.
  palatopharyngeal f.
  paraduodenal f.
  parietocolic f.
  f. pattern
  rectal f's
  right gastropancreatic f.
  rugal f.
  semilunar f's of colon
  semilunar f. of transversalis fascia
  sentinel f.
  sigmoid f's of colon
  spiral f.
  spiral f. of cystic duct
  superior duodenal f.
  transverse f's of rectum
  transverse vesical f.
  Treves f.
  vascular cecal f.
  villous f's of stomach

folding
  f. of proteins

Foley
  F. catheter
  F. Y-V ureteropelvioplasty

folic acid
  f. a. analogue

folinic acid

follicle
  aggregated lymphatic f's of Peyer
  gastric f's

follicle *(continued)*
  intestinal f's
  Lieberkühn f's
  f.-stimulating hormone

follicular
  f. atresia
  f. center cell lymphoma
  f. cholecystitis
  chronic f. gastritis
  f. cystitis
  f. dendritic cells (FDC)
  f. fluid
  f. gastritis
  f. lymphoid hyperplasia

folliculitis
  f. gonorrhoeica

Follmann balanitis

follow-through
  small-bowel f.-t. (SBFT)

followup
  f. evaluation
  f. examination
  f. test

food
  f. addiction
  f. allergen
  f. allergy
  f. ball
  bland f.
  f. bolus
  f. bolus impaction
  f. bolus obstruction
  f. challenge
  cholecystokinetic f.
  fatty f.
  fatty f. intolerance
  f. poisoning
  f.-sensitive enteropathy
  solid f.
  undigested f. in stool

foot
  f. cells
  f. process disease

footprinting
  DNA f.

foramen *pl.* foramina
    Duverney f.
    epiploic f.
    f. epiploicum
    glandular foramina of Littre
    greater sciatic f.
    omental f.
    f. omentale
    foramina papillaria renis
    papillary foramina of kidney
    f. of Winslow

foraminal
    f. hernia

forbidden clone theory

force
    coulombic f.
    electrostatic f.
    hydrophobic f.
    Van der Waals f.

forced
    f. alimentation
    f. feeding

forceps
    ACMI Martin endoscopy f.
    Adair-Allis f.
    Adson f.
    Adson tissue f.
    Adson-Brown tissue f.
    Allis f.
    Barrett intestinal f.
    Behrend cystic duct f.
    Best gallstone f.
    Bevan gallbladder f.
    Billroth f.
    biopsy f.
    Blake gallstone f.
    Buie f.
    Buie pile f.
    Crile bile duct f.
    DeMartel appendix f.
    Dennis f.
    Dennis intestinal f.
    Desjardins gallbladder f.
    Desjardins gallstone f.
    Doyen f.

forceps *(continued)*
    Doyen gallbladder f.
    Doyen intestinal f.
    Elliott gallbladder f.
    fine tissue f.
    fine-toothed f.
    gallstone f.
    Gavin-Miller intestinal f.
    Gemini gall duct f.
    Glenn diverticulum f.
    Haberer intestinal f.
    Halsted f.
    Hasson bullet-tip f.
    Hasson needle-nose f.
    Hasson ring f.
    Hasson spike-tooth f.
    Healy intestinal f.
    hot biopsy f.
    hot flexible f.
    Lillie intestinal f.
    lithotomy f.
    Lockwood-Allis intestinal f.
    McGivney hemorrhoid f.
    Mayo-Blake gallstone f.
    Mayo-Robson intestinal f.
    Medicon-Jackson rectal f.
    Mikulicz peritoneal f.
    Moynihan gall duct f.
    Muir hemorrhoid f.
    Nissen gall duct f.
    Nussbaum intestinal f.
    Ochsner f.
    Orr gall duct f.
    packing f.
    Ratliff-Blake gallstone f.
    f. removal
    Rudd-Clinic hemorrhoidal f.
    Schnidt gall duct f.
    Schoenberg intestinal f.
    tissue f.

forcible feeding

forearm graft arteriovenous fistula

Foregger rigid esophagoscope

foregut

foreign
    anal f. body

foreign *(continued)*
    anorectal f. body
    f. body
    f.-body appendicitis
    f. body removal
    colonic f. body
    duodenal f. body
    esophageal f. body
    gastric f. body
    ingested f. body
    lower GI tract f. body
    Mallory hyaline body
    f. object
    rectal f. body
    upper GI tract f. body

foreshortening of the colon

foreskin
    hooded f.

forestomach

Formad kidney

formalin

formation
    abscess f.
    adhesion f.
    calculous f.
    "false channel" f.
    focus f.
    gallstone f.
    Gothic arch f.
    lattice f.
    pseudoaneurysm f.
    stone granuloma f.

formed stool

forme fruste

formula
    Advance f.
    Enfamil with iron f.
    Ensure Plus f.
    Isomil SF f.
    I-Soyalac f.
    Lofenalac f.
    Lonalac f.
    Nursoy f.
    Nutramigen f.
    Portagen f.

formula *(continued)*
    predigested protein f.
    Pregestimil f.
    Prosobee f.
    Prosobee liquid f.
    RCF f.
    Similac PM 60/40 low-iron f.
    SMA f.
    Soyalac f.
    soy-based f.

fornix *pl.* fornices
    gastric f.
    f. gastricus
    f. of stomach
    f. ventricularis
    f. ventriculi

Foroblique
    50-degree F. optic laparo-
        scope
    F. fiberoptic esophago-
        scope
    F. lens
    F. resectoscope

Forssman
    F. antibody
    F. antigen

Fortison enteral feeding

forward-viewing
    f.-v. endoscope
    f.-v. telescope
    f.-v. video colonoscope

foscarnet

Foss
    F. bifid gallbladder retrac-
        tor
    F. biliary duct retractor
    F. intestinal clamp

fossa *pl.* fossae
    Broesike f.
    f. caecalis
    crural f.
    f. cystidis felleae
    duodenojejunal f.
    femoral f.
    f. of gallbladder

fossa *(continued)*
    Gruber-Landzert f.
    ileocolic f.
    inferior digital f.
    inferior duodenal f.
    inferior ileocecal f.
    inferior f. of omental sac
    infraduodenal f.
    f. intermesocolica transversa
    intersigmoid f.
    f. of Jonnesco
    Landzert f.
    f. for ligamentum teres
    f. longitudinalis hepatis
    Luschka f.
    mesentericoparietal f.
    mesogastric f.
    f. of Morgagni
    navicular f. of male urethra
    f. navicularis urethrae
    f. navicularis urethrae [Morgagnii]
    paraduodenal f.
    parajejunal f.
    f. paravesicalis
    retrocecal f.
    retroduodenal f.
    right longitudinal fossae of liver
    fossae sagittales dextrae hepatis
    fossae sagittales hepatis
    f. sagittalis sinistra hepatis
    splenic f. of omental sac
    subcecal f.
    subsigmoid f.
    superior duodenal f.
    superior ileocecal f.
    superior f. of omental sac
    terminal f.
    f. transversalis hepatis
    f. of Treitz
    f. umbilicalis hepatis
    f. venae cavae
    f. venae umbilicalis
    f. vesicae biliaris
    f. vesicae felleae
    Waldeyer f.

foul-smelling
    f.-s. stool

four
    f. phases of swallowing
    f.-pronged polyp grasper
    f.-quadrant tattooing

Fournier
    F. disease
    F. gangrene

fovea *pl.* foveae
    crural f.
    femoral f.
    f. of Morgagni

foveola *pl.* foveolae
    gastric foveolae
    foveolae gastricae
    foveolae papillae

foveolar
    f. gastric mucosa
    f. hyperplasia

Fowler
    F. position
    F.-Stephens maneuver
    F.-Stephens procedure

fowlpox
    f. virus

Foxy Pouch cover

FPC
    familial polyposis coli

FPG
    fasting plasma glucose

fraction
    alpha-gliadin f.
    anionic IgG 4 f.
    ejection f.
    filtration f.
    gallbladder ejection f.
    mesangial volume f.
    packing f.
    regurgitant f.

fractional weight change

fractionated
  f. diet

fractionation of bilirubin

fragile X syndrome

fragmentary defecation

fragmentation
  DNA f.

fragmentin

framework
  f. regions
  f. segments

Framingham follow-up study

Francisella
  F. tularensis

Franco operation

Frank operation

frank
  f. blood
  f. blood in stool
  f. cirrhosis
  f. pus

Frankfeldt rectal snare

Franz abdominal retractor

Fraser syndrome

Fredet-Ramstedt operation

free
  f. acetate
  f. band of colon
  f. fatty acid
  f. fecal bile acid
  f. hepatic venous pressure
  f. hormone hypothesis
  f. jejunal graft
  f. radical
  f. reflux

freeing up of adhesions

freezing
  gastric f.

Frei test

French
  F. bougie
  F. Cope loop nephrostomy
    catheter
  F. cystoscope
  F. dilator
  F. introducer set
  F. stent
  F. Swan-Ganz balloon
  F. T-tube

Frenta
  F. Mat feeding pump
  F. System II feeding pump

frenulum *pl.* frenula
  f. of ileocecal valve
  f. preputii penis
  f. valvae ilealis
  f. valvae ileocaecalis

frenum *pl.* frena
  f. of Morgagni

frequency
  f. of stool
  urinary f.

Freund's adjuvant

Freyer operation

friable
  f. mucosa

friction-fit adapter

frondlike filling defect

frontal tenderness

frosted liver

frothy

frozen section

Fruchaud
  myopectineal orifice of F.

fructose
  f. tolerance test

fructosuria
  essential f.

FTA test

FTA-ABS test

fugax
proctalgia f.

Fujinon
F. EG-FP series endoscope
F. EVE series endoscope
F. EVG-CT series endoscope
F. EVGFP series endoscope
F. EVG-F series endoscope
F. FP series endoscope
F. UGI-FP series video endoscope

fulguration
electrosurgical f.
endoscopic f.

full
f.-column barium enema
f. liquid diet
f.-lumen esophagoscope
f. range of motion

Fuller
F. operation
F. rectal shield

fullness
abdominal f.
adnexal f.
postprandial f.
pyloric f.

fulminant
f. colitis
f. Crohn disease
f. dysentery
f. hepatic failure
f. hepatitis
f. hepatitis A
f. hepatitis B
f. hepatitis C
f. hepatitis D
f. hepatitis E
f. hepatocellular failure
f. liver failure
f. viral hepatitis

fulminating
f. appendicitis
f. dysentery
f. pancreatitis
f. ulcerative colitis

fumigatus
Aspergillus f.

function
anal sphincter f.
bactericidal f. of phagocytes
bowel f.
effector T cell f.
excretory f.
gallbladder f.
gastric f. test
gastrin cell f.
impaired colonic motor f.
Leydig cell secretory f.
liver f. profile
liver f. test
pharyngoesophageal f.
pudendal nerve f.
rectoanal f.
rectosigmoid f.
sexual f.
sphincter f.
splenic f.
T cell f.

functional
f. bleeding
f. bowel disorder (FBD)
f. bowel distress
f. bowel syndrome
chronic f. constipation
chronic f. symptomatology
f. constipation
f. cystic duct obstruction
f. deletion
f. diarrhea
f. disorder of the stomach
f. dyspepsia
f. hematuria
f. impotence
f. pain
f. prepubertal castrate syndrome

fundal
   f. gastritis
   f. plication
   f. varix

fundectomy

fundic
   f.-antral junction
   f. atrophic gastritis
   f. glands
   f. gland atrophy
   f. gland gastritis
   f. gland heterotopia
   f. gland polyp
   f. mucosa
   f. patch operation
   f. wrapping

fundoplasty
   Gomez f.
   Thallium exercise stress
      test f.

fundoplication
   Belsey Mark IV f.
   Belsey Mark IV 240-de-
      gree f.
   Belsey partial f.
   Belsey two-thirds wrap f.
   floppy type of Nissen f.
   intrathoracic Nissen f.
   Nissen f.
   Nissen 360-degree wrap f.
   Rossetti modification of
      Nissen f.
   slipped Nissen f.
   Toupet f.

fundopyloric mucosal border

fundus *pl.* fundus
   f. of bladder
   f. of gallbladder
   gastric f.
   f. gastricus
   f. glands
   f. of stomach
   f. of urinary bladder
   f. ventricularis

fundus *(continued)*
   f. ventriculi
   f. vesicae biliaris
   f. vesicae felleae
   f. vesicae urinariae

fundusectomy

fungal
   f. abscess
   f. ball
   f. bezoar
   f. disease
   f. esophageal infection
   f. esophagitis
   f. infection
   f. liver abscess
   f. peritonitis
   f. spore

fungating

fungemia

fungi

funguria

fungus *pl.* fungi
   cutaneous f.
   generalized f.
   localized f.
   opportunistic f.
   subcutaneous f.
   systemic f.
   f. testis

funicular
   f. artery
   f. hydrocele
   f. process

funiculitis
   endemic f.
   filarial f.

funiculoepididymitis

funiculopexy

funiculus *pl.* funiculi
   hepatic f.
   f. spermaticus

Furniss anastomosis clamp

Furniss-Clute clamp

furrier suture

furrow
    Liebermeister f's

furuncle

fused kidney

fusible calculus

fusiform
    f. bougie

fusin

fusion fascia

Fv
    fragment variable

FVH
    fulminant viral hepatitis

G
    G cells

gag
    Millard mouth g.
    mouth g.
    g. reflex
    g. response

gagging

gait
    broad-based g.
    spastic g.

galactocele

galactokinase

galactoma

galactorrhea

galactosemia

galacturia

Galeati glands

Galen pore

gall
    g. duct
    g. duct spoon
    Moynihan g. duct forceps

gallbladder
    adenomyoma of g.
    g. bed
    g. bile
    bilobed g.
    calculous g. disease
    g. calculus
    g. carcinoma
    cholesterolosis of g.
    Christie g. retractor
    chronically inflamed g.
    g. contraction
    Courvoisier g.
    Desjardins g. forceps
    Desjardins g. probe
    Desjardins g. scoop
    dilated g.
    g. disease

gallbladder *(continued)*
    g. displacement
    double g.
    Doyen g. forceps
    g. dysmotility
    edematous g.
    g. ejection fraction
    g. ejection rate
    g. emptying-refilling curve
    empyema of g.
    endoscopic transpapillary
      catheterization of the g.
    fat-induced g. contraction
    fish-scale g.
    floating g.
    g. function
    g. fundus
    fundus of g.
    gangrene of g.
    hourglass g.
    g. hydrops
    g. ileus
    inflamed g.
    infundibulum of g.
    mobile g.
    mucocele of g.
    multiseptate g.
    nonvisualization of g.
    notch of g.
    palpable g.
    perforation of g.
    porcelain g.
    sandpaper g.
    g. scan
    g. scoop
    g. sludge
    stasis g.
    g. stone
    strawberry g.
    thickened g. wall
    thick-walled g.
    thin-walled g.
    g. torsion
    g. trauma
    g. trocar
    g. varices
    g. wall
    g. wall abscess
    wandering g.

Gallie transplant

gallium 67

gallium scan

gallstone
    asymptomatic g.
    bilirubin pigment g.
    black pigment g.
    calcified g.
    cholesterol g.
    cholesterol-containing g.
    g. colic
    Desjardins g. forceps
    Desjardins g. probe
    dissolution of g.
    faceted g.
    floating g.
    g. forceps
    g. formation
    g. ileus
    g. incidence
    innocent g.
    intragastric g.
    g. migration
    Moynihan g. probe
    Moynihan g. scoop
    mulberry g.
    g. pancreatitis
    g. pattern
    pigment g.
    pigmented g.
    g. probe
    radiolucent g.
    retained g.
    silent g.
    symptomatic g.

GALT
    gut-associated lymphoid
        tissue

gametocyte

gamma
    g.-activated factor (GAV)
    g.-aminobutyric acid
    g.-aminobutyric acid accu-
        mulation
    g. chain
    g. delta T receptors

gamma *(continued)*
    g. emission
    g. globulins
    g. globulin antibodies
    g. heavy chains
    g. heavy chain disease
    g. heavy chains of immuno-
        globulins
    interferon g.
    g. interferon
    g. transverse colon loop

gammopathy
    monoclonal g.
    polyclonal g.

Gan gastric balloon

ganglia
    plural of ganglion

ganglion *pl.* ganglia
    enteric ganglia
    intramural ganglia

ganglioneuroma

ganglioside

gangosa

gangrene
    Fournier g.
    g. of gallbladder
    gas g.

gangrenosum
    pyoderma g.

gangrenous
    g. appendicitis
    g. appendix
    g. balanitis
    g. bowel
    g. cholecystitis
    g. ischemic colitis
    g. ischemic enterocolitis

Ganser diverticulum

Gant clamp

gap
    anion g.
    g. junction
    stool osmotic g.

gargle
  viscous Xylocaine g.

Garren
  G. gastric bubble
  G.-Edwards balloon
  G.-Edwards gastric bubble

gas
  g. abscess
  arterial blood g.
  g.-bloat syndrome
  blood g.
  bowel g.
  g. chromatography
  colonic g.
  g.-forming pyogenic liver
    infection
  g. gangrene
  hydrogen g.
  g. pains
  g. pattern
  g. peritonitis
  g.-producing food

gaseous
  g. cholecystitis
  g. distention
  g. pericholecystitis

gaseousness

gasless
  g. laparoscopic approach
  g. laparoscopy

Gasser syndrome

gassiness

gassy

gaster

gastradenitis

gastralgia

gastralgokenosis

gastratrophia

gastrectasia

gastrectasis

gastrectomized patient

gastrectomy
  Billroth g.
  Billroth I g.
  Billroth II g.
  distal g.
  esophagoproximal g.
  high subtotal g.
  Horsley g.
  partial g.
  proximal g.
  subtotal g.
  total g.

gastric
  g. accommodation test
  g. achlorhydria
  g. acid
  g. acidity
  g. acidity reduction
  g. acid pump inhibitor
  g. acid rebound
  g. acid secretion
  g. actinomycosis
  g. adenocarcinoma
  g. adenoma
  g. adenopapillomatosis
  g. air bubble
  g. anacidity
  g. analysis
  g. angioma
  g. angiomyolipoma
  g. anisakiasis
  g. anoxia
  anterior g. wall
  antral g. cell
  g. antral erosion
  g. antral sessile polyp
  g. antral vascular ectasia
  g. antrum
  g. arteriovenous malforma-
    tion
  g. aspirate
  g. aspiration
  g. aspiration tube
  g. atony
  g. atresia
  g. atrophy

gastric *(continued)*
  g. bacterial overgrowth
  g. balloon
  g. bezoar
  g. bleeding
  g. bleeding time
  g. body
  g. brush cytology
  g. bypass
  g. calculus
  g. canal
  g. cancer
  g. capacity
  g. carcinoid
  g. carcinoma
  g. carcinosarcoma
  g. channel
  g. chloroma
  circadian g. acidity
  g. coin removal
  g. colic
  g. compression
  g. contents
  crescent g. cardia
  g. cycle
  g. decompression
  Dieulafoy g. erosion
  g. dilatation
  g. dilation
  g. distention
  g. diverticulosis
  Dobbhoff g. decompression
    tube
  g. duplication
  g. dysfunction
  g. dyspepsia
  g. effect
  g. emptying
  g. emptying time
  encephaloid g. carcinoma
  g. epithelium
  excavated g. carcinoma
  g. feeding
  g. fistula
  g. fold
  g. follicles
  g. foreign body
  g. fornix
  g. foveolae

gastric *(continued)*
  g. freezing
  g. function test
  g. fundus
  Garren-Edwards g. bubble
  g. glands
  greater g. curvature
  g. hemorrhage
  g. heterotopia
  g. hyperacidity
  g. hyperemia
  g. hyperplastic polyp
  g. hypersecretion
  g. hypothermia
  g. ileus
  g. impression
  g. impression on liver
  g. indigestion
  infantile hypertrophic g.
    stenosis
  g. inhibitory peptide
  g. inhibitory polypeptide
    (GIP)
  g. insufficiency
  g. juice
  g. Kaposi sarcoma
  g. lavage
  left g. artery
  left g. vein
  left inferior g. artery
  g. leiomyoma
  g. leiomyosarcoma
  g. lesion
  lesser g. curvature
  g. lipoma
  g. lymphoma
  g. malaria
  g. mass
  g. metaplasia
  g. motility
  g. motility disorder
  g. mucosa
  g. mucosal barrier
  g. mucosal damage
  g. mucosal disease
  g. mucosal ectopia in rec-
    tum
  g. mucosal ectopy
  g. mucosal erosion

gastric *(continued)*
- g. mucosal injury
- g. mucosal prolapse
- g. mucus
- g. mycosis
- g. myoelectrical activity
- g. notch
- g. omentum
- g. outlet
- g. outlet obstruction
- g. outline
- g. pacemaker
- papillary g. carcinoma
- g. partitioning
- g. perforation
- g. petechia
- g. pigment
- g. pits
- g. pitting
- g. plexus
- g. polyp
- g. polypectomy
- g. polyposis
- g. pool
- posterior g. artery
- posterior g. wall
- g. pouch
- g. rebound
- g. remnant
- g. resection
- g. residuum
- g. retention
- right g. artery
- right inferior g. artery
- right g. vein
- g. sarcoma
- g. sclerosis
- g. secretion
- g. serosa
- short g. arteries
- short g. veins
- g. stapling
- g. stasis
- g. stump
- superficial g. carcinoma
- g. tear
- g. tetany
- g. transit time
- g. transposition

gastric *(continued)*
- g. trauma
- g. tuberculosis
- g. ulcer
- g. ulceration
- g. urease activity
- g. variceal bleeding
- g. varices
- g. vein
- g. venacaval shunt
- g. vertigo
- g. volvulus
- g. window
- g. xanthoma

gastrin
- antral g.
- g. cell
- g. cell function
- g.-releasing peptide
- g.-secreting cell
- g.-secreting non beta islet cell tumor
- g. secretion

gastrinoma

gastritic

gastritis
- acute erosive g.
- acute hemorrhagic g.
- alcoholic hemorrhagic g.
- alkaline reflux g.
- antral g.
- antral atrophic g.
- antral-predominant g.
- antrum g.
- aspirin-induced g.
- g.-associated peptic ulcer disease
- atrophic g.
- atrophic-hyperplastic g.
- autoimmune g.
- bile reflux g.
- bleeding g.
- catarrhal g.
- chemical g.
- chronic g.
- chronic active g.
- chronic atrophic g.

gastritis *(continued)*
- chronic cystic g.
- chronic erosive g.
- chronic follicular g.
- chronic superficial g.
- cirrhotic g.
- corrosive g.
- diffuse antral g. (DAG)
- diffuse corporal atrophic g.
- drug-induced g.
- emphysematous g.
- endoscopic g.
- endoscopic atrophic g.
- endoscopic enterogastric reflux g.
- endoscopic hemorrhagic g.
- endoscopic raised erosive g.
- endoscopic rugal hyperplastic g.
- eosinophilic g.
- epidemic g.
- erosive g.
- erosive/hemorrhagic g.
- exfoliative g.
- follicular g.
- fundal g.
- fundic atrophic g. (FAG)
- fundic gland g.
- giant hypertrophic g.
- granulomatous g.
- *Helicobacter pylori*-induced g.
- hemorrhagic g.
- histologic chronic active g.
- hypertrophic g.
- idiopathic g.
- idiopathic chronic erosive g.
- interstitial g.
- lymphocytic g.
- multifocal atrophic g.
- nonerosive g.
- nonerosive nonspecific g.
- nonspecific g.
- nonspecific erosive g.
- phlegmonous g.
- polypous g.
- postgastrectomy g.

gastritis *(continued)*
- postoperative g.
- proliferative hypertrophic g.
- pseudomembranous g.
- radiation g.
- reflux g.
- reflux bile g.
- severe g.
- specific g.
- stress g.
- superficial g.
- Sydney classification of g.
- Sydney system g. classification
- syphilitic g.
- toxic g.
- tuberculous g.
- type A g.
- type B g.
- ulcerative g.
- verrucous g.
- viral g.
- zonal g.

gastroadenitis

gastroadynamic

gastroanastomosis

gastroatonia

gastrocamera

gastrocardiac

Gastroccult
- G. test

gastrocele

gastrochronorrhea

gastrocolic
- g. fistula
- g. ligament
- g. omentum
- g. reflex

gastrocolitis

gastrocolostomy

gastrocolotomy

gastrocutaneous
　g. fistula

gastrocystoplasty

gastrodiaphane

gastrodiaphanoscopy

gastrodiaphany

gastroduodenal
　g. artery
　g. carcinoid
　g. Crohn disease
　g. double ulcer
　g. dyspepsia
　g. fistula
　g. lumen
　g. mucosa
　g. mucosal injury
　g. mucosal protection

gastroduodenectomy

gastroduodenitis
　neutrophilic g.

gastroduodenopancreatectomy

gastroduodenoscopy

gastroduodenostomy
　Jaboulay g.

gastrodynia

gastroenteralgia

gastroenteric
　g. fistula

gastroenteritis
　acute g.
　acute infectious g.
　acute infectious nonbacter-
　　ial g.
　astrovirus g.
　calicivirus g.
　coronavirus g.
　endemic nonbacterial in-
　　fantile g.
　eosinophilic g. (EGE)
　epidemic g.
　epidemic nonbacterial g.

gastroenteritis *(continued)*
　infantile g.
　infectious g.
　nonbacterial g.
　Norwalk g.
　rotavirus g.
　viral g.

gastroenteroanastomosis

gastroenterocolitis

gastroenterocolostomy

gastroenterologist

gastroenterology

gastroenteropancreatic

gastroenteropathy
　allergic g.
　eosinophilic g.

gastroenteroplasty

gastroenterostomy
　Balfour g.
　Billroth I g.
　Billroth II g.
　Braun-Jaboulay g.
　Courvoisier g.
　Finney g.
　Heineke-Mikulicz g.
　Hofmeister g.
　Roux-en-Y g.
　Schoemaker g.
　truncal vagotomy and g.
　von Haberer g.
　Wölfler g.

gastroenterotomy

gastroepiploic
　g. artery
　g. blood vessel
　left g. artery
　left g. vein
　right g. artery
　right g. vein

gastroesophageal
　g. hernia
　g. incompetence
　g. junction

gastroesophageal *(continued)*
  g. reflux
  g. reflux disease (GERD)
  g. reflux scan
  g. scintigraphy
  g. scintiscan
  g. sphincter
  g. variceal plexus

gastroesophagitis

gastroesophagostomy

gastrofiberscope

gastrogastrostomy

gastrogavage

gastrogenic
  g. diarrhea

gastrogenous
  g. diarrhea

Gastrografin
  G. contrast medium
  G. enema
  G. GI series
  G. swallow

gastrograph

gastrohepatic
  g. ligament
  g. omentum

gastrohepatitis

gastroileac
  g. augmentation

gastroileal
  g. augmentation
  g. reflex

gastroileitis

gastroileostomy

gastrointestinal (GI)
  g. absorption
  g. assistant (*see* GIA)
  g. bleed
  g. bleeding
  g. cancer
  g. complication

gastrointestinal *(continued)*
  g. disease
  g. endoscopy
  g. endothelium
  g. eosinophilic granuloma
  g. every other sutured
    granuloma
  g. fistula
  g. histoplasmosis
  g. hormone
  g. immunodeficiency syn-
    drome
  g. infection
  g. Kaposi sarcoma
  g. lavage
  g. lesion
  g. manifestations
  g. motility
  g. neurofibroma
  g. polyposis
  g. reflux
  g. smooth muscle
  g. stoma
  g. symptom
  g. system
  g. telangiectasia
  g. tract
  g. tract flora
  g. tract hemorrhage
  g. transit
  upper g.

gastrojejunal
  g. constipation
  g. loop obstruction syn-
    drome

gastrojejunocolic
  g. fistula

gastrojejunoesophagostomy

gastrojejunostomy
  antecolic long-loop isoper-
    istaltic g.
  Billroth II g.
  compression button g.
  loop g.
  Roux-en-Y g.

gastrokinesograph

gastrolavage

gastrolienal
  g. ligament

gastrolith

gastrolithiasis

gastrologist

gastrology

gastrolysis

Gastrolyte oral solution

gastromalacia

gastromegaly

gastromotor
  g. insufficiency

gastromycosis

gastromyotomy

gastromyxorrhea

gastro-omental
  left g. artery
  left g. vein
  right g. vein
  right g. vein

gastropancreatic
  left g. fold
  g. ligament
  g. ligaments of Huschke
  g. reflex
  right g. fold

gastropancreatitis

gastroparalysis

gastroparesis
  diabetic g.
  g. diabeticorum
  idiopathic g.
  nondiabetic g.
  postvagotomy g.
  transient g.

gastroparietal

gastropathic

gastropathy
  aphthous g.
  benign hyperplastic g.
  cardiofundic g.
  congestive g.
  congestive hypertensive g.
  diabetic g.
  erosive g.
  erythematous g.
  hemorrhagic g.
  hypertrophic g.
  idiopathic g.
  idiopathic hypertrophic g.
  portal hypertensive g.
  prolapse g.
  varioliform g.

gastroperiodynia

gastroperitonitis

gastropexy
  Boerema anterior g.
  Hill posterior g.

gastrophotography

gastrophrenic
  g. ligament

gastrophthisis

gastroplasty
  Collis g.
  Eckhout vertical g.
  Gomez horizontal g.
  greater curvature banded g.
  horizontal g.
  Laws g.
  Laws g. with Silastic collar–reinforced stoma
  Mason vertical banded g.
  O'Leary lesser curvature g.
  silicone elastomer ring vertical g.
  Stamm g.
  tubular vertical g.
  unbanded g.
  vertical banded g.
  vertical ring g.
  vertical Silastic ring g.

gastroplegia

gastroplication

gastropneumonic

Gastro-Port II feeding device

gastroptosis

gastropulmonary

gastropylorectomy

gastropyloric

gastrorenal shunt

gastrorrhagia

gastrorrhaphy

gastrorrhea

gastrorrhexis

gastroschisis
    reduction of g.
    Silastic silo reduction of g.
    Silon tent for g.

gastroscope
    ACMI g.
    Benedict g.
    Bernstein g.
    Cameron g.
    Cameron omni-angle g.
    Chevalier Jackson g.
    Eder g.
    Eder-Bernstein g.
    Eder-Chamberlin g.
    Eder-Hufford g.
    Eder-Palmer semiflexible g.
    Ellsner g.
    end-viewing g.
    Ewald g.
    fiberoptic g.
    flexible g.
    Hirschowitz g.
    Housset-Debray g.
    Kelling g.
    Mikulicz g.
    peroral g.

gastroscopic

gastroscopy
    high-magnification g.

gastroselective

gastrosis

gastrospasm

gastrosplenic
    g. ligament
    g. omentum

gastrostaxis

gastrostenosis

gastrostogavage

gastrostolavage

gastrostoma

gastrostomy
    Beck g.
    g. button
    Depage-Janeway g.
    dual percutaneous endo-
        scopic g. (DPEG)
    endoscopic g.
    feeding g.
    g. feeding
    Glassman g.
    Janeway g.
    Kader g.
    Olympus g.
    percutaneous endoscop-
        ic g.
    Partipilo g.
    Russell percutaneous en-
        doscopic g.
    g. scarring
    Stamm g.
    Surgitek One-Step percuta-
        neous endoscopic g.
    g. tube
    g. tube migration
    ultrasound-assisted percu-
        taneous endoscopic g.
    venting percutaneous g.
    Witzel g.

gastrosuccorrhea
    digestive g.

gastrotome

gastrotomy

gastrotonometer

gastrotonometry

gastrotoxin

gastrotropic

gastrotympanites

Gastrovist
  G. contrast medium

Gas-X

GATA-2

Gaucher
  G. cell
  G. disease
  G. splenomegaly

Gauderer Ponsky PEG

gauze pack

GAV
  gamma-activated factor

gavage
  g. feeding

Gavard muscle

Gavin-Miller intestinal
  forceps

Gaviscon

Gay glands

G cells

G-CSF
  granulocyte colony-stimu-
    lating factor

Gee
  G. disease
  G.-Herter disease
  G.-Herter-Heubner disease
  G.-Herter-Heubner syn-
    drome
  G.-Thaysen disease

gel
  agar g.
  agarose g.
  aluminum hydroxide g.
  aluminum phosphate g.
  basic aluminum carbona-
    te g.
  dried aluminum hydroxi-
    de g.
  g. filtration chromatogra-
    phy

gelatinous ascites

Gelfoam

Gély suture

Gemini
  G. gall duct forceps
  G. paired wire helical bas-
    ket

gender

general
  g. anesthesia
  g. endotracheal anesthesia
  g. peritonitis

generalized
  g. distal renal tubular aci-
    dosis
  g. fungus

generative lymphoid organs

genetic
  g. alteration
  g. hemochromatosis

genital
  g. ducts
  external g. differentiation
  g. gland
  g. organs
  g. tract
  g. wart

genitalia
  ambiguous g.
  anomalous g.

genitocrural

genitofemoral

genitourinary
  g. fistula
  g. neoplasm
  g. prolapse
  g. region
  g. system
  g. tract

genome

genomic organization

genotype

gentian

GERD
  gastroesophageal reflux
    disease

geriatric constipation

Gerlach valve

German measles

germinal
  g. cell aplasia
  g. center
  dark zone g. center
  light zone g. center

germinoma

Gerota
  G. capsule
  G. fascia
  fascia of G.

gestation
  ectopic g.

gestational diabetes

GH
  growth hormone
    excess GH

GHRF
  growth hormone–releasing
    factor

GI
  gastrointestinal
    GI bleeding
    GI cocktail
    lower GI bleeding
    occult GI bleeding
    GI tract
    GI tract flora

GIA
  gastrointestinal assistant
    GIA autosuture appa-
      ratus
    GIA autosuture device
    GIA instrument
    GIA stapler

giant
  g. colon
  g. diverticulum
  g. hypertrophic gastritis
  g. peptic ulcer

giant cell
  g. c. adenocarcinoma
  osteoclast-like g. c.

Giardia lamblia

giardiasis

gigantism
  acromegalic g.
  cerebral g.
  eunuchoid g.
  hyperpituitary g.
  normal g.
  pituitary g.

Gilbert
  G. cholemia
  G. disease
  G. sign
  G. syndrome

Gillette suspensory ligament

gingivostomatitis
  herpetic g.

Giordano sphincter

GIP
  gastric inhibitory polypep-
    tide

Giraldés
　　organ of G.

girdle ulcer

girth
　　abdominal g.

GI series
　　Gastrografin GI s.

Gitelman syndrome

glabrous cirrhosis

gland
　　accessory adrenal g.
　　accessory parotid g.
　　accessory thyroid g.
　　acid g's
　　adrenal g.
　　Albarrán g.
　　anal g's
　　anal intramuscular g.
　　anteprostatic g.
　　apocrine g.
　　Aselli's g.
　　g's of bile duct
　　biliary g's
　　g's of biliary mucosa
　　Brunner g's
　　bulbocavernous g.
　　bulbourethral g.
　　cardiac g's
　　circumanal g's
　　Cobelli g's
　　Cowper g.
　　duodenal g's
　　Duverney g.
　　endocervical g.
　　endocrine g.
　　esophageal g's
　　exocrine g.
　　extraparotid lymph g.
　　fundic g's
　　fundus g's
　　Galeati g's
　　gastric g's
　　Gay g's
　　genital g.
　　Gley's g.
　　Guérin g's

gland (continued)
　　g's of Haller
　　hepatic g's
　　heterocrine g.
　　intermediate g's
　　interstitial g.
　　intestinal g's
　　g's of large intestine
　　lenticular g's of stomach
　　g's of Lieberkühn
　　Littre g's
　　mixed g.
　　Morgagni g's
　　mucous g's of duodenum
　　mucus-secreting g.
　　odoriferous g's of prepuce
　　oxyntic g's
　　pancreatic g.
　　parafrenal g's
　　parathyroid g.
　　paraurethral g's
　　peptic g's
　　pineal g.
　　pituitary g.
　　pregnancy g.
　　prehyoid g.
　　preputial g's
　　proper gastric g's
　　prostate g.
　　pyloric g's
　　salivary g's
　　Sandström's g.
　　Schüller g's
　　seminal g.
　　sentinel g.
　　sexual g.
　　Skene g's
　　suprarenal g.
　　g's of small intestine
　　target g.
　　Theile g's
　　thymus g.
　　thyroid g.
　　g's of Tyson
　　urethral g's of female ure-
　　　thra
　　urethral g's of male urethra
　　Virchow's g.
　　Wölfler's g.

glandula *pl.* glandulae
glandulae biliares
g. bulbourethralis
g. bulbourethralis [Cowperi]
glandulae circumanales
glandulae ductus biliaris
glandulae ductus choledo-
chi
glandulae duodenales
glandulae duodenales
[Brunneri]
glandulae esophageae
glandulae hepaticae
glandulae intestinales
glandulae mucosae biliosae
glandulae oesophageae
glandulae pelvis renalis
glandulae preputiales
g. prostatica
glandulae pyloricae
g. seminalis
glandulae urethrales [Lit-
trei]
glandulae urethrales ure-
thrae femininae
glandulae urethrales ure-
thrae masculinae
glandulae urethrales ure-
thrae muliebris
glandulae vesicales vesicae
urinariae
g. vesiculosa

glandular
g. epispadias
g. fever
g. foramina of Littre
g. hypospadias

Glassman gastrostomy

Glauber salt

Gleason
G. grade
G. score

gleet

gleety

Glenn diverticulum forceps

Gley
G. cells
G's gland

gliadin

glial cell

glioma-polyposis syndrome

Glisson
G. capsule
G. cirrhosis
G. sphincter

glissonitis

glitter cells

Globularia

globulin
α-g.
α_2-g.
alpha$_2$ g.
g. antibodies
antihuman g. (AHG)
antihuman g. test (AHG
test)
antilymphocyte g.
β-g.
corticosteroid-binding g.
(CBG)
fluorescein-labeled antihuman g.
γ-g's
gamma g's
intravenous immune g.
(IVIg)
zoster immune g. (ZIG)

globus *pl.* globi
g. major epididymidis
g. minor epididymidis

glomerular
g. basement membrane
g. basement membrane au-
toantibodies
g. basement membrane au-
toimmune disease
g. capillary
g. capsule

glomerular *(continued)*
   g. crescent
   g. disease
   g. epithelium
   g. filtrate
   g. filtration rate
   g. injury
   g. membrane
   g. nephritis
   g. sclerosis

glomerulitis

glomerulocapsular
   g. nephritis

glomerulonephritis
   acute g.
   chronic g.
   chronic hypocomplemen-
     temic g.
   crescentic g.
   diffuse g.
   fibrillary g.
   focal g.
   focal embolic g.
   IgA g.
   immune complex g.
   lobular g.
   lobulonodular g.
   lupus g.
   malignant g.
   membranoproliferative g.
   membranous g.
   mesangial proliferative g.
   mesangiocapillary g.
   nodular g.
   pauci-immune crescentic g.
   pauci-immune rapidly pro-
     gressive g.
   postinfectious g.
   poststreptococcal g.
   rapidly progressive g.
   segmental g.
   subacute g.

glomerulonephropathy

glomerulopathy
   Adriamycin g.
   collapsing g.
   diabetic g.

glomerulopathy *(continued)*
   immunotactoid g.
   microtubular g.
   minimal change g.

glomerulosclerosis
   diabetic g.
   focal g.
   focal segmental g.
   intercapillary g.

glomerulose

glomerulus *pl.* glomeruli
   glomeruli of kidney
   malpighian glomeruli
   renal glomeruli
   glomeruli renis
   Ruysch glomeruli

glossitis

glossodynia

glover suture

glucagon
   g. test

glucagonoma

glucitol

glucocorticoid
   g. receptor

glucogenesis

gluconeogenesis

glucose
   blood g.
   declining g. tolerance
   g.-dependent insulinotropic
     polypeptide
   fasting plasma g. (FPG)
   g. intolerance
   intravenous g.
   g. level
   oral g.
   g.-6-phosphate dehydrogen-
     ase (G6PD)
   g.-sparing
   g. tolerance test (GTT)
   g. transport system

glucosuria

glutamic acid

glutaraldehyde
activated alkaline g.

gluten
g. enteropathy
g.-free diet
rectal g. challenge
g.-sensitive diarrhea
g.-sensitive enteropathy
g. sensitivity

gluteus maximus

GlyCAM-1
glycan-bearing cell adhesion molecule-1

glycan
g.-bearing cell adhesion molecule-1 (GlyCAM-1)

glycemia

L-glycericaciduria

glycerin

glyceryl alcohol

glycine
g. irrigation

glycochenodeoxycholate

glycochenodeoxycholic acid

glycocholate

glycocholic acid

glycogen
g. nephrosis
g.-rich cystadenoma

glycogenesis

glycogenetic

glycogenic
g. acanthosis

glycogenolysis

glycogenosis
brancher deficiency g.

glycogenosis *(continued)*
generalized g.
hepatophosphorylase g.
hepatorenal g.
myophosphorylase deficiency g.

glycogenous

glycolicaciduria

glycolipid

glycolysis
aerobic g.
anaerobic g.

glycolytic pathway

glycoprotein
g. accumulation
g. hormone

glycosuria
alimentary g.
benign g.
nondiabetic g.
nonhyperglycemic g.
normoglycemic g.
orthoglycemic g.
renal g.

glycosylation

glycyl alcohol

glycyltryptophan
g. test

GM-1

Gm allotype

GM-CSF
granulocyte-macrophage colony-stimulating factor

gnawing pain

goblet cell metaplasia

Goldberg Anorectic Attitude scale

Goldblatt
G. clamp

Goldblatt *(continued)*
  G. hypertension
  G. kidney
  G. phenomenon

Goldstein hematemesis

GoLYTELY
  G. bowel prep
  G. solution

Gomco
  G. suction

Gomez
  G. fundoplasty
  G. horizontal gastroplasty

gonacratia

gonad

gonadal
  g. arteries
  g. stromal tumor

gonadoblastoma

gonadotropin
  human chorionic g. (HCG)

gonaduct

gonecyst

gonecystic calculus

gonecystis

gonecystitis

gonecystolith

gonecystopyosis

gonepoiesis

gonepoietic

gonocele

gonococcal
  g. perihepatitis
  g. proctitis

gonophore

gonorrhea
  rectal g.

gonorrheal proctitis

Goodpasture syndrome

Goodsall rule

Goormaghtigh cells

Gore-Tex
  G. graft
  G. soft tissue patch

gorget

goserelin acetate

Gothic arch formation

Gouley catheter

gouty
  g. nephropathy
  g. urethritis

G6PD
  glucose-6-phosphate dehy-
    drogenase

grade
  Gleason g.

graded alcohol

gradient
  acinar g.
  biliary-duodenal pres-
    sure g.
  duodenobiliary pressure g.
  Ficoll g.
  Ficoll-Hypaque g. centrifu-
    gation

grading
  histologic g.

graft
  aortic g.
  aortoenteric g.
  aortohepatic arterial g.
  arteriovenous g.
  g. bed
  bovine g.
  buccal mucosal patch g.
  bypass g.
  chronic g.-versus-host dis-
    ease
  Dacron g.
  Dacron interposition g.

graft *(continued)*
    g.-enteric fistula
    free jejunal g.
    Gore-Tex g.
    g.-versus-host disease
    HLA identical kidney g.
    Impra g.
    interposition g.
    loop forearm g.
    Marlex g.
    omental g's
    mucosal g.
    omental pedicle flap g.
    patch g.
    g. placement
    reduced-size g.
    "scotty dog" g.
    segmental liver g.
    seromuscular intestinal
        patch g.
    g. spatulation
    split-thickness skin g.
    g. survival
    synthetic vascular g.
    g.-versus-host disease

Graham scale for drug-induced
    gastric damage

Gram
    G. stain
    G. stain of stool

gram-negative
    g.-n. bacteria
    g.-n. rod
    g.-n. sepsis

gram-positive
    g.-p. bacteria
    g.-p. sepsis

Grant gallbladder retractor

granular
    g. atrophy of kidney
    g. cast
    g. induration

granulation
    Bright g's

granule
    acidophilic PAS-positive g.
    acrosomal g.
    hemosiderin g.
    juxtaglomerular g's
    Kretz g's
    perichromatin g's
    proacrosomal g.
    seminal g's

granulocyte
    g. colony-stimulating factor
        (G-CSF)
    g.-macrophage colony-stim-
        ulating factor (GM-CSF)

granuloma *pl.* granulomas,
    granulomata
    amebic g.
    barium g.
    eosinophilic g.
    epithelioid g.
    gastrointestinal eosinophil-
        ic g.
    gastrointestinal every other
        sutured g.
    hepatic g.
    noncaseating tubercle-
        like g.
    stone g.
    suture g.
    umbilical g.

granulomatosis
    lipophagic intestinal g.
    Wegener g.

granulomatous
    g. cholangitis
    g. colitis
    g. disease
    g. enteritis
    g. enterocolitis
    g. gastritis
    g. hepatitis
    g. ileitis
    g. peritonitis
    g. prostatitis
    g. transmural colitis

Graser diverticulum

grasp
  palmar g.

grasper
  Allis tooth g.
  four-pronged polyp g.

Gratiola

gravel

gravity-dependent drainage

Grawitz tumor

great
  g. epiploon
  g. lacuna of urethra
  g. pancreatic artery
  g. saphenous vein

greater
  g. curvature banded gastro-
    plasty
  g. curvature of stomach
  g. curvature ulcer
  g. gastric curvature
  g. omentum
  g. peritoneal cavity
  g. peritoneal sac
  g. renal calices
  g. sac of peritoneum
  g. sciatic foramen

green
  g. sputum
  g. stool

Greenen
  G. Endotorque
  G. pancreatic stent

Greenville gastric bypass

Grey Turner
  G. T. sign of retroperito-
    neal hemorrhage

gridiron incision

Griffen Roux-en-Y bypass

griping pain

gripping pain

groin
  g. incision

Grondahl
  G.-Finney esophagogastro-
    plasty
  G.-Finney operation

groove
  anal intersphincteric g.
  esophageal g.
  Liebermeister g's
  oval-form colonic g.
  g. pancreatitis
  spindle colonic g.

Gross disease

gross hematuria

ground-glass
  g.-g. appearance
  g.-g. cell
  g.-g. hepatocyte

Gruber-Landzert fossa

Grynfeltt
  G. hernia
  G. triangle
  triangle of G. and Lesshaft

gryposis
  g. penis

GTT
  glucose tolerance test

guaiac
  g.-negative stool
  g.-positive stool

guarding
  abdominal g.
  involuntary g.
  muscle g.
  voluntary g.

gubernacular

gubernaculum pl. *gubernacula*
  chorda g.
  Hunter g.
  g. testis

Guérin
  G. ducts
  G. fold
  G. glands
  G. sinus
  G. valve

guidance
  choledochoscopic g.
  fluoroscopic g.

guide

guided transcutaneous biopsy

guidewire
  Eder-Puestow g.
  olive over g.

guillotine needle biopsy

gulf
  Lecat g.

Gull renal epistaxis

gullet

gun
  g.-barrel enterostomy
  biopsy g.

gunpowder lesion

gurgle

gurgling bowel sounds

Gussenbauer suture

gut
  artificial g.
  g.-associated lymphoid tissue (GALT)
  blind g.
  chromic g.
  chromicized g.
  nervous g.
  g. rest
  ribbon g.
  surgical g.

Guthrie muscle

gutter
  lateral g.
  left g.
  paracolic g.

Guyon sign

H_2
    histamine$_2$
        H_2 antagonist therapy
        H_2 receptor
        H_2 receptor antagonist
        H_2 receptor antagonist
            therapy
        H_2 receptor blocker
        H_2 receptor–blocking
            drug

habenula *pl.* habenulae
    Haller h.

habenular

Haberer
    H. abdominal spatula
    H. intestinal clamp
    H. intestinal forceps

habit
    bowel h's
    dietary h's
    drinking h.
    eating h's

habitus
    body h.

HAEC
    Hirschsprung-associated
        enterocolitis

Hagner bag

HAI
    histologic activity index

hair
    h. ball
    h. cast

hairball

hairy
    h. leukemia
    h. leukoplakia
    h. tongue

Haley's M-O

half
    h.-normal saline

half *(continued)*
    h.-strength feeding

halitosis

Hallberg biliointestinal bypass

Haller
    H. aberrant duct
    H. cones
    crypts of H.
    glands of H.
    H. habenula
    rete of H.

halo effect

halothane
    h. hepatotoxicity
    h.-induced hepatitis

Halsted
    H. forceps
    H. hemostat
    H. inguinal herniorrhaphy
    H. operation
    H. suture
    H.-Bassini hernia repair
    H.-Bassini herniorrhaphy

hamartoma
    ampullary h.
    angiomatous lymphoid h.
    Brunner gland h.
    cystic h.
    duodenal wall h.
    mesenchymal h.
    pancreatic h.
    Peutz-Jeghers h.

hamartomatous
    h. gastric polyp
    h. lesion
    h. polyp
    h. polyposis

Hamel test

Hamilton-Thorn motility ana-
    lyzer

hammock

hanging panniculus

Hanley rectal bladder procedure

Hanot cirrhosis

H_2 antagonist therapy

Hanta virus

haptocorrin

haptoglobin
    serum h.

haptotoxic range

Hara classification of gallbladder inflammation

hard
    h. adhesion
    h. stool

Har-el pharyngeal tube

Harrington
    H. Deaver retractor
    H. esophageal diverticulectomy

Harris
    H. tube
    H. band

Hartmann
    H. closure of rectum
    H. colostomy
    H. operation
    H. point
    H. pouch
    H. procedure
    H. reconstruction technique

Harvard pump

Hashimoto
    H. struma
    H. thyroiditis

Haslinger esophagoscope

Hasson
    H. bullet-tip forceps
    H. cannula
    H. needle-nose forceps

Hasson *(continued)*
    H. open laparoscopy cannula
    H. ring forceps
    H. spike-tooth forceps

haustral
    h. blunting
    h. fold
    h. indentation
    h. marking
    h. pattern
    h. pouch
    h. segmentation

haustrum *pl.* haustra
    haustra coli
    haustra of colon

HAV
    hepatitis A virus

Havrix

HB
    Tagamet HB

HBAg
    hepatitis B antigen

HBcAg
    hepatitis B core antigen

HBeAG
    hepatitis Be antigen
        HBeAg-positive

HBe antibody

HBIG
    hepatitis B immunoglobulin

HBsAg
    hepatitis B surface antigen

HBV
    hepatitis B virus
        HBV-associated DNA polymerase
        HBV-specific T cell

HBVV
    hepatitis B virus vaccine

HC
    hemochromatosis

HC *(continued)*
    high calorie

HC-1
    Anusol-HC-1

HCA
    hepatocellular adenoma

HCC
    hepatocellular carcinoma

HCG
    human chorionic gonado-
        tropin

HCl
    hydrochloric acid
    hydrochloride

HCN
    high calorie and nitrogen

HCTZ-TA
    hydrochlorothiazide-triam-
        terene

HCV
    hepatitis C virus
        HCV antibody

HD
    hemodialysis

HDAg
    hepatitis D antigen

HDL
    high-density lipoprotein

HDL-C
    high-density lipoprotein
        cholesterol

HDV
    hepatitis delta virus
    hepatitis D virus

HE
    hepatic encephalopathy

H&E
    hematoxylin and eosin

head
    h. of epididymis
    h. of pancreas

head *(continued)*
    h. of penis

healed
    h. yellow atrophy
    h. ulcer

healing
    delayed primary inten-
        tion h.
    h. by primary intention
    h. by secondary intention

Healy intestinal forceps

Heaney clamp

heaped-up edges
    ulcer with h.-u. e.

heart
    h.-kidney transplant
    h.-lung machine

heartburn
    nocturnal h.
    h. of pregnancy

heater
    h. probe
    h. probe coagulation
    h. probe therapy

HeatProbe lavage

heaves
    dry h.

heavy
    h. silk suture

Hegar
    H. bougie
    H. rectal dilator

Heidenhain
    H. cells
    rods of H.

Heimlich
    H. maneuver

Heineke
    H.-Mikulicz gastroenteros-
        tomy
    H.-Mikulicz incision

Heineke *(continued)*
    H.-Mikulicz operation
    H.-Mikulicz principle
    H.-Mikulicz pyloroplasty

Heister
    H. fold
    spiral valve of H.
    H. valve

helical
    h. CT
    h. fashion

Helicobacter
    H.-induced gastric injury
    H. pylori
    H. pylori-induced gastritis

Heller
    H. cardiomyotomy
    H. esophagomyotomy
    H. myotomy
    H. operation

HELLP
    hemolysis, elevated liver
        enzymes, and low platelet
        count
        HELLP syndrome

helminth
    h. infection

helminthemesis

helminthiasis

helminthic
    h. appendicitis
    h. dysentery
    h. pseudotumor

helminthism

Helvetius
    ligaments of H.

hemangioendothelioma
    infantile h.

hemangioma
    cavernous h.
    hepatic h.
    strawberry h.
    vascular h.

hemangiomatosis
    duodenal h.
    splenic capillary h.

hemangiopericytoma
    h. of kidney

hemangiosarcoma

hematemesis
    Goldstein h.

Hematest
    H. test

hematobilia

hematocele
    scrotal h.
    vaginal h.

hematocelia

hematochezia
    pancreatic h.

hematochyluria

hematocoelia

hematocrit
    hemoglobin and h. (H&H)

hematocyturia

hematogenous
    h. micrometastasis
    h. pyelitis
    h. spread of infection

hematologic
    h. abnormality
    h. complication
    h. study

hematoma
    duodenal h.
    esophageal h.
    esophageal intramural h.
    expanding retroperitoneal h.
    intrahepatic h.
    intramural h.
    mesenteric h.
    parenchymal h.
    perianal h.

hematoma *(continued)*
   perirenal h.
   pulsatile h.
   rectus sheath h.
   renal h.
   septal h.
   subcapsular h.

hematonephrosis

hematoperitoneum

hematopoiesis
   hepatic extramedullary h.

hematopoietic
   h. cell
   h. lineage

hematoscheocele

hematospermatocele

hematospermia

hematoxylin
   h. and eosin (H&E)
   h. and eosin stain
   h. stain

hematuresis

hematuria
   benign familial h.
   benign recurrent h.
   h.-dysuria syndrome
   essential h.
   false h.
   functional h.
   gross h.
   idiopathic h.
   macroscopic h.
   microscopic h.
   persistent h.
   primary h.
   renal h.
   urethral h.
   vesical h.

Hema-Wipe
   H. test

heme
   h.-negative stool

heme *(continued)*
   h.-positive NG (nasogastric) aspirate
   h.-positive stool

HemeSelect

hemibladder

hemiblock
   anterior h.

hemicolectomy
   Duecollement h.
   laparoscopy-assisted h.
   left h.
   right h.

hemicolon

hemigastrectomy

hemihepatectomy

hemihypertrophy

heminephrectomy

heminephroureterectomy

hemiparesis

hemiplegia

hemipylorectomy

hemipyonephrosis

hemispherium *pl.* hemispheria
   hemispheria bulbi urethrae

hemoaccess

hemobilia

Hemoccult
   H. II
   H. II test
   H. Sensa
   H. Sensa developer
   H. Sensa slide
   H. Sensa test
   H. test

hemocholecyst

hemocholecystitis

hemochromatosis (HC)
   African h.

hemochromatosis *(continued)*
  Desferal Mesylate challenge for h.
  genetic h.
  idiopathic h.
  precirrhotic h.

hemochromatotic cirrhosis

hemoconcentration

hemoculture

hemodiafiltration

hemodialysis (HD)
  h. access
  h.-associated amyloidosis
  h.-associated ascites
  high efficiency h.
  high flux h.
  h. vascular access

hemodialyzer
  h. membrane

hemofilter

hemofiltration
  continuous arteriovenous h.
  continuous venovenous h.

hemoglobin
  h. cast
  h. content indices
  h. and hematocrit
  mean corpuscular h. (MCH)

hemoglobinemia

hemoglobinocholia

hemolysis
  h., elevated liver enzymes, and low platelet count (HELLP)

hemolytic
  h. anemia
  h. jaundice
  h. splenomegaly
  h. strep
  h. uremic syndrome

hemonephrosis

hemoperfusion
  charcoal h.
  h. with charcoal

hemoperitoneum

hemoproctia

hemoptysis

hemopyelectasis

HemoQuant
  H. assay
  H. fecal blood test

hemorrhage
  acute nonvariceal upper gastrointestinal h.
  colonic h.
  concealed h.
  h. control
  diverticular h.
  exsanguinating h.
  gastric h.
  gastrointestinal tract h.
  Grey Turner sign of retroperitoneal h.
  hepatic h.
  internal h.
  intestinal h.
  intra-abdominal h.
  intramural intestinal h.
  intraperitoneal h.
  lower gastrointestinal h.
  nonvariceal upper gastrointestinal h.
  pancreatitis-related h.
  postgastrectomy h.
  postpolypectomy h.
  renal h.
  stigmata of recent h.
  stress ulcer h.
  subcapsular h.
  subconjunctival h.
  submucosal gastric h.
  upper gastrointestinal h.
  variceal h.

hemorrhaged ascites

hemorrhagic
    h. ascites
    h. capillary toxicosis
    h. colitis
    h. cystitis
    h. dengue
    h. diarrhea
    h. enterocolitis
    erosive/h. gastritis
    h. fever
    h. gastritis
    h. gastropathy
    h. necrotizing pancreatitis
    h. nephritis
    h. pancreatitis
    h. peritonitis
    h. pyelitis
    h. radiation injury

hemorrhoid
    h. banding
    bleeding h.
    combined h.
    cryotherapy for h's
    dilation of h's
    external h.
    internal h.
    laser h. excision
    ligation of h's
    mixed h.
    mucocutaneous h.
    necrotic h's
    prolapsed h.
    prolapsing internal h's
    rubber band ligation of h.
    strangulated h.
    thrombosed h.

hemorrhoidal
    h. banding
    h. cushion
    inferior h. artery
    middle h. artery
    h. plexus
    h. prolapse
    h. sclerotherapy
    superior h. artery
    h. tag
    h. vessels

hemorrhoidal (continued)
    h. zone

hemorrhoidectomy
    ambulatory h.
    closed h.
    laser h.
    Lord h.
    modified Whitehead h.
    open h.
    semi-open h.

HemoSelect test

hemosiderin
    h. deposit
    h. granule

hemosiderosis
    hepatic h.

hemospermia

hemostasis
    endoscopic h.

hemostat
    Crile h.
    Halsted h.
    Ochsner h.

hemostatic
    h. agent
    h. suture

hemothorax

Hemovac drain

hemotympanum

hemp seed calculus

hemuresis

Henle
    H. ampulla
    H. band
    H. canal
    H. loop
    loop of H.
    H. sphincter
    H. tubule

Hennings sign

Henoch
- H. purpura
- H.-Schönlein purpura
- H.-Schönlein syndrome

Hensing
- H. fold
- H. ligament

hepar
- h. adiposum
- h. lobatum

heparin
- h.-induced thrombocytopenia

heparinization

heparinized saline

hepatalgia

hepatatrophia

hepatatrophy

hepatectomize

hepatectomy
- donor h.
- partial h.
- recipient h.
- triple lobe h.

hepatic
- h. abnormality
- h. abscess
- h. adenoma
- h. adhesion
- h. allograft
- h. amebiasis
- h. amyloidosis
- h. angiomatosis
- h. angiosarcoma
- h. architecture
- h. arteriogram
- h. artery
- h. artery aneurysm
- h. artery infusion pump
- h. artery ligation
- h. bed
- h. blood pool scan
- h. calculus

hepatic *(continued)*
- h. candidal infection
- h. capsule
- h. capsulitis
- h. cells
- cell-mediated h. injury
- Child h. dysfunction classification
- h. circulation
- h. cirrhosis
- h. clearance
- h. colic
- h. coma
- common h. artery
- common h. duct
- congenital h. fibrosis (CHF)
- h. copper overload
- h. cords
- h. crisis
- h. cyst
- h. diverticulum
- h. duct
- h. dullness
- h. edge
- h. encephalopathy
- h. extramedullary hematopoiesis
- h. fever
- h. fibrosis
- h. fistula
- h. flexure of colon
- h. function test
- h. funiculus
- h. glands
- h. granuloma
- h. hemangioma
- h. hemorrhage
- h. hemosiderosis
- h. hilar region
- h. hilum
- h. Hodgkin disease
- h. infantilism
- h. insufficiency
- intermediate h. veins
- h. iron index
- left h. duct
- h. leiomyosarcoma
- h. ligament
- h. lipase

hepatic *(continued)*
   h. lobes
   h. lobectomy
   h. lobules
   h. malignancy
   h. mass lesion
   h. metabolism
   h. metastatic disease
   middle h. veins
   h. nevus
   h. osteodystrophy
   h. outflow tract
   h. parenchyma
   h. perfusion index
   h. portal
   proper h. artery
   h. resection
   right h. duct
   h. rupture
   h. sarcoidosis
   h. schistosomiasis
   sclerosing h. carcinoma
   h. sclerosis
   h. siderosis
   h. span
   h. steatosis
   h. subsegmentectomy
   h. telangiectasia
   h. toxemia
   h. trauma
   h. triads
   h. tumor
   h. uptake
   h. vein
   h. vein catheterization
   h. vein thrombosis
   h. vein wedge pressure
   h. venogram
   h. veno-occlusive disease
   h. venous outflow
   h. venous outflow obstruc-
     tion
   h. venous pressure
   h. venule
   h. web
   h. wedge pressure
Hepatic-Aid
   H. powdered feeding

hepaticocholangiojejunostomy

hepaticocholedochostomy

hepaticodochotomy

hepaticoduodenostomy

hepaticoenterostomy

hepaticogastrostomy

hepaticojejunostomy
   Roux-en-Y h.

hepaticolithotomy

hepaticolithotripsy

hepaticopancreatic
   h. duct

hepaticopulmonary

hepaticostomy

hepaticotomy

hepatism

hepatitis *pl.* hepatitides
   h. A
   active chronic h.
   acute h. (AH)
   acute alcohol h.
   acute mononucleosis-like h.
   acute parenchymatous h.
   acute self-limited h.
   acute viral h. (AVH)
   h. A infection
   alcoholic h.
   alcohollike h.
   amebic h.
   anesthetic h.
   anicteric h.
   anicteric viral h.
   autoimmune h.
   h. A virus (HAV)
   h. B
   h. B antigen (HBAg)
   h. B core antigen (HBcAg)
   h. Be antigen (HBeAG)
   h. B immunoglobulin
     (HBIG)

hepatitis *(continued)*
    h. B infection
    h. B surface antigen
      (HBsAg)
    h. B virus (HBV)
    h. B virus–encoded antigen
    h. B virus vaccine (HBVV)
    h. C
    cholangiolitic h.
    cholangitic h.
    cholestatic h.
    cholestatic viral h.
    chronic h.
    chronic active h. (CAH)
    chronic active viral h.
    chronic active viral h., non-
      A, non-B
    chronic active viral h., type
      B
    chronic aggressive h.
      (CAH)
    chronic autoimmune h.
    chronic fibrosing h.
    chronic interstitial h.
    chronic lobar h.
    chronic persistent h.
    chronic persisting h.
    chronic progressive h.
    chronic viral h.
    h. C infection
    h. C viremia
    h. C virus (HCV)
    h. D
    h. D antigen (HDAg)
    delta h.
    delta h. superinfection
    h. delta virus (HDV)
    h. D infection
    drug-induced h.
    h. D superinfection
    h. D virus (HDV)
    h. E
    h. E infection
    enterically transmitted
      non-A, non-B h. (ET-
      NANB)
    epidemic h.
    h. E virus (HEV)
    familial h.

hepatitis *(continued)*
    fatty liver h.
    fulminant h.
    fulminant h. A
    fulminant h. B
    fulminant h. C
    fulminant h. D
    fulminant h. E
    fulminant viral h. (FVH)
    h. G
    granulomatous h.
    halothane-induced h.
    herpetic h.
    homologous serum h.
    idiopathic autoimmune
      chronic h.
    infectious h.
    inoculation h.
    ischemic h.
    La Brea h.
    lobular h.
    long-incubation h.
    lupoid h.
    malarial h.
    mother-to-infant transmis-
      sion of h. C virus
    MS-1 h.
    MS-2 h.
    non-A, non-B h.
    nonspecific reactive h.
    oxacillin-associated anicter-
      ic h.
    persistent chronic h.
    persistent viral h.
    plasma cell h.
    posttransfusion h.
    pseudoalcoholic h.
    serum h.
    short-incubation h.
    subacute h.
    subclinical h.
    superimposed alcoholic h.
    syncytial giant-cell h.
    toxic h.
    transfusion h.
    transfusion-associated h.
    viral h.
    yeast-recombinant h. B

hepatobiliary
  h. capsule
  h. disease
  h. malignancy
  h. manifestation
  h. scan
  h. scintigraphy
  h. tree

hepatoblastoma

hepatobronchial

hepatocanalicular
  h. cholestasis

hepatocarcinogenesis

hepatocarcinogenic

hepatocarcinoma

hepatocele

hepatocellular
  h. adenoma
  h. adnexa
  h. atypia
  h. ballooning
  h. carcinoma
  h. cholestasis
  clear cell h. carcinoma
  h. death
  h. disease
  h. jaundice
  h. necrosis

hepatocholangeitis

hepatocholangiocarcinoma

hepatocholangioduodenostomy

hepatocholangioenterostomy

hepatocholangiogastrostomy

hepatocholangiostomy

hepatocholangitis

hepatocirrhosis

hepatocolic
  h. ligament

hepatocystic
  h. duct

hepatocystocolic
  h. ligament

hepatocyte
  cobblestone pattern of h.
  ground-glass h.
  h. growth factor
  lipid-laden h.
  h. necrosis
  periportal h.
  polygonal h.

hepatoduodenal
  h. ligament
  h.-peritoneal reflection
  h. reflection

hepatoduodenostomy

hepatodynia

hepatoenteric

hepatoenterostomy

hepatofugal

hepatogastric
  h. ligament

hepatogastroduodenal
  h. ligament

hepatogastroenterology

hepatogenic
  h. jaundice

hepatogenous
  h. jaundice
  h. pigment

hepatoid adenocarcinoma

hepato-iminodiacetic acid
  (HIDA)

hepatojugular
  h. reflux

hepatolenticular

hepatolienal

hepatolienomegaly

hepatolith

hepatolithectomy

hepatolithiasis

hepatologist

hepatology

hepatolysis

hepatolytic

hepatoma
    fibrolamellar h.
    malignant h.

hepatomalacia

hepatomegalia

hepatomegaly
    congestive h.

hepatomelanosis

hepatometry

hepatonephric

hepatopancreatic
    h. ampulla
    h. fold

hepatopath

hepatopathy
    radiation h.

hepatoperitonitis

hepatopetal

hepatopexy

hepatophlebitis

hepatopleural
    h. fistula

hepatopneumonic

hepatopoietin A (HPTA)

hepatoportal
    h. sclerosis

hepatoportoenterostomy
    Kasai-type h.

hepatoptosis

hepatopulmonary

hepatorenal
    h. angle
    h. bypass
    h. glycogenosis
    h. ligament
    h. syndrome

hepatorrhagia

hepatorrhaphy

hepatorrhea

hepatorrhexis

hepatoscopy

hepatosis
    serous h.

hepatosolenotropic

hepatosplenitis

hepatosplenomegaly

hepatosplenometry

hepatosplenopathy

hepatostomy

hepatotomy
    transthoracic h.

hepatotoxic

hepatotoxicity
    acetaminophen h.
    anesthetic h.
    anticonvulsant agent h.
    antidepressant drug h.
    antidiabetic agent h.
    antineoplastic drug h.
    antipsychotic drug h.
    antithyroid h.
    carbamazepine h.
    cardiovascular drug h.
    chemotherapeutic agent h
    cocaine h.
    drug h.
    halothane h.
    nitrofurantoin h.

hepatotoxicity *(continued)*
  potentiation of drug h.

hepatotoxin

hepatotropic

hepatoxic

hepatoumbilical
  h. ligament

Heptavax-B

herald bleed

hereditary
  h. amyloidosis
  h. angioedema
  h. hemorrhagic telangiecta-
    sia
  h. nonpolyposis colorectal
    carcinoma
  h. tubulointerstitial nephri-
    tis

heredofamilial amyloidosis

Hering
  canals of H.

hernia
  abdominal h.
  abdominal wall h.
  h. adiposa
  axial hiatal h.
  Barth h.
  Béclard h.
  Bochdalek h.
  cecal h.
  Cloquet h.
  Cooper h.
  crural h.
  diaphragmatic h.
  direct h.
  direct inguinal h.
  diverticular h.
  duodenojejunal h.
  easily reducible h.
  encysted h.
  epigastric h.
  external h.
  extrasaccular h.
  fat h.

hernia *(continued)*
  femoral h.
  foraminal h.
  gastroesophageal h.
  Grynfeltt h.
  Hesselbach h.
  Hey h.
  hiatal h.
  hiatus h.
  Holthouse h.
  incarcerated h.
  h. incarceration
  incisional h.
  indirect h.
  indirect inguinal h.
  infantile h.
  inguinal h.
  inguinocrural h.
  inguinofemoral h.
  inguinoproperitoneal h.
  inguinosuperficial h.
  intermuscular h.
  internal h.
  interparietal h.
  intersigmoid h.
  interstitial h.
  intra-abdominal h.
  intraperitoneal h.
  irreducible h.
  ischiatic h.
  ischiorectal h.
  Krönlein h.
  labial h.
  lateral ventral h.
  Laugier h.
  levator h.
  Littre h.
  lumbar h.
  mesenteric h.
  mesentericoparietal h.
  mesocolic h.
  Morgagni h.
  oblique h.
  obturator h.
  omental h.
  pantaloon h.
  paraesophageal h.
  paraduodenal h.

hernia *(continued)*
    paraesophageal diaphrag-
       matic h.
    paraesophageal hiatal h.
    parahiatal h.
    paraperitoneal h.
    parasaccular h.
    parastomal h.
    parietal h.
    pectineal h.
    perineal h.
    Petit h.
    prevascular h.
    properitoneal h.
    pudendal h.
    reducible h.
    retrocecal h.
    retrograde h.
    retroperitoneal h.
    retrovascular h.
    Richter h.
    Rieux h.
    Rokitansky h.
    rolling h.
    sciatic h.
    scrotal h.
    Serafini h.
    sliding h.
    sliding esophageal hiatal h.
    sliding hiatal h.
    slip h.
    slipped h.
    spigelian h.
    strangulated h.
    Treitz h.
    Velpeau h.
    ventral h.
    vesical h.
    W h.
hernial
    h. canal
    h. hydrocele
    h. sac
herniated
    h. preperitoneal fat
hernioappendectomy
hernioenterotomy

herniolaparotomy
hernioplasty
    tension-free h.
herniopuncture
herniorrhaphy
    Bassini inguinal h.
    Halsted-Bassini h.
    Halsted inguinal h.
    Hill-type hiatus h.
    Lichtenstein h.
    Macewen h.
    McVay h.
    Madden incisional h.
    pants-over-vest h.
    Ponka h.
    Shouldice inguinal h.
    ventral h.
    vest-over-pants h.
herniotome
    Cooper h.
herniotomy
herpangina
herpes
    h. infection
    h. labialis
    h. pharyngitis
    h. simplex
    h. simplex esophagitis
    h. simplex infection
    h. simplex virus
    h. zoster
herpesvirus
herpetic
    h. esophagitis
    h. gingivostomatitis
    h. hepatitis
    h. stomatitis
    h. ulcer
herpetiform
    h. esophagitis
herpetiformis
    dermatitis h.

Herter
  H. disease
  H. infantilism
  H.-Heubner disease

Hesselbach
  H. hernia
  H. ligament

heterochylia

heterocrine gland

heteroduplex analysis

heterogeneous texture

heterolith

heteropancreatism

heterotopia
  gastric h.

heterotopic
  h. gastric mucosa
  h. pancreas
  h. transplantation

Heubner-Herter disease

HEV
  hepatitis E virus

Hey hernia

Heymann nephritis

HGF
  hepatocyte growth factor

H&H
  hemoglobin and hematocrit

H3 histone

hiatal
  axial h. hernia
  h. hernia

hiatus *pl.* hiatus
  diaphragmatic h.
  esophageal h.
  h. esophageus
  h. femoralis
  h. oesophageus
  patulous h.

hiatus *(continued)*
  h. of Winslow

hiccup (*also spelled* hiccough)
  pl. hiccups

Hickman
  H. catheter
  H. percutaneous introducer

HIDA
  hepato-iminodiacetic acid

hidradenitis suppurativa

high
  h. anion-gap metabolic acidosis
  h. bulk, low fat diet
  h. calorie (HC)
  h. calorie diet
  h. calorie and nitrogen (HCN)
  h. carbohydrate diet
  h. cecum
  h.-density
  h.-density lipoprotein
  h.-density lipoprotein cholesterol
  h. efficiency hemodialysis
  h. efficiency membrane
  h. enema
  h. fat diet
  h. flux hemodialysis
  h. flux membrane
  h.-grade
  h.-grade cholestasis
  h.-grade dysplasia
  h.-grade obstruction
  h. intermuscular abscess
  h. ligation
  h. lithotomy
  h. magnification
  h.-magnification colonoscopy
  h.-magnification endoscopy
  h.-magnification gastroscopy
  h.-pitched bowel sounds
  h.-power field
  h. protein diet

high *(continued)*
    h. roughage diet
    h. small-bowel obstruction
    h. subtotal gastrectomy

highly selective vagotomy

hilar
    h. cholangiocarcinoma
    h. mass

Hill
    H. antireflux operation
    H. hiatus hernia repair
    H. posterior gastropexy
    H. rectal retractor
    H. repair
    H.-type hiatus herniorrha-
        phy
    H.-Ferguson rectal retrac-
        tor

hill diarrhea

hillock
    seminal h.

Hilton white line

hilum *pl.* hila
    hepatic h.
    h. hepatis
    h. of kidney
    liver h.
    h. renale
    splenic h.
    h. stimulation

hilus *(variant of* hilum)

hindgut
    h. carcinoid

Hinkle-James rectal speculum

Hinman syndrome

Hirschmann
    H. anoscope
    H. pile clamp
    H. speculum

Hirschowitz
    H. endoscope
    H. gastroduodenal fiber-
        scope

Hirschowitz *(continued)*
    H. gastroscope

Hirschsprung
    H.-associated enterocolitis
    H. disease

hirsutism
    adrenal h.

hirsutoid
    h. papilloma
    h. papillomas of penis

His
    angle of H.

Histalog test

histamine
    h.$_2$
    h.$_2$ receptor antagonist
    h.-resistant achlorhydria
    h. test

histiocytic lymphoma

histochemical
    h. pattern
    h.-ultrastructural analysis

histocompatibility antigen

histologic
    h. activity index
    h. chronic active gastritis
    h. cirrhosis
    h. damage
    h. diagnosis
    h. esophagitis
    h. grading

histological

histone
    H3 h.

histoplasmosis
    disseminated h.
    gastrointestinal h.
    intestinal h.
    mediastinal h.
    recurrent colonic h.

hitch
    psoas h.

HIV
> human immunodeficiency
> virus
>> HIV-associated ne-
>> phropathy
>> HIV infection

H⁺,K⁺-ATPase

H^+,K^+-ATPase

HLA
> HLA antigens
> HLA identical kidney graft

HN feeding

hobnail liver

Hochenegg operation

hockey-stick incision

Hodge planes

Hodgkin disease
> hepatic H. d. (hepatic infan-
> tiliom)

Hoehn and Yahr stage

Hofmeister
> H. anastomosis
> H. gastroenterostomy
> H. operation
> H. procedure
> H. technique
> H.-Polya anastomosis

Holinger esophagoscope

Hollister urostomy bag

hollow viscus

holmium:YAG laser

Holthouse hernia

homeostasis

home parenteral nutrition

homogeneous
> h. ablation
> h. texture

homologous
> h. restriction factor

homologous (continued)
> h. serum hepatitis
> h. serum jaundice

homotopic transplantation

homovanillic acid (HVA)

homozygous sickle cell anemia

hook
> Barr fistula h.
> Crile nerve h.
> Loughnane h.

Hopkins rod-lens system for
rigid choledochoscope

horizontal
> h. folds of rectum
> h. gastroplasty
> h. plane

hormonal
> h. fever

hormone
> adrenocorticotropic h.
> (ACTH)
> h. antagonist
> antidiuretic h. (ADH)
> follicle-stimulating h.
> gastrointestinal h.
> glycoprotein h.
> growth h. (GH)
> excess growth h.

Horn sign

horseshoe
> h. abscess
> h. fistula
> h. kidney

Horsley
> H. anastomosis
> H. gastrectomy
> H. suture

hortobezoar

hose-pipe appearance of terminal ileum

hot
> h. appendix

hot *(continued)*
    h. biopsy
    h. biopsy forceps
    h. biopsy technique
    h. flexible forceps
    h. spot

hourglass
    h. constriction of gallbladder
    h. deformity
    h. gallbladder
    h. narrowing
    h. stomach
    h. stricture

House advancement anoplasty

House flap anoplasty

Houston
    H. muscle
    H. valves

Howship-Romberg sign

hpf
    high-power field

HPTA
    hepatopoietin A

HPV
    human papillomavirus

HPV 16
    human papillomavirus 16

H_2 receptor
    H_2 r. antagonist
    H_2 r. antagonist therapy
    H_2 r. blocker
    H_2 r.–blocking drug

H-shaped ileal pouch-anal anastomosis

5-HT4 agonist

Hueter maneuver

Hufford esophagoscope

Huggins operation

Huhner test

human
    h. adenovirus 12
    h. gut bacteria
    h. immunodeficiency virus–associated nephropathy
    h. papillomavirus (HPV)
    h. papillomavirus 16 (HPV 16)
    h. serum jaundice

hump
    dromedary h.

hunger
    h. pain

Hunner
    H. stricture
    H. ulcer

Huschke
    gastropancreatic ligaments of H.
    H. ligament

Hutch diverticulum

HVA
    homovanillic acid

hyalin
    alcoholic h.

hyaline
    h. arteriolar nephrosclerosis
    h. arteriolosclerosis
    h. cast

hyaluronic acid

hybrid
    F1 h.

hydatid
    h. of Morgagni
    sessile h.

HydraClense sitz bath

hydraeroperitoneum

hydragogue

hydramnios
    acute h.

hydraulic abdominal concus-
    sion

hydremic ascites

hydrepigastrium

hydroappendix

hydrobilirubin

hydrocalycosis

hydrocalyx

hydrocele
    abdominoscrotal h.
    chylous h.
    communicating h.
    congenital h.
    cord h.
    diffused h.
    Dupuytren h.
    encysted h.
    funicular h.
    hernial h.
    noncommunicating h.
    postoperative h.
    h. renalis
    scrotal h.

hydrocelectomy

hydrochloretic drug

hydrochloric acid (HCl)

hydrochloride (HCl)

hydrochlorothiazide
    h.-triamterene (HCTZ-TA)

hydrocholecystis

hydrocholeresis

hydrocholeretic

hydrocirsocele

hydrocortisone
    h. acetate
    h. enema

hydrodiuresis

hydrogen
    h. gas
    h. peroxide
    h. peroxide enema

hydrohematonephrosis

hydronephrosis
    closed h.
    open h.

hydronephrotic

hydroperinephrosis

hydrophobic
    h. force

hydrophorograph

hydropic nephrosis

hydropneumoperitoneum

hydrops
    gallbladder h.

hydropyonephrosis

hydrosarcocele

hydrostatic pressure

hydrothorax
    cirrhotic h.

hydroureter

hydroureteronephrosis

hydroureterosis

hydrouria

hydroxyzine
    h. hydrochloride
    h. pamoate

hydruria

hydruric

hymenal valve of male urethra

hyoscyamine
    h. hydrobromide
    h. sulfate

Hypaque
    H. contrast medium
    H. swallow

hypazoturic nephropathy

hyperabsorption

hyperacidity
  gastric h.

hyperactive
  h. bowel sounds

hyperacute rejection

hyperalgesia
  colonic h.

hyperalimentation
  central h.
  intravenous h.
  parenteral h.
  peripheral h.

hyperbilirubinemia
  h. I
  congenital h.
  conjugated h.
  constitutional h.
  neonatal h.
  unconjugated h.

hypercalciuria
  absorptive h.

hypercatharsis

hypercathartic

hyperchloremic metabolic acidosis

hyperchlorhydria

hypercholesterolemia
  biliary h. xanthomatosis
  familial h.
  familial h. with hyperlipidemia

hypercholesterolia

hypercholia

hyperchylia

hyperchylomicronemia
  familial h.
  familial h. with hyperprebetalipoproteinemia

hyperdiuresis

hyperdynamic
  h. ileus

hyperemesis

hyperemetic

hyperemia
  gastric h.

hyperfiltration

hyperfunction
  antral gastrin cell h.

hyperhepatia

hyperhydrochloria

hyperhydrochloridia

hyperinsulinism
  alimentary h.

hyperkalemia

hyperkaliemia

hyperkeratosis
  esophageal h.

hyperlipidemia
  familial fat-induced h.
  idiopathic h.

hyperlipoproteinemia
  acquired h.
  familial h.

hypermobile
  h. kidney

hypermotility

hypernatremic
  h. dehydration

hypernephroid carcinoma

hypernephroma

hyperosmolar perfusate

hyperosmotic feeding

hyperoxaluria
  absorptive h.
  acquired h.

hyperoxaluria *(continued)*
  enteric h.
  primary h.

hyperpancreorrhea

hyperpepsia

hyperpepsinia

hyperperistalsis

hyperpituitary
  h. gigantism

hyperplasia
  adenomatous h. (AH)
  adrenal h.
  antral G-cell h.
  atypical adenomatous h.
  benign prostatic h.
  bilobar h.
  congenital adrenal h. (CAH)
  ductal epithelial h.
  focal nodular h. (FNH)
  follicular lymphoid h.
  foveolar h.
  nodular h.
  nodular lymphoid h.
  nodular h. of the prostate
  nodular regenerative h.
  papillary h.

hyperplastic
  h. adenomatous polyp
  h. arteriolar nephrosclero-
    sis
  h. arteriolitis
  h. cholecystosis
  h. epithelial gastric polyp
  h. gastric polyp
  h. nodule
  h. obesity
  h. polyp
  h. polyposis

hyperpotassemia

hyperprebetalipoproteinemia
  familial h.

hyperreflexia
  detrusor h.

hyperresonant abdomen

hypersecretion
  gastric h.

hypersensitivity
  cholestatic h.

hypertension
  accelerated h.
  allograft-mediated h.
  ductal h.
  Goldblatt h.
  noncirrhotic portal h.
  pancreatic ductal h.
  portal h.
  renal h.
  renovascular h.
  splenoportal h.

hypertensive
  h. nephrosclerosis

hyperthyroxinemia
  familial dysalbuminemic h.
    (FDH)
  familial isolated h.

hypertriglyceridemia
  familial h.

hypertrophic
  h. cirrhosis
  h. gastritis
  h. gastropathy
  h. obesity
  h. pyloric stenosis

hypertrophy
  benign prostatic h.
  Billroth h.
  bilobar h.
  rugal h.

hypoactive bowel sounds

hypobilirubinemia

hypocarbonemia

hypochlorhydria

hypochlorohydric
  hypochlorhydric cirrhosis

hypochondriac
    h. region

hypochondrium *pl.* hypochon-
    dria

hypochylia

hypodiaphragmatic

hypoechoic
    h. cancer
    h. lesion
    h. periphery
    h. ringed layer

hypogammaglobulinemic
    h. sprue

hypoganglionosis

hypogastric
    h. artery
    h. region

hypogastrium

hypohepatia

hypohydrochloria

hypokalemia

hypokalemic
    h. nephrosis

hypokaliemia

hypokinetic renal tubular acido-
    sis

hypolactasia
    adult h.

hyponatremia
    depletional h.
    dilutional h.

hypopancreatism

hypopancreorrhea

hypopepsia

hypopepsinia

hypoperistalsis

hypopharyngeal diverticulum

hypophrenic

hypophrenium

hypoplasia
    bile duct h.
    oligomeganephronic re-
    nal h.

hypopotassemia

hypopotassemic

hypospadia

hypospadiac

hypospadias
    balanic h.
    balanitic h.
    female h.
    glandular h.
    penile h.
    penoscrotal h.
    perineal h.
    pseudovaginal h.

hyposthenuria
    tubular h.

hypothermia
    gastric h.

hypothesis
    free hormone h.

hypotonia
    rectal h.

hypotonic
    h. syndromes

hypouresis

hypourocrinia

hypoventilation
    benzodiazepine-induced h.

hypovolemic
    h. anemia
    h. shock

Hyrtl sphincter

hysterical vomiting

iatrogenic
  i. coagulopathy
  i. colitis
  i. immunodeficiency syn-
    drome
  i. malabsorption
  i. pancreatic trauma
  i. pneumothorax
  i. trauma

IBD
  inflammatory bowel dis-
    ease

IBS
  inflammatory bowel syn-
    drome
  irritable bowel syndrome

IBW
  ideal body weight

iced
  i. intestine
  i. lactated Ringer solution
  i. saline lavage

ice-water swallow

icing liver

icteric
  i. sclera
  i. skin
  i. sputum

icteritious

icterogenic

icterogenicity

icterohematuria

icterohematuric

icterohemoglobinuria

icterohepatitis

icteroid

icterus
  benign familial i.
  i. neonatorum

identification
  lesion i.

idiopathic
  i. achalasia
  i. ascites
  i. autoimmune cholangitis
  i. autoimmune chronic hep-
    atitis
  chronic i. constipation
  i. chronic erosion
  i. chronic erosive gastritis
  chronic i. intestinal
    pseudo-obstruction
  chronic i. jaundice
  i. colitis
  i. constipation
  i. diffuse ulcerative non-
    granulomatous enteritis
  i. edema
  i. enteropathy
  i. esophageal ulcer
  i. fibrosing pancreatitis
  i. gastric acid secretion
  i. gastritis
  i. gastroparesis
  i. gastropathy
  i. hematuria
  i. hemochromatosis
  i. hyperlipidemia
  i. hypertrophic gastropathy
  i. inflammatory bowel dis-
    ease
  i. intestinal pseudo-ob-
    struction
  i. megacolon
  i. obstruction
  i. pancreatitis
  i. proctitis
  i. proctocolitis
  i. recurrent pancreatitis
  i. retroperitoneal fibrosis
  i. steatorrhea
  i. varices
  i. volvulus

IDL
  intermediate-density lipo-
    protein

IF
    intrinsic factor

Ig
    immunoglobulin

IgA
    immunoglobulin A
        IgA glomerulonephritis
        IgA nephropathy
        IgA neuropathy

IgA1

IgA2

IgD
    immunoglobulin D

IgE
    immunoglobulin E

IgG
    immunoglobulin G

IgG1

IgG2

IgM
    immunoglobulin M
        IgM-HA antibody
        IgM anti-HAV antibody
        IgM anti-HBc antibody
        anti-*Helicobacter pylori* IgM
        anti-hepatitis A-IgM immunological study
        IgM nephropathy

ileac

ileal
    i. arteries
    i. biopsy
    i. bladder
    i. blood vessel
    i. conduit
    i. crypt
    i. duplication cyst
    i. inflow tract
    i. interposition
    i. J-pouch
    i. loop

ileal *(continued)*
    i. neobladder
    i. orifice
    i. outflow tract
    i. papilla
    i. pouch
    i. pouch–anal anastomosis
    i. pouch–distal rectal anastomosis
    i. pull-through
    i. resection
    i. reservoir
    i. sleeve
    i. S-pouch
    i. spout
    i. stasis
    i. varix
    i. veins
    i. W-pouch

ileectomy

ileitis
    Crohn i.
    distal i.
    granulomatous i.
    Meckel i.
    obstructive dysfunctional i.
    pouch i.
    regional i.
    terminal i.

ileoanal
    i. anastomosis
    i. endorectal pull-through
    i. pouch
    i. pull-through
    i. pull-through anastomosis
    i. pull-through procedure
    i. reservoir

ileoascending colostomy

ileocecal
    i. bladder
    i. continent urinary reservoir
    i. fat pad
    i. fold
    i. incompetence
    inferior i. fossa
    i. insufficiency

ileocecal *(continued)*
  i. intussusception
  i. junction
  i. opening
  i. papilla
  i. pouch
  i. region
  i. reservoir
  i. segment
  i. sphincter
  superior i. fossa
  i. syndrome
  i. tuberculosis
  i. valve

ileocecocystoplasty

ileocecostomy

ileocecum

ileococcygeus muscle

ileocolectomy

ileocolic
  i. artery
  ascending i. artery
  i. disease
  i. fold
  i. fossa
  i. intussusception
  i. plexus
  i. resection
  i. urinary diversion
  i. valve
  i. vein
  i. vessel

ileocolitis
  Crohn i.
  transmural i.
  tuberculous i.
  i. ulcerosa chronica

ileocolonic
  i. bladder
  i. Crohn disease
  i. neobladder
  i. pouch urinary diversion

ileocolostomy
  end-loop i.
  LeDuc-Camey i.

ileocolotomy

ileoconduit

ileocystoplasty
  Camey i.
  clam i.
  LeDuc-Camey i.

ileocystostomy

ileogastric
  i. reflex

ileoileal intussusception

ileoileostomy

ileojejunitis

ileopexy

ileoproctostomy

ileorectal
  i. anastomosis

ileorectostomy

ileorenal
  iliorenal bypass

ileorrhaphy

ileosigmoid
  i. colostomy
  i. fistula
  i. knot

ileosigmoidostomy

ileostogram

ileostomy
  anal i. with preservation of
    sphincter
  i. bag
  blow-hole i.
  Brooke i.
  i. closure
  continent i.
  Dennis-Brooke i.
  i. diarrhea
  diversionary i.
  diverting loop i.
  double-barrel i.
  i. effluent

ileostomy *(continued)*
   end i.
   end-loop i.
   incontinent i.
   Kock i.
   loop i.
   permanent loop i.
   pouched i.
   split i.
   i. stoma
   temporary loop i.
   terminal i.
   Turnbull end-loop i.

ileotomy

ileotransverse
   i. colon anastomosis
   i. colostomy

ileotransversostomy

ileovesical
   i. anastomosis
   i. fistula

ileum
   antimesenteric border of
     distal i.
   duplex i.
   hose-pipe appearance of
     terminal i.
   neoterminal i.
   i. nipple
   terminal i.

ileus
   adhesive i.
   adynamic i.
   colonic i.
   dynamic i.
   focal i.
   gallbladder i.
   gallstone i.
   gastric i.
   hyperdynamic i.
   mechanical i.
   meconium i.
   occlusive i.
   paralytic i.
   i. paralyticus

ileus *(continued)*
   spastic i.
   verminous i.

iliac
   anterior i. artery
   i. artery
   i. colon
   common i. artery
   external i. artery
   internal i. artery
   i. mesocolon
   i. roll
   small i. artery
   i. vein

iliofemoral
   i. triangle

iliohypogastric
   i. nerve

ilioinguinal
   i. nerve
   i. ring

iliolumbar
   i. artery

iliopsoas
   i. ring
   i. sign
   i. test

ilium *pl.* ilia

image
   i. analysis
   longitudinal i.

imbalance
   acid-base i.

imbibe

imbricate

imbrication
   cecal i. procedure

iminoglycinuria

Imlach fat plug

immune
  i. response
  i. response gene

immune complex
  i. c. glomerulonephritis

immunity
  cell-mediated i.
  cellular i.

immunoassay
  Abbott TDx monoclonal fluorescence polarization i.

immunodeficiency
  acquired i.
  gastrointestinal i. syndrome

immunoglobulin
  i. A (IgA)
  i. D (IgD)
  i. E (IgE)
  i. G (IgG)
  i. G1
  i. G2
  hepatitis B i.
  i. M (IgM)
  i. neuropathy

immunologic
  i. abnormality

immunomodulatory
  i. action

immunoproliferative
  i. small intestine disease

immunosuppressive regimen

immunotactoid
  i. glomerulopathy

impacted
  i. ampullary stone
  i. calculus
  i. cystic duct
  i. feces
  i. stone
  i. stool

impaction
  endoscope i.
  fecal i.
  food bolus i.
  meat i.
  rectal i.
  stone i.

impaired
  i. colonic motor function
  i. gastric absorption

imperforate
  i. anus

implant
  Lifecath peritoneal i.
  penile i.

implantation
  LeDuc i.
  i. metastasis
  metastatic i.

impotence
  diabetic i.
  endocrinologic i.
  functional i.
  neurogenic i.
  organic i.
  primary i.
  psychic i.
  psychogenic i.
  secondary i.
  vasculogenic i.

impotency

Impra graft

impressio *pl.* impressiones
  i. cardiaca hepatis
  i. colica hepatis
  i. duodenalis hepatis
  i. esophagea hepatis
  i. gastrica hepatis
  i. gastrica renis
  i. hepatica renis
  i. muscularis renis
  i. oesophagea hepatis
  i. renalis hepatis

impressio *(continued)*
    i. suprarenalis hepatis

impression
    cardiac i.
    colic i. of liver
    digastric i.
    duodenal i. of liver
    esophageal i. of liver
    gastric i.
    gastric i. of liver
    renal i. of liver
    suprarenal i. of liver

inacidity

inadequate
    i. bowel prep
    i. dilation

inanition
    i. fever

incarcerated
    i. bowel
    i. hernia
    i. omentum

incarceration
    colon i.
    hernia i.
    i. symptom

incidence
    angle of i.
    gallstone i.

incidental
    i. adenoma
    i. appendectomy
    i. splenectomy

incision
    apron skin i.
    Bevan abdominal i.
    bilateral subcostal i.
    bilateral transabdominal i.
    bucket-handle i.
    buttonhole i.
    celiotomy i.
    chevron i.
    choledochotomy i.

incision *(continued)*
    circumumbilical i.
    cruciate i.
    darting i.
    i. and drainage
    eleventh rib flank i.
    elliptical i.
    endoscopic i.
    epigastric i.
    fish-mouth i.
    flank i.
    gridiron i.
    groin i.
    Heineke-Mikulicz i.
    hockey-stick i.
    infraumbilical i.
    inguinal i.
    inverted-U abdominal i.
    LaRoque herniorrhaphy i.
    i. line
    lower abdominal trans-
      verse i.
    low-transverse i.
    McBurney i.
    median i.
    midabdominal transverse i.
    midline i.
    midline lower abdominal i.
    midline upper abdominal i.
    muscle-splitting i.
    Nagamatsu i.
    oblique i.
    omega-shaped i.
    paramedian i.
    pararectus i.
    perineal i.
    Pfannenstiel i.
    relaxing i.
    Rockey-Davis i.
    smiling i.
    stable i.
    stepladder i. technique
    subcostal i.
    subcostal flank i.
    subcostal transperitoneal i.
    surgical i.
    thoracoabdominal i.
    transpubic i.

incision *(continued)*
    transverse i.
    transverse semilunar skin i.
    unilateral subcostal i.
    vertical midline i.
    xiphoid-to-pubis midline
      abdominal i.
    xiphoid-to-umbilicus i.
    Y-shaped i.

incisional
    i. biopsy
    i. hernia

incisura *pl.* incisurae
    i. angularis
    i. angularis gastris
    i. angularis ventriculi
    i. cardiaca gastris
    i. cardiaca ventriculi
    i. cardialis
    i. interlobaris hepatis
    i. ligamenti teretis
    i. pancreatis
    i. umbilicalis

incisure
    angular i. of stomach
    cardiac i. of stomach
    umbilical i.

incompetence
    gastroesophageal i.
    ileocecal i.
    neurogenic sphincteric i.

incompetent
    i. ileocecal valve
    i. sphincter
    i. valve

incomplete
    i. cirrhosis
    i. epispadias

incontinence
    anterior fecal i.
    bowel i.
    fecal i.
    i. of the feces
    intermittent i.
    ischemic fecal i.
    overflow i.

incontinence *(continued)*
    paradoxical i.
    passive i.
    rectal i.
    secondary i.
    stool i.
    stress i.
    urge i.
    urgency i.
    urinary i.
    i. of urine

incontinent
    i. ileostomy

incontinentia
    i. alvi
    i. urinae

incrusted cystitis

indentation
    haustral i.

index *pl.* indexes, indices
    biliary saturation i.
    Crohn disease activity i.
      (CDAI)
    Crohn Disease Endoscopic
      I. of Severity
    fever i.
    hemoglobin content in-
      dices
    hepatic perfusion i.
    histologic activity i.
    juxtaglomerular i.
    nutritional i.
    obesity i.
    penile brachial i.

indigestion
    acid i.
    fat i.
    gastric i.
    intestinal i.
    nervous i.
    sugar i.

indigitation

indigo calculus

indirect
    i. bilirubin

indirect *(continued)*
    i. hernia
    i. inguinal hernia

indurated
    i. appendix

induration
    cyanotic i.
    granular i.
    penile i.
    plastic i.

indurative nephritis

indwelling
    i. catheter

inertia
    colonic i.

infant esophagoscope

infantile
    i. celiac disease
    i. colic
    i. diarrhea
    i. embryonal carcinoma
    i. gastroenteritis
    i. hemangioendothelioma
    i. hernia
    i. hypertrophic gastric stenosis
    i. hypertrophic pyloric stenosis
    i. liver

infantilism
    celiac i.
    hepatic i.
    Herter i.
    intestinal i.
    renal i.

infarct
    Brewer i's
    small-bowel i.
    i. of Zahn

infarcted bowel

infarction
    acute nonocclusive bowel i.
    intestinal i.
    mesenteric i.

infarction *(continued)*
    myocardial i.
    nonocclusive i.
    nonocclusive intestinal i.
    nonocclusive mesenteric i.
    occlusive i.
    omental i.
    small intestinal i.
    total i.

infected
    i. bile duct
    i. necrosis
    i. pseudocyst
    i. tract

infection
    active systemic bacterial i.
    adenovirus i.
    antifungal esophageal i.
    antifungal-resistant opportunistic i.
    Aspergillus i.
    bacterial i.
    blood stream i.
    i. calculus
    candidal i.
    CMV i.
    coxsackievirus i.
    cryptosporidial i.
    cytomegalovirus i.
    deep-seated fungal i.
    dengue hemorrhagic fever i.
    disseminated CMV i.
    enteric i.
    Epstein-Barr viral i.
    esophageal i.
    esophageal fungal i.
    exit site i.
    fungal i.
    gas-forming pyogenic liver i.
    gastrointestinal i.
    helminth i.
    hematogenous spread of i.
    hepatic candidal i.
    hepatitis A i.
    hepatitis B i.
    hepatitis C i.

infection *(continued)*
    hepatitis D i.
    hepatitis E i.
    herpes i.
    herpes simplex i.
    HIV i.
    intestinal i.
    intra-abdominal i.
    liver cyst i.
    monilial i.
    multiple hepatitis virus i.
    Mycobacterium i.
    necrotizing i.
    nematode i.
    nosocomial i.
    nosocomial fungal i.
    opportunistic i.
    parasitic i.
    perianal i.
    perineal i.
    peristomal i.
    peritoneal fungal i.
    pneumococcal i.
    postsplenectomy i.
    retrovirus i.
    rotavirus i.
    i. stone
    tunnel i.
    urinary tract i.
    varicella zoster i.
    viral i.
    whipworm i.
    wound i.

infectious
    i. colitis
    i. complication
    i. diarrhea
    i. esophagitis
    i. gastroenteritis
    i. hepatitis
    i. jaundice
    i. mononucleosis
    i. splenomegaly

infective
    i. jaundice
    i. splenomegaly

inferior
    i. aberrant ductule

inferior *(continued)*
    i. angle of duodenum
    i. border of body of pan-
        creas
    i. border of liver
    i. border of pancreas
    i. capsular artery
    i. duodenal fold
    i. duodenal fossa
    i. epigastric artery
    i. epigastric vein
    i. flexure of duodenum
    i. fossa of omental sac
    i. hemorrhoidal artery
    i. ileocecal fossa
    i. layer of pelvic diaphragm
    i. ligament of epididymis
    i. lip of ileocecal valve
    i. mesenteric artery
    i. mesenteric vein
    i. pancreatic artery
    i. pancreaticoduodenal ar-
        teries
    i. part of duodenum
    i. pole of kidney
    i. pole of testis
    i. rectal artery
    i. rectal veins
    i. right colic artery
    i. segment
    i. segmental artery of kid-
        ney
    i. suprarenal artery
    i. thoracic aperture
    i. vesical artery

inferomedial

infertile

infertilitas

infertility

infestation
    biliary i.

infiltrating adenocarcinoma

infiltration
    bacterial mucosal i.
    cellular i.
    colonic i.

COLOR PLATES

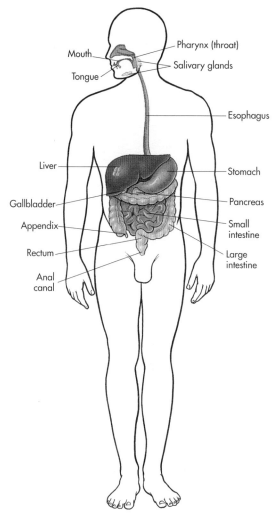

Digestive system. (From Thibodeau, GA, Patton, KT: Structure & Function of the Body, 11th ed. St. Louis, Mosby, Inc., 2000.)

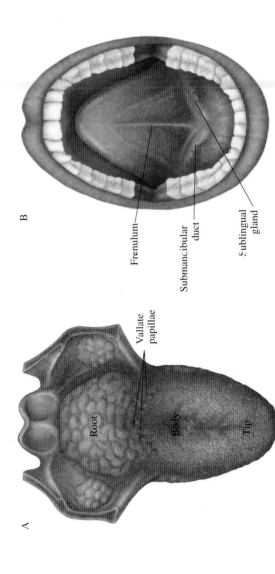

The tongue. A. Surface. B, Mouth cavity showing the undersurface of the tongue (From Thibodeau, GA, Patton, KT: Structure & Function of the Body, 11th ed. St. Louis, Mosby, Inc., 2000.)

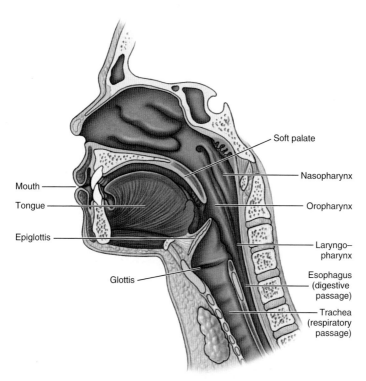

Soft palate

Nasopharynx

Mouth

Tongue

Oropharynx

Epiglottis

Laryngo–
pharynx

Glottis

Esophagus
(digestive
passage)

Trachea
(respiratory
passage)

Eating and swallowing, from mouth to pharynx to esophagus. Food follows a path as it is ingested and swallowed. Note the epiglottis, the structure that prevents the entrance of food into the respiratory passages. (From Herlihy, B, Maebius, NK: The Human Body in Health and Illness. Philadelphia, W.B. Saunders Company, 2000.)

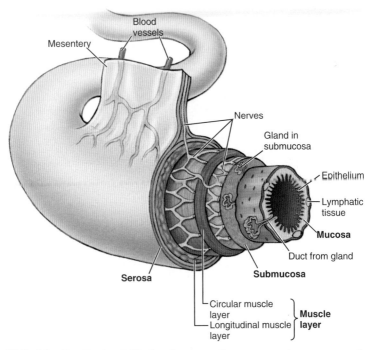

Wall of the digestive tract. The four layers are the mucosa, submucosa, muscle layer, and serosa. Note that the glands empty their secretions into the lumen of the digestive tract by way of ducts. Note also that the serosa extends as the mesentery. Peristalsis resembles the movement of toothpaste as it is squeezed through the tube. (From Herlihy, B, Maebius, NK: The Human Body in Health and Illness. Philadelphia, W.B. Saunders Company, 2000.)

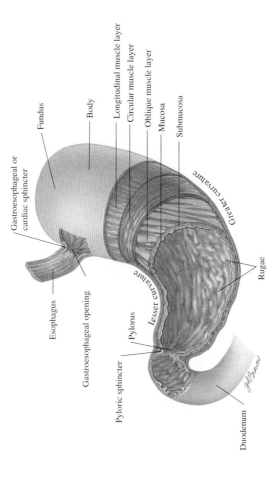

Stomach. A portion of the anterior wall has been cut away to reveal the muscle layers of the stomach wall. Notice that the mucosa lining the stomach forms folds called rugae. (From Thibodeau, GA, Patton, KT: Structure & Function of the Body, 11th ed. St. Louis, Mosby, Inc., 2000.)

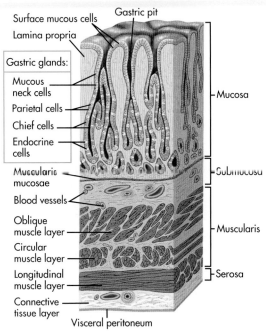

Surface mucous cells

Gastric pit

Lamina propria

Gastric glands:

Mucous neck cells

Parietal cells

Chief cells

Endocrine cells

Muscularis mucosae

Blood vessels

Oblique muscle layer

Circular muscle layer

Longitudinal muscle layer

Connective tissue layer

Visceral peritoneum

Mucosa

Submucosa

Muscularis

Serosa

Gastric pits and gastric glands. Gastric pits are depressions in the epithelial lining of the stomach. At the bottom of each pit is one or more tubular gastric glands. Chief cells produce the enzymes of gastric juice, and parietal cells produce stomach acid. (From Thibodeau, GA, Patton, KT: Anthony's Textbook of Anatomy & Physiology, 16th ed. St. Louis, Mosby, Inc., 1999.)

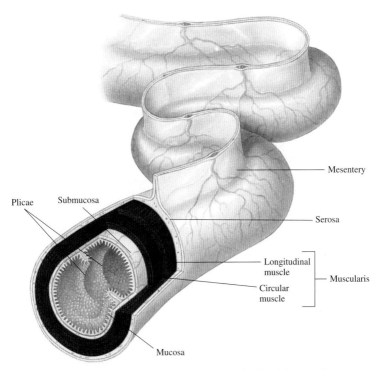

Plicae

Submucosa

Mesentery

Serosa

Longitudinal
muscle

Circular
muscle

Muscularis

Mucosa

Section of the small intestine. The four layers typical of walls of the gastrointestinal tract are shown. Circular folds of mucous membrane called plicae increase the surface area of the lining coat. (From Thibodeau, GA, Patton, KT: Structure & Function of the Body, 11th ed. St. Louis, Mosby, Inc., 2000.)

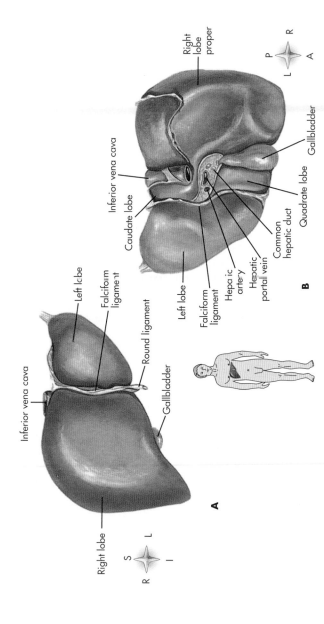

Gross structure of the liver. *A*, Anterior view. *B*, Inferior view. (From Thibodeau, GA, Patton, KT: Anthony's Textbook of Anatomy & Physiology, 16th ed. St. Louis, Mosby, Inc., 1999.)

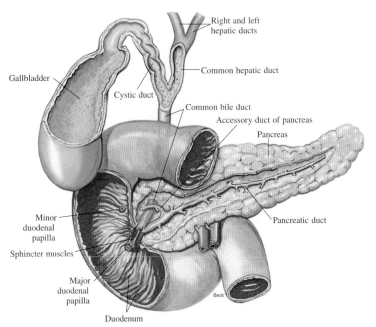

Gallbladder

Cystic duct

Right and left hepatic ducts

Common hepatic duct

Common bile duct

Accessory duct of pancreas

Pancreas

Minor duodenal papilla

Pancreatic duct

Sphincter muscles

Major duodenal papilla

Beck

Duodenum

The gallbladder and bile ducts. Obstruction of the hepatic or common bile duct by stone or spasm blocks the exit from the liver, where bile is formed, and prevents it from being ejected into the duodenum. (From Thibodeau, GA, Patton, KT: Structure & Function of the Body, 11th ed. St. Louis, Mosby, Inc., 2000.)

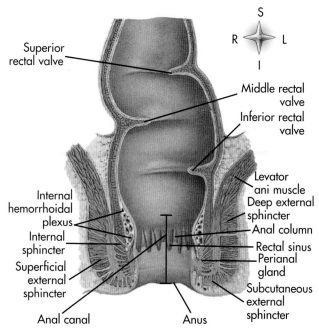

Superior rectal valve

Middle rectal valve

Inferior rectal valve

Levator ani muscle

Deep external sphincter

Anal column

Rectal sinus

Perianal gland

Subcutaneous external sphincter

Internal hemorrhoidal plexus

Internal sphincter

Superficial external sphincter

Anal canal

Anus

S
R — L
I

The rectum and anus. (From Thibodeau, GA, Patton, KT: Anthony's Textbook of Anatomy & Physiology, 16th ed. St. Louis, Mosby, Inc., 1999.)

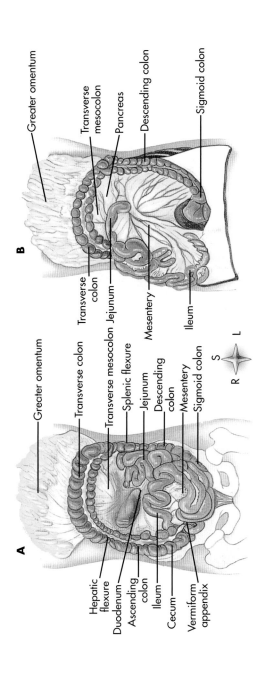

Projections of the peritoneum. *A,* Abdominal viscera from the front. The transverse colon and the greater omentum are elevated to reveal the flexures of the colon and the loops of the small intestine. *B,* The transverse colon and greater omentum are raised and the small intestine is pulled to the side to show the transverse mesocolon and mesentery. (From Thibodeau, GA, Patton, KT: Anthony's Textbook of Anatomy & Physiology, 16th ed. St. Louis, Mosby, Inc., 1999.)

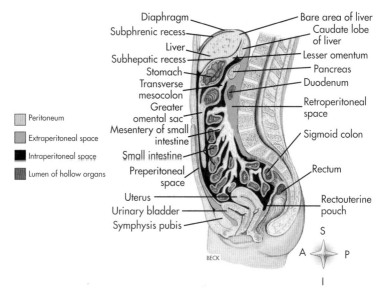

Peritoneum. Sagittal view of the abdomen showing the peritoneum and its reflections. Intraperitoneal spaces are shown in red and extraperitoneal spaces in green. The portion of the extraperitoneal space along the posterior wall of the abdomen is often called the retroperitoneal space. (From Thibodeau, GA, Patton, KT: Anthony's Textbook of Anatomy & Physiology, 16th ed. St. Louis, Mosby, Inc., 1999.)

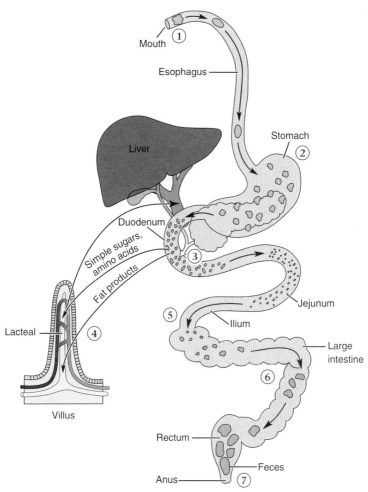

Digestion and absorption. The food is mechanically and chemically digested and pushed through the various parts of the digestive tract. The nutrients are absorbed from the upper small intestine, primarily the duodenum, into the blood capillaries and lacteals. Blood that is rich in digestive end-products flows to the intestinal tract. The undigestible or nonabsorbable food particles accumulate in the rectum as waste. (From Herlihy, B, Maebius, NK: The Human Body in Health and Illness. Philadelphia, W.B. Saunders Company, 2000.)

infiltration *(continued)*
    fatty i. of liver
    focal fatty i. of liver
    neutrophilic i.
    urinous i.

infiltrative lymphoma

inflamed
    i. appendix
    i. gallbladder
    i. mucosa

inflammation
    interstitial i.

inflammatory
    i. bowel disease (IBD)
    i. bowel syndrome
    chronic i. disease
    i. colitis
    i. diarrhea
    i. polyp

influenza virus

infracolic

infraduodenal fossa

infrarenal chemolysis

infraumbilical
    i. incision
    i. mound

infravesical

infrequent defecation

infundibula *(plural of* infundibulum)

infundibuliform fascia

infundibulopelvic

infundibulum *pl.* infundibula
    i. of bile duct
    i. of gallbladder
    infundibula of kidney
    infundibula renum
    i. of urinary bladder

ingested foreign body

ingestion
    acid i.

ingestion *(continued)*
    alkali i.

inguinal
    i. adenopathy
    anterior i. ligament
    i. arteries
    i. bulge
    i. canal
    i. crease
    deep i. ring
    external i. ring
    i. floor
    i. hernia
    i. incision
    internal i. ligament
    internal i. ring
    i. ligament of Blumberg
    posterior i. ligament
    i. sphincter
    superficial i. ring

inguinocrural
    i. hernia

inguinofemoral
    i. hernia

inguinoperitoneal

inguinoproperitoneal
    i. hernia

inguinoscrotal

inguinosuperficial
    i. hernia

inhaler
    Allis i.

inhibiting factor

inhibitor
    alpha-glucosidase i.
    angiotensin-converting enzyme i. (ACEI)
    gastric acid pump i.
    proton pump i.
    rectoanal i.

inhibitory
    gastric i. peptide
    gastric i. polypeptide (GIP)

initial cells

injection
    i. sclerosis
    tangential colonic submu-
        cosal i.

injury
    acid i.
    alkaline i.
    antecedent pancreatic i.
    cell-mediated hepatic i.
    drug-induced acute hepa-
        tic i.
    duodenal i.
    gastric mucosal i.
    gastroduodenal mucosal i.
    hemorrhagic radiation i.
    obstetric i.
    open i.
    pancreatic i.
    radiation i.
    rectal i.
    splenic i.

inlet
    esophageal i.

inner
    i. medulla of kidney
    i. stripe
    i. zone of renal medulla

innocent gallstone

innocuous

innominate

inoculation hepatitis

insertion
    flatus tube i.
    tube i.

insipidus
    diabetes i.

in situ

insorption

inspissated
    i. bile

inspissated *(continued)*
    i. bile syndrome
    i. feces

instability
    detrusor i.

institutional dysentery

instrument
    biopsy i.
    GIA i.
    oblique-forward-viewing i.

instrumentation
    biliary i.

insufficiency
    gastric i.
    gastromotor i.
    hepatic i.
    ileocecal i.
    progressive renal i.
    pyloric i.
    renal i.
    vascular i.

insula *pl.* insulae
    insulae of Peyer

insular
    i. lobe

insulin
    i.-dependent
    i.-dependent diabetes
    i.-dependent diabetes melli-
        tus

insulinoma

insult
    ischemic i.

intake and output (I&O)

intention
    delayed primary i.
    healing by primary i.
    healing by secondary i.

interaction
    cell–cell i.

intercalated cells

intercapillary
    i. cells
    i. glomerulosclerosis
    i. nephrosclerosis

intercolonoscopy

intercolumnar
    i. fascia
    i. fibers

intercostal
    i. scan
    i. space
    i. supraclavicular space

intercrural
    i. fibers

interdeferential

interdialytic

interesophageal variceal pressure

interferon
    i. alfa-2a
    i. alfa-2b
    i. alfa-2b, recombinant
    i. alfa-n1
    i. alfa-n3
    i. alpha
    alpha i.
    basal i.-gamma
    beta i.
    i. beta
    i. beta-1a
    i. beta-1b
    i. beta-2
    gamma i.
    i. gamma
    i. gamma-1a
    i. gamma-1b
    recombinant i. alfa-2a
    recombinant human alpha i.
    i. therapy
    i. treatment

interlobar
    i. arteries of kidney

interlobar *(continued)*
    i. notch
    i. veins of kidney

interlobular
    i. arteries of kidney
    i. arteries of liver
    i. bile ducts
    i. biliary canals
    i. ductules
    i. veins of kidney

interlocking ligature

interloop
    i. abscess

intermediate
    i. colic vein
    i. glands
    i. hepatic veins
    i. part of male urethra

intermesenteric
    i. abscess

intermittent
    i. diarrhea
    i. drip feeding
    i. hepatic fever
    i. incontinence
    i. obstruction
    i. pain
    i. peritoneal dialysis
    i. suctioning

intermuscular hernia

internal
    i. abdominal ring
    i. absorption
    i. anal sphincter
    aponeurosis of i. oblique
    i. biliary lavage
    i. crus of anterior inguinal ring
    i. genital organs
    i. hemorrhage
    i. hemorrhoid
    i. hernia
    i. iliac artery
    i. inguinal ligament

internal *(continued)*
    i. inguinal ring
    i. margin of testis
    i. oblique aponeurosis
    i. oblique fascia
    i. oblique muscle of abdo-
        men
    i. orifice of urethra
    i. procidentia
    i. proctotomy
    i. pudendal artery
    i. pudendal vein
    i. spermatic fascia
    i. sphincter muscle of anus
    i. sphincterotomy
    i. urethral orifice
    i. urethrotomy

interosseous ligament of pubis
  (of Winslow)

interparietal
    i. hernia

interposition
    colonic i.
    i. graft
    ileal i.

interrenal

intersigmoid
    i. fossa
    i. hernia

intersphincteric
    i. abscess
    i. anal fistula
    i. anorectal space
    i. perirectal abscess
    i. space

interstitial
    acute i. nephritis
    i. cells
    i. cells of Cajal
    i. cells of Leydig
    i. cell tumor
    chronic i. cystitis
    chronic i. hepatitis
    i. fibrosis

interstitial *(continued)*
    i. gastritis
    i. gland
    i. hernia
    i. inflammation
    i. nephritis
    i. pancreatitis
    i. rejection

intersymphyseal bar

interureteral
    i. ligament

interureteric
    i. fold
    i. ridge

interval
    i. appendectomy

intervention
    angiographic i.

intestina *(plural of* intestinum)

intestinal
    i. absorption
    i. absorptive cell
    i. amebiasis
    i. anastomosis
    i. angina
    i. arteries
    i. atony
    i. atresia
    i. bacteria
    i. bag
    i. bypass
    i. calculus
    i. canal
    chronic i. dysmotility
    chronic i. ischemic syn-
        drome
    i. clamp
    closed-loop i. obstruction
    i. colic
    i. contents
    i. decompression
    i. diverticulum
    i. dyspepsia
    i. emphysema

intestinal *(continued)*
  i. endoscopy
  i. fistula
  i. fixation
  i. flora
  i. follicles
  i. glands
  i. hemorrhage
  i. histoplasmosis
  i. indigestion
  i. infantilism
  i. infarction
  i. infection
  i. intoxication
  i. intussusception
  i. ischemia
  i. juice
  i. lamina propria
  i. lipodystrophy
  i. loop
  i. lumen
  i. lymphangiectasia
  i. metaplasia
  i. motility disorder
  i. mucosa
  i. myiasis
  i. necrosis
  i. obstruction
  i. parasite
  i. peptide
  i. perforation
  i. perfusion
  i. peritoneum
  i. permeability measure-
    ment
  i. pneumatosis
  i. polyposis
  i. prolapse
  i. pseudo-obstruction
  i. schistosomiasis
  i. sling
  i. stasis
  i. steatorrhea
  i. stricture
  i. strongyloidiasis
  i. surgery
  i. tract
  i. tuberculosis

intestinal *(continued)*
  i. viability
  i. villus
  i. volvulus
  i. web

intestinalization

intestine
  blind i.
  Crohn small i.
  empty i.
  folds of large i.
  iced i.
  jejunoileal i.
  large i.
  malrotation of i.
  mesenterial i.
  milking of i.
  segmented i.
  small i.
  straight i.

intestinointestinal
  i. reflex

intestinum *pl.* intestina
  i. caecum
  i. crassum
  i. ileum
  i. jejunum
  i. rectum
  i. tenue
  i. tenue mesenteriale

intolerance
  fatty food i.
  glucose i.

intoxication
  intestinal i.
  water i.

intra-abdominal
  i. abscess
  i. adhesion
  i. bile leakage
  i. hemorrhage
  i. ileal reservoir
  i. infection
  i. mass

intra-abdominal *(continued)*
  i. pressure
  i. sepsis
  i. viscus

intra-anal
  i. pressure
  i. wart

intra-appendicular

intra-arterial
  i. digital subtraction angiography

intracavernosal

intracellular
  i. canaliculi of parietal cells
  i. acidity

intracholedochal pressure

intracolic

intractable
  i. constipation
  i. diarrhea
  i. ulcerative colitis
  i. vomiting

intradialytic

intraductal pressure

intraduodenal

intraepithelial cysts

intraesophageal peristaltic pressure

intragastric
  i. acidity
  i. balloon
  i. bubble
  i. gallstone
  i. pressure

intrahepatic
  i. abscess
  i. AV fistula
  i. bile duct
  i. bile duct carcinoma
  i. biliary cystic dilation
  i. biliary stricture
  i. cholangiojejunostomy

intrahepatic *(continued)*
  i. cholelithiasis
  i. cholestasis
  i. ductal dilation
  i. hematoma
  i. portal obstruction
  i. radicle
  i. sclerosing cholangitis
  i. shunt
  i. spontaneous arterioportal fistula

intraintestinal

intralobular
  i. biliary canals

intraluminal
  i. clot
  i. cysts
  i. duodenal diverticulum
  i. esophageal pressure
  i. filling defect
  i. pouch
  i. pressure
  i. proliferation
  i. stapler
  i. stone

intramesenteric
  i. abscess

intramucosal
  i. cancer
  i. carcinoma
  i. metastasis

intramural
  i. atheromatous disease
  i. colonic air
  i. diverticulum
  i. fistulous tract
  i. ganglia
  i. hematoma
  i. intestinal hemorrhage
  i. lesion

intraoperative
  i. biliary endoscopy
  i. endoscopy

intraoperative
  i. antibiotic

intraoperative *(continued)*
    i. ultrasonography and an-
       giography

intrapancreatic
    i. bile duct
    i. nerve

intrapapillary terminus

intrapelvic

intraperitoneal
    i. abscess
    i. adhesion
    i. cavity
    i. chemotherapy
    i. hemorrhage
    i. hernia
    i. perforation
    i. viscus

intraprostatic

intrarectal

intrarenal
    i. arteries
    i. reflux

intrascrotal

intratesticular

intrathecal
    i. chemotherapy

intrathoracic
    i. esophagogastroscopy
    i. Nissen fundoplication

intraureteral

intraurethral

intravenous
    i. cholangiogram
    i. cholangiography
    i. drug
    i. drug abuse
    i. feeding
    i. glucose
    i. hyperalimentation

intravesical
    i. anastomosis
    i. chemotherapy

intrinsic
    i. enzymatic activity
    i. factor
    i. rhabdosphincter

introducer
    Hickman percutaneous i.

introgastric

introsusception

intubation
    catheter-guided endoscop-
      ic i. (CAGEIN)
    endotracheal i.
    esophageal i.
    i. failure
    nasogastric i.
    nasotracheal i.
    oral i.
    orotracheal i.

intussusception
    agonic i.
    appendiceal i.
    bowel i.
    cecocolic i.
    colocolic i.
    ileocecal i.
    ileocolic i.
    ileoileal i.
    intestinal i.
    jejunogastric i.
    jejunojejunocolic i.
    postmortem i.
    retrograde i.
    triple i.

intussusceptum

intussuscipiens

inulin
    i. clearance test

invagination

invasive
    i. adenocarcinoma
    i. colorectal polyp

inversion
    i. appendectomy

inverted
    i. sigmoid diverticulum
    i. testis
    i.-U abdominal incision

inverting suture

in vitro

in vivo

involuntary
    i. guarding
    i. reflex rigidity

I&O
    intake and output

iodinated contrast agent

ipecac
    i. abuse
    i.-induced vomiting
    i. syrup

ipsilateral adrenalectomy

iris *pl.* irides

iron
    i.-deficiency anemia
    hepatic i. index
    i. liver
    oral i.

irradiation
    i. colitis
    i. effect
    i. failure

irreducible
    i. hernia

irregularity
    sawtooth i. of bowel con-
        tour

irretrievable object

irrigate

irrigation
    acetohydroxamic acid i.
    Coloplast ostomy i. set
    i. colostomy
    Dansac ostomy i. set

irrigation *(continued)*
    glycine i.
    rectum i.
    sodium chloride i.
    i.-suction drainage
    i. test

irrigator

irritability
    i. of the bladder
    i. of the stomach

irritable
    i. bladder
    i. bowel syndrome
    i. colon
    i. colon syndrome
    constipation-predominant i.
        bowel syndrome
    i. stricture

irritative
    i. diarrhea

ischemia
    colonic i.
    intestinal i.
    mesenteric i.
    mucosal i.
    myocardial i.
    i. necrosis
    nonocclusive mesenteric i.
    visceral i.

ischemic
    i. bowel
    i. bowel disease
    i. colitis
    i. fecal incontinence
    i. hepatitis
    i. insult
    i. necrosis
    i. nephropathy

ischiatic
    i. hernia

ischiocavernous
    i. muscle

ischiocele

ischioprostatic
i. ligament

ischiorectal
i. abscess
i. anorectal space
i. aponeurosis
i. fascia
i. fossa plane
i. hernia
i. perirectal abscess
i. space

ischuretic

ischuria
i. paradoxa
i. spastica

island
i. pedicle flap

islet
i's of Langerhans
pancreatic i's

islet cell
i. c. adenoma
i. c. antibody
i. c. carcinoma
i. c. of Langerhans
non-alpha, non-beta pancreatic i. c.
pancreatic i. c.
pancreatic i. c. carcinoma

isoamyl alcohol

Isocal HCN liquid feeding

isodose contour

isoperistaltic
i. anastomosis
i. ileal reservoir

isorrhea

isorrheic

isosmotic lavage

isosthenuria

Isotein HN feeding

isotonic
i. contraction
i. feeding

isthmus *pl.* isthmi
i. prostatae
i. urethrae

isuria

Ito cells

IVIg
intravenous immune globulin

Ivor Lewis two-stage subtotal esophagectomy

Jaboulay
J. button
J. gastroduodenostomy
J. pyloroplasty

Jackson
J. esophageal bougie
J. esophagoscope
J. membrane
J. veil
J.-Pratt drain

Jacobs-Palmer laparoscope

Jadassohn test

Jamaican vomiting sickness

Jamshidi liver biopsy needle

Janeway
J. gastroscope
J. gastrostomy

Japanese
J. classification of cancer
J. dysentery
J. schistosomiasis

Jarvis
J. hemorrhoid clamp
J. pile clamp

Jasbee esophagoscope

Jatrox *Helicobacter pylori* test

jaundice
acholuric j.
benign postoperative j.
black j.
Budd j.
cholestatic j.
chronic idiopathic j.
congenital familial nonhemolytic j.
congenital nonhemolytic j.
Crigler-Najjar j.
epidemic j.
familial chronic idiopathic j.
familial nonhemolytic j.
hemolytic j.

jaundice *(continued)*
hepatocellular j.
hepatogenic j.
hepatogenous j.
homologous serum j.
human serum j.
infectious j.
infective j.
latent j.
leptospiral j.
malignant obstructive j.
mechanical j.
nonhemolytic j.
obstructive j.
parenchymal j.
regurgitation j.
retention j.
shrapnel-induced obstruc-
tive j.

jaundiced skin

Javorski *(variant of* Jaworski)

Jaworski *(spelled also* Javorski)
J. bodies
J. corpuscles
J. test

jaw wiring

jejunal
j. arteries
j. bypass
j. limb
j. loop
j. syndrome
j. ulcer
j. veins
j. villus

jejunectomy

jejunitis

jejunocecostomy

jejunocolic fistula

jejunocolostomy

jejunogastric intussusception

jejunoileal
j. bypass
j. intestine
j. shunt

jejunoileitis

jejunoileostomy
Roux-en-Y distal j.

jejunojejunocolic intussusception

jejunojejunostomy

jejunorrhaphy

jejunostomy
j. elemental diet feeding
loop j.
j. tube feeding

jejunotomy

jejunum

Jenckel cholecystoduodenostomy

Jesberg esophagoscope

jet
water-j.

jetlike bleeding

Jevity isotonic liquid nutrition

JFB III endoscope

Johnson esophagogastroscopy

Jones and Cantarow test

Jonnesco
fossa of J.

J-pexy
omental J-p.

J pouch
colonic J-p.

J-scope esophagoscope

J-shaped
J-s. endoscope

J-shaped *(continued)*
J-s. ileal pouch–anal anastomosis
J-s. reservoir

juice
acid-peptic j.
gastric j.
intestinal j.
pancreatic j.

junctio *pl.* junctiones
j. anorectalis

junction
anorectal j.
cardioesophageal j.
choledochopancreatic ductal j.
duodenojejunal j.
esophagogastric j.
gap j.
gastroesophageal j.
ileocecal j.
pancreaticobiliary j.
pancreaticobiliary ductal j.
patulous gastroesophageal j.
pharyngoesophageal j.
rectosigmoid j.
ureteropelvic j.
ureterovesical j.

junctional tubule

juvenile
acute j. cirrhosis
j. cirrhosis
j. embryonal carcinoma
j. intestinal polyposis
j. nephronophthisis–medullary cystic disease complex
j. polyps
j. polyposis
j. polyposis syndrome

juxta-anal
j. colostomy

juxtaglomerular
- j. apparatus
- j. cells
- j. cell tumor
- j. complex
- j. granules
- j. index
- j. tumor

juxtapapillary duodenal diverticulum

juxtapyloric

juxtavesical

J-Vac closed wound drainage

J-Vac suction reservoir

Kader
K. gastrostomy
K. operation

kaladana

kaliopenia

kaliopenic

kaliuresis

Kalk esophagoscope

kaluresis

kamala

kanyemba

Kaopectate

Kaposi
appendiceal K. sarcoma
gastric K. sarcoma
gastrointestinal K. sarcoma
intracolonic K. sarcoma
K. sarcoma

Karaya ring ileostomy appliance

Karl Storz endoscope

Kasai
K. operation
K.-type hepatoportoenterostomy

Kasugai classification

Kayexalate enema

Kegel exercises

Kelling gastroscope

Kelly
K. operation
K. sign
K. speculum
K. sphincteroscope

kelotomy

Keofeed feeding tube

Kerckring (*spelled also* Kerkring)
circular folds of K.
K. folds (*of small intestine*)
K. valves

Kerkring (*variant of* Kerckring)

keto acid

ketoacidosis
diabetic k.

keyhole deformity

kidney
abdominal k.
k. abscess
k. allograft
amyloid k.
Armanni-Ebstein k.
arteriosclerotic k.
artificial k.
atrophic k.
cadaver k.
cake k.
cicatricial k.
clump k.
congested k.
contracted k.
cortex of k.
crush k.
cyanotic k.
cystic k.
disk k.
doughnut k.
ectopic k.
k. failure
fatty k.
flea-bitten k.
floating k.
Formad k.
k. function test
fused k.
Goldblatt k.
hilum of k.
horseshoe k.
hypermobile k.
lardaceous k.
large red k.

231

kidney *(continued)*
  lumbar k.
  lump k.
  medullary sponge k.
  mortar k.
  movable k.
  mural k.
  myelin k.
  myeloma k.
  pelvic k.
  polycystic k's
  k. punch
  putty k.
  Rose-Bradford k.
  sacciform k.
  sigmoid k.
  sponge k.
  k. stone
  supernumerary k.
  surgical k.
  thoracic k.
  wandering k.
  waxy k.

Kiernan spaces

Kimmelstiel
  K.-Wilson lesion
  K.-Wilson nodule
  K.-Wilson syndrome

kinetics
  urea k.

kink in bowel

Kirchner diverticulum

Kirschner abdominal retractor

kissing ulcers

kit
  Abbott HCV E1A 2nd gener-
    ation k.
  Abbott HCV 2.0 test k.
  Moss PEG k.

Klatskin tumor

Klebs disease

kneeling-squatting position

knife
  k. blade
  Desmarres paracentesis k.
  Lempert paracentesis k.
  skin k.

knifelike pain

knot
  ileosigmoid k.

knuckle of colon

Kobelt tubules

Kocher
  K. dilatation ulcer
  K. maneuver
  K. operation

kocherization

Kock
  K. ileostomy
  K. pouch
  K. procedure

Kohlrausch
  K. folds
  K. valves

Kollmann dilator

kolypeptic

König syndrome

Kraske operation

Krause ligament

Kretz granules

Kron
  K. bile duct dilator
  K. gall duct dilator

Krönlein hernia

krypton laser

Kt/V

Kulchitsky cell
  Kulchitsky-cell carcinoma

Külz
  K. cast

Külz *(continued)*
    K. cylinder

Kunkel syndrome

Kupffer
    K. cell sarcoma
    K. cells

Kussmaul endoscope

label
  fluorescent l's

labia (*plural of* labium)

labial
  l. hernia

labialis
  herpes l.

labium *pl.* labia
  l. inferius valvulae coli
  l. superius valvulae coli
  l. urethrae

La Brea hepatitis

labyrinth
  cortical l.
  Ludwig l's

laceration
  longitudinal l.
  rectal l.

lacis
  l. cells

Lactaid

lactate
  l. dehydrogenase (LDH)

lactated Ringer solution

lactic
  l. acid
  l. acidosis

Lactobacillus acidophilus

lactobezoar

lactose
  l.-associated diarrhea
  l.-free diet
  l.-free feeding
  l. malabsorption

lactulose
  l. concentrate
  l. enema
  l.-mannitol ratio
  l. solution

lactulose *(continued)*
  l. syrup

lacuna *pl.* lacunae
  great l. of urethra
  l. magna
  lacunae of Morgagni
  lacunae Morgagnii urethrae
    muliebris
  lacunae of urethra
  urethral lacunae
  lacunae urethrales
  urethral lacunae of Mor-
    gagni

lacunar
  l. abscess

Ladd
  L. bands
  L. procedure

Laënnec
  L. cirrhosis
  L. disease

Lahey liver transplant bag

Laird-McMahon anorectoplasty

lake
  bile l.

Lallemand
  L. bodies
  L.-Trousseau bodies

lambliasis

lamina *pl.* laminae
  l. densa
  intestinal l. propria
  l. muscularis mucosae coli
  l. muscularis mucosae
    esophagi
  l. muscularis mucosae gas-
    tris
  l. muscularis mucosae in-
    testini crassi
  l. muscularis mucosae in-
    testini recti
  l. muscularis mucosae in-
    testini tenuis

lamina *(continued)*
    l. muscularis mucosae oes-
        ophagi
    l. muscularis mucosae recti
    l. muscularis mucosae ven-
        triculi
    l. parietalis tunicae vagi-
        nalis propriae testis
    l. parietalis tunicae vagi-
        nalis testis
    l. rara
    l. rara externa
    l. rara interna
    submucous l. of stomach
    vascular l. of stomach
    l. visceralis tunicae vagi-
        nalis propriae testis
    l. visceralis tunicae vagi-
        nalis testis

laminar

Lancereaux nephritis

Landzert fossa

Lane
    L. bands
    L. disease
    L. operation

Langerhans
    L. cells
    islet cell of L.

Langhans cell

Lanz point

lapactic

laparocele

laparocholecystotomy

laparocolectomy

laparocolostomy

laparocolotomy

laparocystectomy

laparocystotomy

laparoenterostomy

laparoenterotomy

laparogastroscopy

laparogastrostomy

laparogastrotomy

laparohepatotomy

laparoileotomy

laparonephrectomy

laparorrhaphy

laparoscope
    50-degree Foroblique op-
        tic l.
    Jacobs-Palmer l.

laparoscopic
    l. biopsy
    l. cholecystectomy
    l. clip application
    l. colectomy
    l. vagotomy
    l. varix ligation

laparoscopist

laparoscopy
    l.-assisted hemicolectomy
    l. cannula
    flexible l.
    gasless l.
    l.-guided subhepatic chole-
        cystectomy
    Hasson open l. cannula
    laser l.
    therapeutic l.

laparotome

laparotomy
    emergency l.
    exploratory l.
    l. pad cover
    second-look l.
    staging l.

laparotyphlotomy

Lapwall laparotomy sponge

lardaceous kidney

large
l. bowel
l. bowel carcinoma
l. bowel obstruction
l.-diameter bougie
l.-droplet fatty liver
l. intestine
l.-particle biopsy
l. red kidney
l. regenerative nodule
l.-volume paracentesis

large-bore
l.-b. biliary endoprosthesis
l.-b. cannula
l.-b. catheter
l.-b. gastric lavage tube
l.-b. rigid esophagoscope

LaRoque herniorrhaphy incision

Larry rectal probe

larval nephrosis

laryngeal
l. carcinoma
l. edema

laryngopharyngectomy

laryngoscope

laryngoscopy
direct l.

laryngospasm

larynx

laser
l. ablation
argon l.
carbon dioxide l.
l. hemorrhoidectomy
l. hemorrhoid excision
holmium:YAG l.
krypton l.
KTP l.
l. laparoscopy
neodymium:yttrium-aluminum-garnet (Nd:YAG) l.

late
l. dumping syndrome

late *(continued)*
l. graft dysfunction
l.-onset hepatic failure

latent
l. jaundice

lateral
l. crus of superficial inguinal ring
l. decubitus position
l. gutter
l. internal pelvic reservoir
l. ligament of colon
l. ligaments of liver
l. lithotomy
l. lobes of prostate gland
l. margin of kidney
l. oblique fascia
l. pancreaticojejunostomy
l. reflection of colon
l. sacral arteries
l. sacral veins
l. segmental artery of liver
l. ventral hernia
l. window technique

lateral-lateral pouch

latex allergy

latissimus dorsi muscle

lattice
l. formation

Laubry-Soulle syndrome

Laugier hernia

Lauren gastric carcinoma classification

lavage
abdominal l.
colonic l.
Easi-Lav l.
external biliary l.
gastric l.
gastrointestinal l.
HeatProbe l.
iced saline l.
internal biliary l.
isosmotic l.
nasogastric l.

lavage *(continued)*
 oral l.
 PEG l.
 peritoneal l.
 rapid colonic l.
 l. solution
 stomach l.
 l. and suction

law
 Courvoisier l.

Laws gastroplasty

laxation

laxative
 l. abuse
 anthracene-type l.
 bulk l.
 bulk-forming l.
 contact l.
 lubricant l.
 osmotic l.
 saline l.
 stimulant l.

LaxCaps
 Phillips L.

layer
 Bernard glandular l.
 circular l. of muscular coat of colon
 circular l. of muscular coat of rectum
 circular l. of muscular coat of small intestine
 circular l. of muscular coat of stomach
 deep l. of triangular ligament
 fascial l.
 hypoechoic ringed l.
 inferior l. of pelvic diaphragm
 longitudinal l. of muscular coat of colon
 longitudinal l. of muscular coat of rectum
 longitudinal l. of muscular coat of small intestine

layer *(continued)*
 longitudinal l. of muscular coat of stomach
 parietal l. of pelvic fascia
 parietal l. of tunica vaginalis of testis
 submucous l. of bladder
 submucous l. of colon
 submucous l. of esophagus
 submucous l. of small intestine
 submucous l. of stomach
 submucous l. of urinary bladder
 subserous l. of gallbladder
 subserous l. of liver
 subserous l. of peritoneum
 subserous l. of small intestine
 subserous l. of stomach
 subserous l. of urinary bladder
 superficial l. of fascia of perineum
 superficial l. of triangular ligament
 superior l. of pelvic diaphragm
 visceral l. of pelvic fascia
 visceral l. of tunica vaginalis of testis
 Zeissel l.

LDH
 lactate dehydrogenase

LDL
 low-density lipoprotein

LDL-C
 low-density lipoprotein cholesterol

LDS stapler

lead
 chronic l. poisoning
 l. citrate
 l. colic
 l.-pipe colon

leaflike villus

leakage
  anastomotic l.
  bile l.
  biliary l.
  cystic duct l.
  intra-abdominal bile l.
  postoperative biliary l.

leak pressure

leather bottle stomach

leaves of mesentery

Le Bag pouch reservoir

Lecat gulf

LeDuc
  L. implantation
  L. technique
  L.-Camey ileocolostomy
  L.-Camey ileocystoplasty

Le Fort sound

left
  l. colectomy
  l. colic artery
  l. colic vein
  l. colon
  l. colonic flexure
  l. epiploic vein
  l. flexure of colon
  l. gastric artery
  l. gastric vein
  l. gastroepiploic artery
  l. gastroepiploic vein
  l. gastro-omental artery
  l. gastro-omental vein
  l. gastropancreatic fold
  l. gutter
  l. hemicolectomy
  l. hepatic duct
  l. hepatic vein
  l. inferior gastric artery
  l. lateral decubitus position
  l. lobe of liver
  l. lower quadrant
  l. mesocolon
  l. pancreaticogastric fold
  l. suprarenal vein

left *(continued)*
  l.-to-right subtotal pancrea-
    tectomy
  l. triangular ligament of
    liver
  l. trisegmentectomy
  l. upper quadrant

left-sided
  l.-s. appendicitis
  l.-s. clonus
  l.-s. colitis

leiomyoblastoma

leiomyoma
  bizarre l.
  epithelioid l.

leiomyosarcoma
  gastric l.
  hepatic l.
  renal l.

Leishmania
  L. donovani
  L. esophagitis

leishmanial enteritis

leishmaniasis

leishmaniosis

Lembert suture

Lempert paracentesis knife

Lennhoff sign

lens
  Foroblique l.

lenticular glands of stomach

leptospiral jaundice

leptospirosis

lesion
  acetowhite l.
  acute gastric mucosal l.
  anal l.
  angiodysplastic l.
  aphthous-type l.
  apple-core l.

lesion *(continued)*
    Armanni-Ebstein l.
    Baehr-Löhlein l.
    bilobed polypoid l.
    bleeding l.
    bull's eye l.
    cauda equina l.
    colonic l.
    colonic vascular l.
    cutaneous l.
    Dieulafoy l.
    Ebstein l.
    ectatic vascular l.
    extramural l.
    fingertip l.
    flat depressed l.
    flat elevated l.
    florid duct l.
    gastric l.
    gastrointestinal l.
    gunpowder l.
    hamartomatous l.
    hepatic mass l.
    hypoechoic l.
    l. identification
    intramural l.
    Kimmelstiel-Wilson l.
    localized l.
    Löhlein-Baehr l.
    macroscopic l.
    Mallory-Weiss l.
    mesenteric vascular l.
    metastatic l.
    minute l.
    minute polypoid l.
    mulberry l.
    nodular l.
    nonerosive gastric mucos-
      al l.
    nonneoplastic l.
    onionskin l.
    pancreatic l.
    papillary l.
    plaquelike l.
    polypoid l.
    precancerous l.
    preoperative l.
    satellite l.
    semipedunculated l.

lesion *(continued)*
    sessile l.
    short-segment l.
    skip l.
    space-occupying l.
    stenotic l.
    stress l.
    subglottic l.
    submucosal l.
    synchronous l.
    target l.
    traumatic l.
    tubulovillous l.
    vascular l.
    vasculitic l.

lesser
    l. gastric curvature
    l. curvature of stomach
    l. curvature ulcer
    l. epiploon
    l. omentum
    l. pancreas
    l. peritoneal cavity
    l. peritoneal sac
    l. sac of peritoneal cavity

Lesshaft
    L. space
    L. triangle
    triangle of Grynfeltt and L.

Lester Martin modification of
    Duhamel operation

leukemia
    acute myelomonocytic l.
    chylous l.
    hairy l.
    l. inhibitory factor

leukocyte
    l. cast
    fecal l.

leukopenia
    acute l.

leukoplakia
    hairy l.
    oral l.

leukotactic factor

leukourobilin

leuprolide acetate

levator
  l. ani
  l. ani muscle
  l. hernia
  l. muscle of prostate
  l. span
  l. syndrome

LeVeen
  L. ascites shunt
  L. peritoneal shunt
  L. valve

level
  air/fluid l.
  glucose l.

Levin tube

Leyden disease

Leydig
  L. cells
  L. cell adenoma
  L. cell secretory function
  L. cell tumor
  interstitial cells of L.

LFT
  liver function test

Lich technique

lichen
  l. sclerosus
  l. sclerosus et atrophicus

Lichtenstein
  L. hernial repair
  L. herniorrhaphy
  L. repair

Liddle syndrome

lidocaine
  l. topical anesthetic
  viscous l.

Lieberkühn
  L. ampulla

Lieberkühn *(continued)*
  crypts of L.
  L. follicles
  glands of L.

Liebermeister
  L. furrows
  L. grooves

lienopancreatic

lienophrenic
  l. ligament

lienorenal
  l. ligament

lienteric
  l. diarrhea
  l. stool

lientery

Lieutaud
  L. body
  L. triangle
  L. uvula

life
  quality of l.

Lifecath peritoneal implant

lifelong obesity

lift-and-cut biopsy

Ligaclip

ligament
  anterior l. of colon
  anterior inguinal l.
  anterior true l. of bladder
  Arantius l.
  basal pelviprostatic l.
  broad l. of liver
  Camper l.
  Carcassone l.
  cholecystoduodenal l.
  Cloquet l.
  l's of colon
  coronary l. of liver
  costocolic l.
  cysticoduodenal l.
  duodenohepatic l.

ligament *(continued)*
- duodenorenal l.
- external l.
- falciform l. of liver
- fundiform l. of penis
- gastrocolic l.
- gastrohepatic l.
- gastrolienal l.
- gastropancreatic l.
- gastropancreatic l's of Huschke
- gastrophrenic l.
- gastrosplenic l.
- Gillette suspensory l.
- l's of Helvetius
- Hensing l.
- hepatic l's
- hepatocolic l.
- hepatocystocolic l.
- hepatoduodenal l.
- hepatogastric l.
- hepatogastroduodenal l.
- hepatorenal l.
- hepatoumbilical l.
- Hesselbach l.
- Huschke l.
- inferior l. of epididymis
- inguinal l.
- inguinal l. of Blumberg
- interfoveolar l.
- internal inguinal l.
- interosseous l. of pubis (of Winslow)
- interureteral l.
- ischioprostatic l.
- Krause l.
- lateral l. of colon
- lateral l's of liver
- left triangular l. of liver
- lienophrenic l.
- lienorenal l.
- mesocolic l. of colon
- pelviprostatic capsular l.
- perineal l. of Carcassone
- phrenicocolic l.
- phrenicolienal l.
- phrenicosplenic l.
- phrenocolic l.

ligament *(continued)*
- posterior inguinal l.
- Poupart l.
- preurethral l. of Waldeyer
- puboischiadic l. of prostate gland
- puboprostatic l.
- puborectal l.
- pubovesical l.
- right triangular l. of liver
- splenocolic l.
- splenogastric l.
- splenophrenic l.
- splenorenal l.
- superior l. of epididymis
- suspensory l. of bladder
- suspensory l. of liver
- suspensory l. of penis
- suspensory l. of spleen
- transverse pelvic l.
- transverse l. of pelvis
- transverse perineal l.
- l. of Treitz
- triangular l. of Colles
- triangular l. of urethra
- Tuffier inferior l.
- venous l. of liver
- vesicopubic l.

ligamenta *(plural of* ligamentum)

ligamentum *pl.* ligamenta
- l. coronarium hepatis
- l. duodenorenale
- l. epididymidis inferius
- l. epididymidis superius
- l. falciforme hepatis
- l. fundiforme penis
- l. gastrocolicum
- l. gastrolienale
- l. gastrophrenicum
- l. gastrosplenicum
- ligamenta hepatis
- l. hepatocolicum
- l. hepatoduodenale
- l. hepatogastricum
- l. hepatorenale
- l. interfoveolare

ligamentum *(continued)*
    l. interfoveolare Hesselbachi
    l. lienorenale
    l. phrenicocolicum
    l. phrenicolienale
    l. phrenicosplenicum
    l. puboprostaticum
    l. pubovesicale
    l. pubovesicale laterale
    l. pubovesicale medium
    ligamenta pylori
    l. splenorenale
    l. suspensorium penis
    l. teres hepatis
    l. transversum pelvis
    l. transversum perinei
    l. triangulare dextrum hepatis
    l. triangulare sinistrum hepatis
    l. venosum
    l. venosum Arantii

ligand-gated channel

ligated
    doubly l.
    suture l.

ligation
    band l.
    Barron l.
    bidirectional l.
    bile duct l.
    elastic band l.
    endoscopic band l.
    endoscopic variceal l.
    l. of hemorrhoids
    hepatic artery l.
    high l.
    laparoscopic varix l.
    open retroperitoneal high l.
    rubber band l.
    stump l.
    transesophageal l. of varix
    transgastric l.
    tubal l.
    variceal band l.
    varix l.

ligator
    Barron rubber band l.

ligature
    elastic l.
    interlocking l.
    pursestring l.
    l. sign
    Surgiwip suture l.
    suture l.

light chain nephropathy

Lightwood syndrome

Lignac
    L. syndrome
    L.-Fanconi syndrome

Lillie intestinal forceps

limb
    afferent l.
    ascending l.
    blind l.
    l. deformity
    descending l.
    efferent l.
    jejunal l.
    Roux l.
    Roux-en-Y jejunal l.
    thick ascending l.
    thin ascending l.

limiting isorrheic concentration

limy bile

line
    anocutaneous l.
    anorectal l.
    anterior axillary l.
    Brödel white l.
    colonic mucosal l.
    Conradi l.
    dentate l.
    Hilton white l.
    incision l.
    mesenteric l.
    middle l. of scrotum
    pararectal l.
    pectinate l.

line *(continued)*
 transverse umbilical l.
 white l. of pelvis

linea *pl.* lineae
 l. alba
 l. alba abdominis
 l. anocutanea
 l. anorectalis

lineage
 hematopoietic l.

linear erosion

linguiform lobe

linitis
 l. plastica

Linton shunt

lip
 inferior l. of ileocecal valve
 superior l. of ileocecal
  valve

liparocele

lipase
 hepatic l.
 pancreatic l.
 l. test

lipectomy
 suction l.

lipid
 biliary l.
 l.-laden clear cell
 l.-laden hepatocyte
 l.-lowering drug
 l. nephrosis
 l.-to-protein ratio

lipocele

lipodystrophia
 l. intestinalis

lipodystrophy
 intestinal l.

lipoid
 l. nephrosis

lipoma
 colonic l.
 gastric l.

lipomalike tissue

lipomatosis
 renal l.
 l. renis

lipomatous
 l. tissue

liponephrosis

lipophagia
 l. granulomatosis

lipophagic
 l. intestinal granulomatosis

lipoprotein
 high-density l. (HDL)
 high-density l. cholesterol
  (HDL-C)
 intermediate-density l.
  (IDL)
 low-density l. (LDL)

liquefactive necrosis

liquid
 l. diarrhea
 l. food dysphagia
 l. stool

liquor *pl.* liquors, liquores
 l. entericus
 l. gastricus
 l. pancreaticus
 l. prostaticus
 l. seminis

lithagogue

lithectasy

lithectomy

lithiasis
 appendicular l.
 pancreatic l.
 uric acid l.

lithiasis *(continued)*
    urinary l.

lithocholate

lithocholic acid

lithocholylglycine

lithocholyltaurine

lithoclast

lithocystotomy

lithodialysis

lithogenesis

lithogenic
    l. bile

lithogenous

litholapaxy

lithology

litholysis
    chemical l.

litholytic

lithometer

lithonephritis

lithoscope

lithotome

lithotomist

lithotomy
    bilateral l.
    l. forceps
    high l.
    lateral l.
    median l.
    mediolateral l.
    perineal l.
    prerectal l.
    rectal l.
    rectovesical l.
    suprapubic l.
    vaginal l.
    vesicovaginal l.

lithotony

lithotresis

lithotripsy
    biliary l.
    blind l.
    external shock wave l.

lithotripter

lithotriptic

lithotriptor

lithotriptoscope

lithotriptoscopy

lithotrite

lithotrity

lithuresis

littoral cell

Littre
    crypts of L.
    L. glands
    glandular foramina of L.
    L. hernia

littritis

Livaditis circular myotomy

liver
    l. abscess
    l. acinus
    acute fatty l.
    acute fatty l. of pregnancy
      (AFLP)
    albuminoid l.
    alcoholic fatty l.
    amyloid l.
    autologous l. cell
    ballotable l.
    l. bed
    biliary cirrhotic l.
    l. biopsy
    l. breath
    brimstone l.
    l. cancer
    capsular cirrhosis of l.

liver *(continued)*
   l. capsule
   caudate lobe of l.
   l. cells
   l. cell adenoma
   centrilobular region of l.
   Child classification of l. disease
   Child l. criterion
   l. cirrhosis
   cirrhosis of l.
   cirrhotic l.
   cholestatic l. disease
   chronic active l. disease
   chronic cholestatic l. disease
   chronic l. disease
   cut surface of l.
   l. cyst infection
   l. death
   degraded l.
   diaphragmatic surface of l.
   l.-directed autoreactivity
   l. disease
   dome of l.
   l. dullness
   l. eater
   echogenic l.
   l. edge
   l. engorgement
   l. enzyme
   l. failure
   fatty l.
   fatty infiltration of l.
   fatty l. disease
   fatty l. of pregnancy
   finely fatty foamy l.
   l. flap
   floating l.
   l. fluke
   foamy l.
   focal fatty infiltration of l.
   focal nonfatty infiltration of l.
   frosted l.
   l. function profile
   l. function test
   l. hilus
   hobnail l.

liver *(continued)*
   icing l.
   infantile l.
   iron l.
   l.-kidney microsomal antibody
   l., kidneys, spleen
   l.-kidney syndrome
   large-droplet fatty l.
   lobular architecture of l.
   l. lymphoma
   macrovesicular fatty l.
   l. membrane antigen
   modified l. diet
   nodular l.
   l. nodule
   noncirrhotic l.
   nonparasitic cyst of l.
   nutmeg l.
   l. parenchyma
   phlegmonous alcoholic fatty l.
   pigmented l.
   polycystic l.
   polycystic disease of l.
   polylobar l.
   potato l.
   quadrate lobe of l.
   l. resection
   l. rot
   sago l.
   segmentectomy of l.
   shock l.
   shrunken l.
   small-droplet fatty l.
   l. span
   shock l.
   l.-specific antigen
   l./spleen scan
   l. stasis
   subacute fatty l. of pregnancy
   sugar-icing l.
   tender l.
   l. transplant
   l. transplantation
   l. trauma
   undersurface of l.
   l. volume

liver *(continued)*
    wandering l.
    waxy l.
    yellow atrophy of l.

living
    l. donor transplant
    l. nonrelated donor
    l. nonrelated donor trans-
       plantation
    l. related donor
    l. related donor transplan-
       tation
    l. unrelated donor
    l. unrelated donor trans-
       plantation

Livingston triangle

livor mortis

Lloyd
    L. sign
    L.-Davis sigmoidoscope

lobar

lobate

lobation
    renal l.

lobe
    appendicular l.
    caudate l.
    caudate l. of liver
    hepatic l's
    insular l.
    "kissing" prostatic l's
    lateral l's of prostate gland
    left l. of liver
    linguiform l.
    median l. of prostate
    l's of prostate
    quadrate l. of liver
    renal l's
    Riedel l.
    right l. of liver
    spigelian l.

lobectomy
    hepatic l.

lobular
    l. architecture of liver
    l. glomerulonephritis
    l. hepatitis

lobulated
    l. mass

lobulation
    portal l.

lobule
    cortical l's of kidney
    l's of epididymis
    hepatic l's
    l's of liver
    l. of pancreas
    portal l.
    l's of testis

lobulonodular
    l. glomerulonephritis

lobulose

lobulous

lobulus *pl.* lobuli
    lobuli corticales renis
    lobuli epididymidis
    lobuli hepatis
    lobuli testis

lobus *pl.* lobi
    l. caudatus hepatis
    l. caudatus [Spigeli]
    l. hepatis dexter
    l. hepatis sinister
    l. medius prostatae
    lobi prostatae dexter et sin-
       ister
    l. quadratus hepatis
    lobi renales
    l. spigelii

local
    l. anesthesia
    l. scarring

localization
    bleeding site l.
    pancreatic tumor l.

localized
  l. fungus
  l. lesion
  l. pain
  l. peritonitis

localizing tenderness

lock-stitch suture

Lockwood-Allis intestinal forceps

Löhlein-Baehr lesion

loin pain

Lomotil

Lonalac
  L. feeding
  L. formula

long-incubation hepatitis

long intestinal tube

longitudinal
  l. bands of colon
  l. choledochotomy
  l. enterotomy
  l. esophageal stricture
  l. fasciculi of colon
  l. fissure
  l. fold of duodenum
  l. image
  l. laceration
  l. layer of muscular coat of colon
  l. layer of muscular coat of rectum
  l. layer of muscular coat of small intestine
  l. layer of muscular coat of stomach
  l. myotomy
  l. pancreaticojejunostomy
  l. plane
  l. view

loop
  afferent l.
  air-filled l.

loop *(continued)*
  blind l.
  bowel l.
  l. choledochojejunostomy
  closed afferent l.
  closed efferent l.
  colonic l.
  contiguous l.
  dilated l's of bowel
  l. diuretic
  duodenal l.
  duodenal C-l.
  efferent l.
  l. esophagojejunostomy
  l. forearm graft
  gamma transverse colon l.
  l. gastrojejunostomy
  Henle l.
  l. of Henle
  ileal l.
  l. ileostomy
  intestinal l.
  jejunal l.
  l. jejunostomy
  ostomy l.
  l. ostomy bridge
  l's of redundant colon
  Roux-en-Y l.
  sentinel l.
  l. stoma
  l. suture
  transverse l.
  l. transverse colostomy

loopogram

loose stool

Lopez enteral valve

LoPresti
  L. endoscope
  L. fiberoptic esophagoscope

Lord hemorrhoidectomy

lordosis

Losec

Loughnane hook

l.-density lipoprotein (LDL)
l.-density lipoprotein cholesterol (LDL-C)
l.-grade dysplasia
l.-grade fever
l. intermittent suction
l.-pitched bowel sounds
l. residue feeding
l. small bowel obstruction
l.-transverse incision

lower
l. abdominal transverse incision
l. esophageal sphincter
l. esophageal sphincter pressure
l. esophageal sphincter tone
l. gastrointestinal hemorrhage
l. GI (gastrointestinal) bleeding
l. GI tract foreign body
l. nephron nephrosis

Lowsley operation

Lubarsch crystals

lubricant
l. cathartic
l. laxative

Ludwig
L. labyrinths
L. plane

lumbar
l. appendicitis
l. arteries
ascending l. vein
l. hernia
l. kidney
l. nephrectomy
l. nephrotomy
l. veins

lumboabdominal

lumbocolostomy

lumbocolotomy

lumbocrural

lumboinguinal

lumbosacral fascia

lumen *pl.* lumina, lumens
bile duct l.
duodenal l.
esophageal l.
gastroduodenal l.
intestinal l.

luminal
l. acid
l. narrowing

luminalis

lump kidney

Lundh test

lung
farmer's l.

lupoid hepatitis

lupus
l. glomerulonephritis
l. nephritis

Luschka
L. crypts
L. ducts
L. fossa

Lütkens sphincter

lymph
l. channel
l. node
l. node metastasis

lymphadenectomy
inguinal lymphadenopathy
retroperitoneal l.

lymphadenitis
mesenteric l.

lymphangiectasia
intestinal l.
pancreatic l.

lymphatic
  aggregated l. follicles of
    Peyer

lymphenteritis

lymph node
  l. n. adenopathy
  celiac l. n.

lymphocytic
  l. colitis
  l. gastritis

lymphoid
  l. cholangitis

lymphoid *(continued)*
  l. nodule
  l. polyps

lymphoma
  Burkitt l.
  colorectal l.
  duodenal l.
  gastric l.
  liver l.

lymphomatous nodule

lysis of adhesions

lytic cocktail

Macalister
  valve of M.

McBurney
  M. incision
  M. operation
  M. point
  M. retractor
  M. sign

MacConkey agar

Macdonald test

Macewen
  M. hernia operation
  M. herniorrhaphy
  M. operation

McGill operation

McGivney hemorrhoid forceps

Machida choledochoscope

machine
  Accuson-128 color flow
    Doppler m.
  Belzer m.
  heart-lung m.

Mackenzie point

McLean pile clamp

MacLean-de Wesselow test

McNeer classification

McNemar ascites test

macrocolon

macrocyst
  adrenocortical m.

macronodular
  m. cirrhosis

macro-orchidism

macrophage
  bile-laden m.
  m. migration inhibitory factor

macrophallus

macroregenerative nodule

macroscopic
  m. hematuria
  m. lesion
  m. liver cyst

macrosigmoid

macrovesicular fatty liver

macula *pl.* maculae
  maculae albidae
  m. densa
  maculae lacteae
  maculae tendineae

McVay
  M. herniorrhaphy
  M. operation
  M. repair

Madden incisional herniorrhaphy

magenstrasse

Magnacal liquid feeding

magnesia
  citrate of m.
  milk of m. (MOM)
  Phillips Milk of M.

magnesium
  m. citrate oral solution

magnetic resonance
  m. r. angiography
  m. r. imaging (MRI)

magnification
  high m.
  high-m. colonoscopy
  high-m. endoscopy
  high-m. gastroscopy

magnifying
  m. endoscope

MAGPI procedure
  meatal advancement and
    glanuloplasty

Maisonneuve urethrotome

major
    m. caruncle of Santorini
    m. duodenal papilla
    m. renal calices

majus
    omentum m.

malabsorption
    bile acid m.
    m. disease
    folate m.
    iatrogenic m.
    lactose m.
    vitamin B_{12} m.

malabsorptive
    m. diarrhea

malacoplakia
    renal m.
    m. vesicae

Malakit *Helicobacter pylori*
Biolab

malaria
    bilious remittent m.
    dysenteric algid m.
    falciparum m.
    gastric m.
    malignant tertian m.
    pernicious m.

malarial
    m. cirrhosis
    m. dysentery
    m. hepatitis

Malassez disease

malassimilation

maldigestion

maldigestive
    m. diarrhea

male
    m. escutcheon
    m. feminization
    m. genital organs

male *(continued)*
    m. reproductive organs

Malecot
    M. catheter
    M. gastrostomy tube
    M. nephrostomy tube
    M. reentry catheter

malemission

malformation
    anorectal m.
    arteriovenous m.
    Chiari m.
    cloacal m.
    Dieulafoy vascular m.
    gastric arteriovenous m.
    vascular m.

malignancy
    de novo m.
    esophageal m.
    hepatic m.
    hepatobiliary m.
    pancreaticobiliary m.
    peritoneal m.

malignant
    m. arteriolar nephrosclero-
      sis
    m. ascites
    m. biliary obstruction
    m. cachexia
    m. dysentery
    m. dysplasia
    m. glomerulonephritis
    m. hepatoma
    m. jaundice
    m. malnutrition
    m. melanoma
    m. mesenchymal tumor
    m. nephrosclerosis
    m. obstructive jaundice
    m. pheochromocytoma
    m. polyp
    m. potential
    m. seeding
    m. stenosis
    m. stricture

malignant *(continued)*
    m. teratoma
    m. tertian malaria
    m. ulcer

malleable blade

Mallory
    M. bodies
    M. hyaline body
    M.-Weiss lesion
    M.-Weiss mucosal rupture
    M.-Weiss syndrome
    M.-Weiss tear

malnutrition
    malignant m.
    protein-calorie m.

malnutrition-related diabetes
    mellitus

malodorous stool

Malpighi
    pyramids of M.

malpighian
    m. bodies of kidney
    m. capsule
    m. corpuscles of kidney
    m. glomeruli

malrotation of intestine

MALT
    mucosa-associated lym-
      phoid tissue
        MALT lymphoma

management
    mechanical endoscopic m.

maneuver
    Duecollement m.
    Fowler-Stephens m.
    Heimlich m.
    Hueter m.
    Kocher m.
    peroral m.
    Valsalva m.

manifestation
    gastrointestinal m's
    hepatobiliary m.
    otolaryngologic m.

manipulation
    pancreatic duct m.

mannitol

manometer

manometric finding

manometry
    anal m.
    anorectal m.
    biliary m.
    endoscopic m.
    ERCP m.
    esophageal m.
    rectosigmoid m.
    sphincter of Oddi m.

Manson schistosomiasis

mapping
    anal m.

margin
    anterior m. of testis
    cell-positive m.
    convex m. of testis
    dentate m.
    external m. of testis
    internal m. of testis
    lateral m. of kidney
    medial m. of kidney
    posterior m. of testis
    straight m. of testis
    superior m. of pancreas

margo *pl.* margines
    m. anterior corporis pan-
      creatis
    m. anterior hepatis
    m. anterior testis
    m. inferior corporis pan-
      creatis
    m. inferior hepatis
    m. lateralis renis
    m. medialis renis
    m. posterior corporis pan-
      creatis
    m. posterior testis
    m. superior corporis pan-
      creatis

Marion disease

marker
    fecal m.
    Sitz M.

marking
    haustral m.

Marlex
    M. band
    M. graft
    M. hernial repair
    M. mesh
    M. mesh abdominal recto-
        pexy
    M. plug technique

maroon-colored stool

marrow transplant recipient

Marseille pancreatitis classifica-
    tion

Marshall-Marchetti-Krantz oper-
    ation

marshmallow
    barium-impregnated m.
    m. bolus

marsupia (*plural of* marsupium)

marsupialization

marsupium *pl.* marsupia

Martel clamp

Martin
    M. anoplasty
    M. speculum
    M. and Davy speculum

Mason vertical banded gastro-
    plasty

mass
    abdominal m.
    abdominal wall m.
    adnexal m.
    appendiceal m.
    appendix m.
    asymptomatic m.

mass *(continued)*
    colonic m.
    cul-de-sac m.
    discrete m.
    duodenal m.
    esophageal m.
    exophytic m.
    expansile abdominal m.
    extramucosal m.
    extrinsic m.
    flank m.
    fluctuant m.
    gastric m.
    hilar m.
    intra-abdominal m.
    lobulated m.
    mediastinal m.
    mushroom-shaped m.
    palpable m.
    parovarian m.
    periampullary m.
    perirectal m.
    m. peristalsis
    phlegmonous m.
    pleural m.
    polypoid m.
    pulsatile m.
    rectal m.
    salivary m.
    scrotal m.
    soft tissue m.
    submucosal m.

massa *pl.* massae
    m. innominata

massive hepatic necrosis

mast cell

Masters
    M. intestinal clamp
    M.-Schwartz liver clamp

material
    anastomotic m.
    coffee-ground m.
    extravasated contrast m.
    fecal m.
    proteinaceous cast m.
    purulent m.
    suture m.

Mathews speculum

matrix calculus

matted node

maturing of stoma

maximal tubular excretory capacity

maximum *pl.* maxima
    transport m. for glucose
    tubular m.
    m. urinary concentration

Maydl operation

Mayo
    M. abdominal clamp
    M. abdominal retractor
    M. common duct probe
    M. common duct scoop
    M. common duct spoon
    M. gallstone scoop
    M. needle
    M. operation
    M. scissors
    M.-Adams appendectomy
        retractor
    M.-Blake gallstone forceps
    M.-Robson clamp
    M.-Robson intestinal clamp
    M.-Robson intestinal forceps
    M.-Robson position

MCH
    mean corpuscular hemoglobin

meal
    barium m.
    Ewald test m.
    retention m.
    fatty m.
    opaque m.
    test m.

mean
    m. arterial pressure
    m. colonic transit
    m. corpuscular hemoglobin
        (MCH)

mean *(continued)*
    m. venous outflow

measles
    German m.

measurement
    anorectal m.
    anthropometric m.
    Doppler ultrasound intestinal blood flow m.
    intestinal permeability m.
    planimetric m.
    plasma bile acid m.
    pressure m.
    RigiScan m.
    serum bile acid m.

meat impaction

meatome

meatometer

meatoplasty

meatorrhaphy

meatoscope

meatoscopy

meatotome

meatotomy

meatus *pl.* meatus
    fish-mouth m.
    m. urinarius

mechanical
    m. assist system
    m. biliary obstruction
    m. cystitis
    m. diarrhea
    m. duct obstruction
    m. endoscopic management
    m. extrahepatic obstruction
    m. ileus
    m. intestinal obstruction
    m. jaundice
    m. small-bowel obstruction
    m. ventilation

mechanism
    antireflux flap-valve m.
    cell-mediated m.
    countercurrent m.
    deglutition m.
    flap-valve m.
    Mitrofanoff m.
    sphincteric m.
    swallowing m.

Meckel
    M. diverticulitis
    M. diverticulum
    M. ileitis

meconium
    m. ileus
    m. peritonitis
    m. plug

medial
    m. crus of superficial inguinal ring
    m. margin of kidney
    m. segmental artery of liver

median
    m. bar
    m. incision
    m. lithotomy
    m. lobe of prostate
    m. plane
    m. raphe of perineum
    m. sacral artery

mediastinal
    anterior m. arteries
    anterior m. cavity
    m. histoplasmosis
    m. mass
    middle m. cavity
    posterior m. arteries
    posterior m. cavity
    m. shift
    superior m. cavity
    m. thickening
    m. veins

mediastinoscope

mediastinoscopic

mediastinoscopy

mediastinotomy

mediastinum *pl.* mediastina
    m. testis

medical vagotomy

medically-induced achlorhydria

medication
    m. allergy
    m. bezoar

Medicon-Jackson rectal forceps

mediolateral lithotomy

medionodular cirrhosis

medorrhea

medroxyprogesterone acetate

medulla *pl.* medullae
    inner m. of kidney
    m. of kidney
    m. nephrica
    outer m. of kidney
    renal m.
    m. renalis
    m. renis

medullary
    m. collecting duct
    m. collecting tubule
    m. cystic disease
    m. cystic kidney disease
    m. rays
    m. sponge kidney
    m. substance of kidney

megabladder

megacalycosis

megacecum

megacholedochus

megacolon
    acquired m.
    acquired functional m.
    acute m.
    aganglionic m.
    congenital m.
    m. congenitum

megacolon *(continued)*
    idiopathic m.
    toxic m.

megacystis
    m.-megaureter syndrome
    m.-microcolon–intestinal
        hypoperistalsis syndrome
        (MMIHS)

megaduodenum

megaesophagus
    chagasic m.

megaloblastic anemia

megalocystis

megaloesophagus

megalogastria

megalohepatia

megalopenis

megaloureter
    congenital m.
    primary m.
    reflux m.

megarectum

megasigmoid

megaureter

megestrol acetate

MEGX test

melanemesis

melanoma
    malignant m.

melanosis
    m. coli

melanotic

melanuresis

melanuria

melanuric

melena
    m. vera

melenic
    m. stool

Meltzer sign

membrana *pl.* membranae
    m. abdominis
    m. mucosa vesicae felleae
    m. perinei

membranaceous

membrane
    abdominal m.
    antral m.
    glomerular m.
    hemodialyzer m.
    high efficiency m.
    high flux m.
    Jackson m.
    mucous m.
    mucous m. of esophagus
    mucous m. of gallbladder
    mucous m. of large intes-
        tine
    mucous m. of rectum
    mucous m. of small intes-
        tine
    mucous m. of stomach
    mucous m. of ureter
    mucous m. of urinary blad-
        der
    pericolic m.
    perineal m.
    pyloric m.
    slit m.
    submucous m. of stomach
    Toldt m.

membranectomy

membranoproliferative glomer-
    ulonephritis

membranous
    m. glomerulonephritis
    m. nephropathy
    m. part of male urethra
    m. pericolitis
    m. urethra

Ménétrier disease

Menghini needle

Mercier
  M. bar
  M. valve

Meritene liquid feeding

Mersilene mesh

mesalamine
  m. enema

mesangial
  m. angle
  m. cells
  m. proliferative glomerulo-
    nephritis
  m. volume fraction

mesangiocapillary
  m. glomerulonephritis

mesangiolysis

mesangium
  extraglomerular m.

mesaraic

mesenchymal
  m. change
  m. hamartoma
  m. tumor

mesenterectomy

mesenterial
  m. intestine

mesenteric
  m. adenitis
  m. apoplexy
  m. arterial embolism
  m. arterial thrombosis
  m. arteriovenous fistula
  m. cyst
  m. fistula
  m. hematoma
  m. hernia
  m. infarction
  inferior m. artery
  inferior m. vein
  m. ischemia
  m. line

mesenteric *(continued)*
  m. lymphadenitis
  superior m. artery
  superior m. artery syn-
    drome
  superior m. vein
  m. tear
  m. triangle
  m. varix
  m. vascular lesion
  m. vascular occlusion
  m. venous thrombosis
  m. window

mesentericoparietal
  m. fossa
  m. hernia

mesenteriolum
  m. appendicis vermiformis
  m. processus vermiformis

mesenteriopexy

mesenteriorrhaphy

mesenteriplication

mesenteritis
  retractile m.

mesenterium

mesenteroaxial gastric volvulus

mesenterorenal
  m. bypass

mesentery
  m. of ascending part of co-
    lon
  m. of descending part of
    colon
  leaves of m.
  m. of rectum
  m. of sigmoid colon
  small intestine m.
  m. of transverse part of co-
    lon
  m. of vermiform appendix

mesentorrhaphy

mesh
  Dacron m.

mesh *(continued)*
Dexon polyglycolic acid m.
Marlex m.
Mersilene m.
polypropylene m.
m. stent
synthetic m.

meso-appendicitis

mesoappendix

mesobilirubin

mesobilirubinogen

mesobiliviolin

mesocaval
m. anastomosis
m. shunt

mesocecal

mesocecum

mesocolic
m. band
m. hernia
m. ligament of colon
m. shelf

mesocolon
m. ascendens
m. descendens
iliac m.
left m.
pelvic m.
right m.
m. sigmoideum
m. transversum

mesocolopexy

mesocoloplication

mesocyst

mesoepididymis

mesogastric
m. fossa

mesoileum

mesojejunum

mesonephric remnant

meso-omentum

mesopexy

mesophilic bacteria

mesorchial

mesorchium

mesorectum

mesorrhaphy

mesosigmoid

mesosigmoiditis

mesosigmoidopexy

mesostenium

mesothelial metaplasia

mesothelioma
benign cystic m.
benign m. of genital tract
m. of testis
m. of tunica vaginalis

Messerklinger endoscope

metabolic
m. balance
m. calculus
chronic m. acidosis
m. cirrhosis
m. effect

metabolism
bacterial m. in intestines
drug m.
hepatic m.

metachronous adenoma

metaduodenum

metaicteric

metallic embolus

Metamucil

metanephric
m. duct
m. tubules

metaplasia
Barrett m.

metaplasia *(continued)*
    columnar m.
    gastric m.
    goblet cell m.
    intestinal m.
    mesothelial m.
    myeloid m.
    nephrogenic m.
    osseous m.
    pseudopyloric m.

metaplasia-dysplasia-carcinoma
    sequence

metaplastic polyp

metastasis *pl.* metastases
    brain m.
    colonic m.
    cutaneous m.
    diffuse m.
    duodenal m.
    extrahepatic m.
    extralymphatic m.
    implantation m.
    intramucosal m.
    lymph node m.
    neoplasm m.

metastatic
    m. adenocarcinoma
    m. cancer
    m. carcinoma
    m. cholangiocarcinoma
    m. disease
    m. dissemination
    m. implantation
    m. lesion

meteorism

methicillin
    m.-resistant *Staphylococcus
    aureus* (MRSA)

Methocel

method
    Beck m.
    Credé m.
    Parks m. of anal fistulo-
      tomy
    Siffert m.

methylcellulose

methylene blue enema

methylprednisolone acetate

methyltestosterone-induced
    cholestasis

Meyenburg complexes

Michaelis-Gutmann bodies

microalbuminuria

microanastomosis

microcalix

microcalyx

microcolon

microcystometer

microgastria

microhamartoma
    biliary m.

microhepatia

micrometastasis
    hematogenous m.

micronodular cirrhosis

micro-orchidia

micro-orchidism

micropenis

microphallus

micropuncture

microrchidia

microscope
    fluorescent m.

microscopic
    m. colitis
    m. hematuria
    m. urine examination

microscopy
    fluorescent m.

microspherolith

microtubular glomerulopathy

miction

micturate

micturition
    m. bag
    m. reflex

midabdominal
    m. abscess
    m. transverse incision
    m. wall

middle
    m. adrenal artery
    m. capsular artery
    m. colic artery
    m. colic vein
    m. hemorrhoidal artery
    m. hepatic veins
    m. line of scrotum
    m. mediastinal cavity
    m. perineal fascia
    m. rectal artery
    m. rectal veins
    m. suprarenal artery

midepigastric
    m. area

midepigastrium

midesophageal diverticulum

midesophagus

midline
    m. abdominal crease
    m. incision
    m. lower abdominal incision
    m. upper abdominal incision

midpelvic
    m. plane

midrectal
    m. area

midriff

midsagittal
    m. plane

midsigmoid
    m. colon

midstomach

migraine
    abdominal m.

migration
    calculus m.
    gallstone m.
    gastrostomy tube m.
    m. inhibitory factor
    retrograde m.

Mik
    Mikulicz

Mikulicz (Mik)
    M. clamp
    M. colostomy
    M. drain
    M. gastroscope
    M. operation
    M. pack
    M. peritoneal forceps
    M. pyloroplasty
    M. retractor

Miles
    M. abdominoperineal resection
    M. operation

miliary
    m. pyuria
    m. tuberculosis

milk
    acidophilus m.
    m. of bismuth
    m. of calcium bile
    m. of magnesia (MOM)
    Phillips M. of Magnesia
    m. protein antibody
    m.-sensitive colitis
    m. spots

milking
    m. of intestine

milky ascites

Millard mouth gag

Miller
    M.-Abbott tube

Millin-Read operation

Ming gastric carcinoma classification

minilaparoscopic cholecystectomy

minilaparotomy

minimal
    m. change disease
    m. change glomerulopathy
    m. change nephropathy
    m. change nephrotic syndrome
    m. isorrheic concentration

minor
    m. duodenal papilla
    m. pancreatic duct
    m. renal calices

minus
    omentum m.

minute
    m. lesion
    m. polypoid lesion

mitogenic factor

mitotic activity

Mitrofanoff
    M. appendicovesicostomy
    M. catheterization channel
    M. conduit
    M. mechanism
    M. principle
    M. procedure
    M. stoma
    M. technique
    M. valve

mittelschmerz

mixed
    m. cirrhosis
    m. gland
    m. hemorrhoid

mixture
    amino acid–glucose mixture

MMIHS
    megacystis-microcolon–intestinal hypoperistalsis syndrome

mobile
    cecum m.
    m. cecum
    m. gallbladder

mobilization

modeling
    urea kinetic m.

moderate distress

moderately differentiated adenoma

modification
    Lester Martin m. of Duhamel operation
    Rossetti m. of Nissen fundoplication

modified
    m. barium swallow
    m. liver diet
    m. Whitehead hemorrhoidectomy

Moersch esophagoscope

molecular genetic alteration

molecule
    adhesion m.

MOM
    milk of magnesia

monilial
    m. esophagitis
    m. infection

monitoring
    ambulatory m.
    ambulatory pH m.
    esophageal pH m.

monoacinar regenerative nodule

monobasic
m. potassium phosphate
m. sodium phosphate

monoclonal
m. gammopathy
m. immunoglobulin deposi-
tion disease

monoethylglycinexylidide
m. test

monomicrobial non-neutrocytic
bacterascites

mononuclear cell

mononucleosis
infectious m.

monopolypoid adenoma

monorchia

monorchid

monorchidic

monorchidism

monorchis

monorchism

mons *pl.* montes
m. ureteris

Montezuma's revenge

moon facies

morbidity
operative m.

morbid obesity

Morgagni
M. appendix
M. caruncle
columns of M.
crypt of M.
fossa of M.
fovea of M.
frenum of M.

Morgagni *(continued)*
M. glands
M. hernia
hydatid of M.
semilunar valves of M.
urethral lacunae of M.
M. valves

morgagnian
m. caruncle
m. cyst

morning diarrhea

mortar kidney

mosaic duodenal mucosal pattern

Moschcowitz operation

Mosher esophagoscope

Moss
M. gastrostomy tube
M. PEG kit
M. tube

mother/daughter endoscope

mother-to-infant transmission
of hepatitis C virus

motility
colonic m.
m. disorder
esophageal m.
esophageal m. disorder
gastric m.
gastric m. disorder
gastrointestinal m.
intestinal m. disorder
nonspecific esophageal m.
disorder (NEMD)
reduced m.
sequential m.

motor
m. activity
m. paralytic bladder

mound
infraumbilical m.

mouse
peritoneal m.

mouth
Ceylon sore m.
m. gag

movable kidney

movement
pendular m.
segmentation m.
tongue m.
vermicular m's

Moynihan
M. bile duct probe
M. clamp
M. gall duct forceps
M. gallstone probe
M. gallstone scoop
M. test

MRI
magnetic resonance imaging
rectal coil MRI

MRSA
methicillin-resistant *Staphylococcus aureus*

MS-1 hepatitis

MS-2 hepatitis

mucin

mucinous
m. adenocarcinoma
m. adenoma
m. cystadenoma
m. cystic neoplasm

mucin-producing
m.-p. adenocarcinoma

mucocele
m. of gallbladder

mucociliary
m. clearance

mucoclasis

mucocolitis

mucocutaneous hemorrhoid

mucoenteritis

mucoid
m. secretion
m. stool

mucolytic agent

mucomembranous enteritis

mucoprotein
Tamm-Horsfall m.

mucosa
antral m.
m.-associated lymphoid tissue (MALT)
biopsy of gastric m.
buccal m.
colorectal m.
duodenal m.
ectopic gastric m.
esophageal m.
foveolar gastric m.
friable m.
fundic m.
gastric m.
gastroduodenal m.
heterotopic gastric m.
inflamed m.
intestinal m.
multifocal ectopic gastric m.
normal-appearing m.
rectal m.
sloughing of m.

mucosal
m. abnormality
m. adenocarcinoma
m. angiography
m. biopsy
m. bridge
cecal m. nodule
colonic m. line
colonic m. pattern
m. diverticulum
m. dysplasia
m. fatty acid
m. graft
m. ileal diaphragm

mucosal *(continued)*
    m. ischemia
    m. nodularity
    m. pallor
    m. pattern
    m. polyp
    m. tear
    m. tongue
    m. ulcerative colitis
    m. web

mucosa-to-mucosa anastomosis

mucosectomy
    endoanal m.
    rectal m.

mucous
    m. cast
    m. colitis
    m. crypts of duodenum
    m. depletion
    m. diarrhea
    m. enteritis
    m. fistula
    m. folds of rectum
    m. gel thickness
    m. glands of duodenum
    m. membrane
    m. membrane of esophagus
    m. membrane of gallbladder
    m. membrane of large in-
      testine
    m. membrane of rectum
    m. membrane of small in-
      testine
    m. membrane of stomach
    m. membrane of ureter
    m. membrane of urinary
      bladder
    m. neck cells
    m. patch
    m. sinuses of male urethra
    m. stool

mucus
    excess m.
    gastric m.

mucus-secreting
    m.-s. cell
    m.-s. gland

mud
    biliary m.

Muir hemorrhoid forceps

mulberry
    m. calculus
    m. gallstone
    m. lesion
    m. stone

Müller capsule

müllerian
    m. capsule
    persistent m. duct

multiacinar regenerative nodule

multicentricity

multicystic renal dysplasia

multidrug regimen

multifocal
    m. atrophic gastritis
    m. ectopic gastric mucosa

multiforme
    erythema m.

multilobar

multilobular
    m. cirrhosis

multiorgan
    m. system failure

multiple
    m. endocrine neoplasia
    m. familial polyposis
    m. hepatitis virus infection
    m. nodule
    m. organ failure
    m. polyps
    m. recurrent renal colic
    m. sclerosis

multiseptate gallbladder

mumu

mural
    m. kidney

mural *(continued)*
    m. thrombus

Murphy
    M. button
    M. common duct dilator
    M. drip
    M. gallbladder retractor
    M. sign

muscarinic cholinergic agonist

muscle
    adductor brevis m.
    adductor longus m.
    Bell m.
    bronchoesophageal m.
    bulbocavernous m.
    circular Santorini m's
    compressor m. of urethra
    cremaster m.
    cricopharyngeal m.
    cricopharyngeus m.
    dartos m.
    dartos m. of scrotum
    detrusor m. of bladder
    detrusor urinae m.
    erector m. of penis
    external oblique m. of abdomen
    external sphincter m. of anus
    gastrointestinal smooth m.
    Gavard m.
    m. guarding
    Guthrie m.
    Houston m.
    interfoveolar m.
    internal oblique m. of abdomen
    internal sphincter m. of anus
    ischiocavernous m.
    latissimus dorsi m.
    levator ani m.
    levator m. of prostate
    obturator internus m.
    Ochsner m.
    Oddi m.
    pectineal m.

muscle *(continued)*
    m's of pelvic diaphragm
    perineal m's
    m's of perineum
    pubicoperitoneal m.
    pubococcygeal m.
    puboprostatic m.
    puborectal m.
    pubovaginal m.
    pubovesical m.
    pyloric sphincter m.
    rectococcygeal m.
    rectourethral m.
    rectouterine m.
    rectovesical m.
    rectus abdominis m.
    Riolan m.
    sphincter m. of bile duct
    sphincter m. of hepatopancreatic ampulla
    sphincter m. of membranous urethra
    sphincter m. of pylorus
    sphincter m. of urethra
    sphincter urethrae m.
    sphincter m. of urinary bladder
    m.-splitting incision
    suspensory m. of duodenum
    transversus abdominis m.
    m. of Treitz
    trigonal m.
    m's of urogenital diaphragm
    Wilson m.

muscular

muscularis
    m. mucosae

musculocutaneous

musculus *pl.* musculi
    musculi abdominis
    m. bronchooesophageus
    m. bulbocavernosus
    m. bulbospongiosus
    musculi colli
    m. compressor urethrae

musculus *(continued)*
m. cremaster
m. dartos
m. detrusor vesicae
musculi diaphragmatis pelvis
musculi diaphragmatis urogenitalis
m. ischiocavernosus
m. latissimus dorsi
m. levator ani
m. levator prostatae
m. obliquus externus abdominis
m. obliquus internus abdominis
m. pectineus
musculi perineales
musculi perinei
m. prostaticus
m. puboprostaticus
m. puborectalis
m. pubovaginalis
m. pubovesicalis
m. rectococcygeus
m. rectourethralis
m. rectovesicalis
m. rectus abdominis
m. sphincter ampullae hepatopancreaticae
m. sphincter ani externus
m. sphincter ani internus
m. sphincter ductus biliaris
m. sphincter ductus choledochi
m. sphincter pylori
m. sphincter pyloricus
m. sphincter urethrae
m. sphincter urethrae membranaceae
m. sphincter vesicae urinariae
m. suspensorius duodeni
m. transversus perinei profundus
m. transversus perinei superficialis

mushroom-shaped mass

mushy stool

musical bowel sounds

mutated colorectal carcinoma

mutation
germ cell m.

myasthenia
m. gastrica

Mycobacterium
M. infection

mycosis

mycotic
m. aneurysm

myectomy
anorectal m.

myelin
m. kidney
gastric mycosis

myeloid metaplasia

myelolipoma
adrenal m.

myeloma
m. kidney

myenteric
m. ganglion cell
m. reflex

myenteron

myiasis
intestinal m.

myocardial
m. infarction
m. ischemia

myochosis

myocutaneous flap

myoelectric activity
gastric m. a.

nabilone

Nagamatsu incision

nagging pain

naris *pl.* nares

narrow
  n. albumin gradient ascites
  n. pelvic plane

narrowing
  hourglass n.
  luminal n.

nasal
  n. cannula
  n. discharge
  n. feeding
  n. intubation

nasobiliary
  n. drain
  n. drainage
  n. tube

nasoduodenal feeding tube

nasoenteric feeding tube

nasogastric (NG)
  n. aspirate
  n. decompression
  n. drainage
  n. feeding tube
  n. intubation
  n. lavage
  n. suction
  n. tube

nasoileal tube

nasojejunal
  n. feeding
  n. tube

nasopancreatic
  n. catheter
  n. drainage

nasopharyngeal
  n. angiofibroma

nasopharyngeal *(continued)*
  n. reflux

nasotracheal intubation

native renal biopsy

natriuresis

natruresis

nausea
  epidemic n.
  n. epidemica
  postprandial n.
  n. and vomiting

nauseant

nauseate

nauseous

navicular
  n. abdomen
  n. fossa of male urethra

neck
  bladder n.
  n. of gallbladder
  n. of glans penis
  n. of pancreas
  n. of urinary bladder

necrosis *pl.* necroses
  acute sclerosing hyaline n.
  acute tubular n.
  avascular n.
  Balser fatty n.
  biliary piecemeal n.
  bowel n.
  bridging n.
  cell n.
  central n.
  coagulation n.
  colonic n.
  electrocoagulation n.
  ethanol-induced tumor n.
  fatty n.
  fibrinoid n.
  fibrosing piecemeal n.
  hepatocellular n.
  hepatocyte n.

necrosis *(continued)*
    infected n.
    intestinal n.
    ischemic n.
    liquefactive n.
    massive hepatic n.
    papillary n.
    patchy n.
    peripheral n.
    piecemeal n.
    postischemic tubular n.
    pressure n.
    n. of renal papillae
    renal papillary n.
    spinal cord n.
    sterile pancreatic n.
    strangulation n.
    subacute n.
    subacute hepatic n.
    submassive hepatic n.
    tissue n.
    tubular n.
    tumor n.

necrospermia

necrospermic

necrotic
    n. cirrhosis
    n. hemorrhagic colitis
    n. hemorrhoids
    n. tissue
    n. ulceration

necroticans
    enteritis n.

necrotizing
    n. amebic colitis
    n. amebic pancolitis
    n. arteriolitis
    n. bowel vasculitis
    n. enterocolitis
    n. fasciitis
    n. infection
    n. nephrosis
    n. pancreatitis
    n. papillitis
    n. renal papillitis
    n. vasculitis

necrozoospermia

needle
    n. biopsy
    blunt n.
    Chiba n.
    fine-n.
    flexible aspiration n.
    Mayo n.
    Menghini n.

negative
    n. laparotomy
    n. nitrogen balance

Nélaton
    N. catheter
    N. fold
    N. sphincter

nematode infection

NEMD
    nonspecific esophageal mo-
    tility disorder

neo-anal sphincter

neobladder
    Camey n.
    ileal n.
    ileocolonic n.

neodymium:yttrium-aluminum-
    garnet (Nd:YAG) laser

Neoloid

neonatal
    n. cholestasis
    n. hepatitis
    n. hyperbilirubinemia
    n. jaundice

neonatorum
    icterus n.

neoplasia
    cervical intraepithelial n.
    colonic n.
    multiple endocrine n.
    prostatic intraepithelial n.

neoplasm
  colorectal n.
  genitourinary n.
  n. metastasis
  mucinous cystic n.
  periampullary n.
  prostatic n.
  retroperitoneal n.
  n. staging
  stomach n.

neoplastic
  n. cell proliferation
  n. disease
  n. lesion
  n. polyp
  n. potential
  n. tissue
  n. transformation

neorectal emptying

neorectum

neostomy

neoterminal ileum

nephradenoma

nephralgia

nephralgic

nephrapostasis

nephrauxe

nephrectasia

nephrectasis

nephrectasy

nephrectomize

nephrectomy
  abdominal n.
  anterior n.
  lumbar n.
  paraperitoneal n.
  posterior n.
  radical n.

nephredema

nephrelcosis

nephremia

nephric
  n. colic
  n. duct

nephritic
  n. calculus

nephritides *pl.* nephritides

nephritis
  acute n.
  acute focal bacterial n.
    (AFBN)
  acute interstitial n.
  acute suppurative n.
  allergic interstitial n.
  arteriosclerotic n.
  azotemic n.
  bacterial n.
  Balkan n
  capsular n.
  n. caseosa
  caseous n.
  cheesy n.
  chloro-azotemic n.
  chronic n.
  chronic parenchymatous n.
  chronic suppurative n.
  degenerative n.
  n. dolorosa
  dropsical n.
  exudative n.
  fibrolipomatous n.
  fibrous n.
  glomerular n.
  glomerulocapsular n.
  n. gravidarum
  hemorrhagic n.
  hereditary tubulointersti-
    tial n.
  Heymann n.
  indurative n.
  interstitial n.
  Lancereaux n.
  lupus n.
  parenchymatous n.

nephritis *(continued)*
    pneumococcus n.
    potassium-losing n.
    n. of pregnancy
    productive n.
    n. repens
    salt-losing n.
    scarlatinal n.
    subacute n.
    suppurative n.
    syphilitic n.
    transfusion n.
    tubal n.
    tuberculous n.
    tubular n.
    tubulointerstitial n.
    vascular n.

nephritogenic

nephroabdominal

nephroangiosclerosis

nephroblastoma

nephroblastomatosis

nephrocalcinosis

nephrocardiac

nephrocele

nephrocolic

nephrocystanastomosis

nephrocystitis

nephrocystosis

nephrogastric

nephrogenic
    n. adenoma
    n. ascites
    n. metaplasia
    n. zone

nephrogenous

nephrogram
    delayed n.

nephrohemia

nephrohydrosis

nephrohypertrophy

nephrolith

nephrolithiasis
    familial juvenile n.

nephrolithotomy
    percutaneous n.

nephrologist

nephrology

nephrolysis

nephrolytic

nephroma
    congenital mesoblastic n.
    embryonal n.

nephromalacia

nephromegaly

nephron

nephronophthisis
    familial juvenile n.

nephropathia

nephropathic

nephropathy
    acute urate n.
    acute uric acid n.
    analgesic n.
    Balkan n.
    chronic urate n.
    chronic uric acid n.
    diabetic n.
    epidemic n.
    gouty n.
    HIV-associated n.
    human immunodeficiency
        virus–associated n.
    hypazoturic n.
    IgA n.
    IgM n.
    ischemic n.
    light chain n.

nephropathy *(continued)*
  membranous n.
  minimal change n.
  overt n.
  potassium-losing n.
  reflux n.
  sickle cell n.
  thin basement membrane n.
  urate n.
  uric acid n.
  vasomotor n.

nephropexy

nephrophagiasis

nephrophthisis
  familial juvenile n.

nephropoietic

nephroptosia

nephroptosis

nephropyelitis

nephropyelolithotomy

nephropyeloplasty

nephropyosis

nephrorrhagia

nephrorrhaphy

nephrosclerosis
  arteriolar n.
  benign n.
  benign arteriolar n.
  hyaline arteriolar n.
  hyperplastic arteriolar n.
  hypertensive n.
  intercapillary n.
  malignant n.
  malignant arteriolar n.
  senile n.

nephroscope

nephroscopy

nephroses

nephrosis *pl.* nephroses
  acute n.

nephrosis *(continued)*
  Adriamycin-induced n.
  amyloid n.
  cholemic n.
  chronic n.
  Epstein n.
  familial n.
  glycogen n.
  hydropic n.
  hypokalemic n.
  larval n.
  lipid n.
  lipoid n.
  lower nephron n.
  necrotizing n.
  osmotic n.
  toxic n.
  vacuolar n.

nephrosonephritis

nephrospasis

nephrostolithotomy

nephrostomic
  n. cavity

nephrostomy
  n. tube

nephrotic
  n. edema
  n. syndrome

nephrotomy
  abdominal n.
  anatrophic n.
  lumbar n.

nephrotoxic
  n. acute renal failure

nephrotoxicity

nephrotoxin

nephrotropic

nephrotuberculosis

nephroureterectomy

nephroureterocystectomy

nephrydrosis

nephrydrotic

nerve
    iliohypogastric n.
    ilioinguinal n.
    intrapancreatic n.
    vagus n.

nervosa
    anorexia n.
    bulimia n.
    dysphagia n.

nervous
    n. bladder
    n. dyspepsia
    n. gut
    n. indigestion
    n. vomiting

nest
    Brunn epithelial n's

Neubauer and Fischer test

neuroendocrine
    n. cell

neurofibroma
    duodenal n.
    gastrointestinal n.
    von Recklinghausen gastric n.

neurofibromatosis
    von Recklinghausen n.

neurogastric

neurogenic
    n. bladder
    n. impotence
    n. intestinal obstruction
    n. sphincteric incompetence

neuron
    adrenergic n.
    facilitator n.

neuronal
    n. colonic dysplasia
    n. intestinal dysplasia

neuronephric

neuropathy
    autonomic n.
    diabetic n.
    IgA n.
    immunoglobulin n.
    vasculitic n.
    visceral n.

neutrocytic ascites

neutrophil

neutrophilic
    n. gastroduodenitis
    n. infiltration

Neville tracheal reconstruction prosthesis

nevus *pl.* nevi
    hepatic n.
    spider n.

newborn
    n. hepatitis
    n. jaundice

NG
    nasogastric
        NG aspirate
        heme-positive NG aspirate

nicotinic agonist

NIDDM
    non–insulin-dependent diabetes mellitus

Niemeier gallbladder perforation

nil disease

nipple
    ileum n.

nippled stoma

Nissen
    N. antireflux operation
    N. 360-degree wrap fundoplication
    N. fundoplication
    N. gall duct forceps
    N. operation

Nissen *(continued)*
    N. repair
    Rossetti modification of N.
      fundoplication
    slipped N. repair
    tight N. repair

nitremia

nitrofurantoin hepatotoxicity

nitrogen
    n. balance
    high calorie and n. (HCN)
    n. overload
    positive n. balance

Noble
    N. bowel plication
    N. position

noctalbuminuria

nocturia

nocturnal
    n. acid reflux
    n. diarrhea
    n. gastric reflux
    n. heartburn
    n. pain
    n. regurgitation

node
    celiac lymph n.
    lymph n.
    matted n.
    sentinel n.
    shotty lymph n.
    subcarinal n.

nodular
    n. glomerulonephritis
    n. hyperplasia
    n. hyperplasia of the prostate
    n. lesion
    n. liver
    n. lymphoid hyperplasia
    n. lymphoma
    n. pancreatitis
    n. regenerative hyperplasia
    sessile n. carcinoma

nodular *(continued)*
    n. transformation
    n. transformation of the
      liver

nodularity
    coarse n.
    mucosal n.
    surface n.

nodulated

nodulation

nodule
    cecal mucosal n.
    cirrhotic n.
    colonic lymphoid n.
    dysplastic n.
    hyperplastic n.
    Kimmelstiel-Wilson n.
    large regenerative n.
    liver n.
    lymphoid n.
    lymphomatous n.
    macroregenerative n.
    monoacinar regenerative n.
    multiacinar regenerative n.
    multiple n.
    peritoneal n.
    prostatic n.
    regenerative n.
    regenerative cirrhotic n.
    surface n.
    thyroid n.
    yellow n.

nodule-in-nodule pattern

nodulous

noma

non-A, non-B hepatitis

nonalcoholic steatohepatitis

non-alpha, non-beta pancreatic
    islet cell

non–anion-gap metabolic acidosis

nonantibiotic colitis

non–antigen-expressing target cell

nonazotemic cirrhosis

nonbacterial gastroenteritis

nonbilious vomitus

nonbloody stool

noncardiac chest pain

noncaseating tubercle-like granuloma

nonchylous ascites

noncirrhotic
n. liver
n. portal fibrosis
n. portal hypertension

noncleaved B cell

noncommunicating
n. biliary cyst
n. diverticulum
n. hydrocele

noncrushing bowel clamp

nondiabetic
n. gastroparesis
n. glycosuria

nondilating reflux

nondistended abdomen

nondistensible

nonerosive
n. gastric mucosal lesion
n. gastritis
n. nonspecific gastritis

nonfamilial
n. gastrointestinal polyposis
n. intestinal pseudo-obstruction

nonfluctuant

non–gas-forming liver abscess

non–germ cell carcinoma

nongonococcal urethritis

nongranulomatous jejunitis

nonhealing ulcer

nonhemolytic
congenital n. jaundice
congenital familial n. jaundice
familial n. jaundice
n. jaundice

nonhemolyzed blood

non-Hodgkin lymphoma

nonhyperglycemic glycosuria

nonicteric
n. sclera
n. skin

non–insulin-dependent diabetes mellitus (NIDDM)

nonneoplastic
n. lesion

nonnephrotoxic drug

nonneurogenic neurogenic bladder

nonobstructive
n. hepatic parenchymal disease
n. jaundice

nonocclusive
n. infarction
n. intestinal infarction
n. mesenteric infarction
n. mesenteric ischemia
n. mesenteric thrombosis

nonoliguric
n. acute renal failure

nonorganic dyspepsia

nonparasitic
n. cyst of liver

nonparasitic *(continued)*
   n. splenic cyst

nonperforated
   n. appendicitis
   n. appendix

nonplicated appendicocystostomy

nonpolyposis colorectal cancer

nonreflex bladder

nonreflux esophagitis

nonspecific
   n. colitis
   n. erosive gastritis
   n. esophageal motility disorder (NEMD)
   n. esophagitis
   n. gas pattern
   n. gastritis
   n. granulomatous prostatitis
   n. reactive hepatitis
   n. ulcerative proctitis
   n. urethritis

nonsuppurative
   chronic n. destructive cholangitis
   n. destructive cholangitis
   progressive n. cholangitis

nonsteroidal antiinflammatory drug (NSAID)

nontransected pancreatic duct

nontropical sprue

nontyphoidal salmonella

nontyphoidal salmonellosis

nonulcer
   n. dyspepsia
   n. dysplasia

nonvariceal upper GI hemorrhage

nonviable tissue

nonvisualization of gallbladder

no rejection

normal
   n. appendix
   n. caliber duct
   n. carrier hepatitis
   n. flora
   n. gigantism
   palpably n.
   n. saline solution
   visibly n.

normal-appearing mucosa

normoactive bowel sounds

normochlorhydria

normoglycemic
   n. glycosuria

normospermic

normosthenuria

Northern blot analysis

Norwalk gastroenteritis

Norwood rectal snare

nosocomial
   n. fungal infection
   n. infection

nostril blood

notch
   angular n. of stomach
   cardiac n. of stomach
   cardial n.
   n. of gallbladder
   gastric n.
   interlobar n.
   n. for ligamentum teres
   pancreatic n.
   splenic n.
   umbilical n.

Nothnagel bodies

NSAID
   nonsteroidal antiinflammatory drug

nubecula

nuchal rigidity

Nuck
    canal of N.
    N. diverticulum

nuclear
    n. matrix alteration
    n.-tagged cell

nucleocapsid core factor

nucleus *pl.* nuclei
    sanded n.

NuLYTELY
    N. enema

Nupercainal
    N. ointment

Nuport PEG tube

nurse cells

nursing cells

Nursoy formula

Nussbaum
    N. intestinal clamp
    N. intestinal forceps

nutcracker esophagus

nutmeg liver

Nutramigen formula

nutrient enema

nutrition
    enteral n.
    home parenteral n.
    Jevity isotonic liquid n.
    Nutri-Vent liquid n.
    parenteral n.
    Peptamen liquid n.
    perioperative n.
    Replete liquid n.
    support parenteral n.
    total enteral n.
    total parenteral n. (TPN)

nutritional
    n. cirrhosis
    n. deficiency
    n. dropsy
    n. index
    n. pancreatitis
    n. status
    n. support
    n. therapy

Nutri-Vent liquid nutrition

Nutromat Pad S feeding pump

nycturia

Nyhus classification

oat cell
  o. c. carcinoma

O'Beirne
  O'B. sphincter
  O'B. valve

OB-10 Comfort bite block

obesity
  adult-onset o.
  alimentary o.
  endogenous o.
  exogenous o.
  hyperplastic o.
  hypertrophic o.
  o. hypoventilation syn-
    drome
  o. index
  lifelong o.
  morbid o.

object
  foreign o.
  irretrievable o.
  radiolucent o.

objective vertigo

oblique
  aponeurosis of external o.
  aponeurosis of internal o.
  external o.
  external o. muscle of abdo-
    men
  o. fibers of stomach
  o.-forward-viewing instru-
    ment
  o. hernia
  o. incision
  internal o.
  internal o. muscle of abdo-
    men
  o. obturator
  o.-viewing endoscope

obliterans
  appendicitis o.
  endophlebitis hepatica o.

obliterated varices

obliteration
  endoscopic extirpation ci-
    catricial o.
  Okuda transhepatic o. of
    varix
  percutaneous transhepa-
    tic o.
  o. of the psoas shadow

obstetric injury

obstipation

obstipum abdomen

obstructed
  o. defecation
  o. pelvis
  o. testis

obstructing carcinoma

obstruction
  adynamic intestinal o.
  airflow o.
  airway o.
  o. of bile flow
  biliary tract o.
  bowel o.
  cerumen o.
  closed-loop o.
  closed-loop intestinal o.
  colonic o.
  common bile duct o.
  complete bowel o.
  duodenal o.
  esophageal o.
  extrahepatic o.
  extrahepatic bile duct o.
  extrahepatic biliary o.
  false colonic o.
  fecal o.
  food bolus o.
  functional cystic duct o.
  gastric outlet o.
  hepatic venous outflow o.
  high-grade o.
  high small-bowel o.

obstruction *(continued)*
  idiopathic o.
  intermittent o.
  intestinal o.
  intrahepatic portal o.
  large-bowel o.
  low small bowel o.
  malignant biliary o.
  mechanical biliary o.
  mechanical duct o.
  mechanical extrahepatic o.
  mechanical intestinal o.
  mechanical small-bowel o.
  neurogenic intestinal o.
  outlet o.
  outlet o. constipation
  paralytic colonic o.
  paralytic intestinal o.
  partial bile outflow o.
  partial bowel o.
  pyloric o.
  pyloric outlet o.
  pyloroduodenal o.
  shrapnel-induced biliary o.
  simple mechanical o.
  small-bowel o.
  strangulated bowel o.
  ureteropelvic junction o.
  urethral o.
  urodynamic o.

obstructive
  acute o. cholangitis
  acute o. suppurative cho-
    langitis
  o. anuria
  o. appendicitis
  o. biliary cirrhosis
  o. dysfunctional ileitis
  o. gastroduodenal Crohn
    disease
  o. jaundice
  o. nephropathy
  o. pancreatitis
  o. uropathy

obtunded

obturation

obturator
  blunt-tipped o.

obturator *(continued)*
  o. hernia
  o. internus muscle
  oblique o.
  Optiview o.
  o. sign
  o. test

occlusion
  o. balloon
  balloon o. cholangiography
  enteromesenteric o.
  mesenteric vascular o.
  o. of TIPS (transjugular in-
    trahepatic portosystemic
    shunt)
  tourniquet o.

occlusive
  o. clamp
  o. collodion dressing
  o. dressing
  o. ileus
  o. infarction

occult
  o. bleeding
  o. blood
  o. GI (gastrointestinal)
    bleeding
  o. hepatitis
  o. spinal dysraphism

occupational toxin exposure

OCG
  oral cholecystogram

Ochsner
  O. flexible spiral gallstone
    probe
  O. forceps
  O. gallbladder probe
  O. gallbladder trocar
  O. hemostat
  O. muscle
  O. ring

OCL bowel prep

octreotide
  o. acetate
  o. effect

octreotide-induced hepatic toxicity

OCTT
    orocecal transit time

Oddi
    O. muscle
    sphincter of O.
    tumor of O.

odditis

odynophagia

oesophagus

Ogilvie syndrome

O'Hanlon intestinal clamp

oil
    aromatic castor o.
    castor o.
    cottonseed o.
    olive o.
    peppermint o.
    o. retention enema
    ricinus o.

oily stool

ointment
    Nupercainal o.
    Tucks o.

OK cell

Okuda transhepatic obliteration of varix

Oldfield syndrome

O'Leary lesser curvature gastroplasty

olestra fat substitute

oligakisuria

oligoanuria

oligocholia

oligochylia

oligochymia

oligocilia

oligohydramnios

oligohydruria

oligomeganephronia

oligomeganephronic
    o. renal hypoplasia

oligonecrospermia

oligopepsia

oligophosphaturia

oligospermatism

oligospermia

oligozoospermatism

oligozoospermia

oliguresis

oliguria

oliguric
    o. renal failure

olive
    Eder-Puestow o.
    expandable o.
    o. oil
    o. over guidewire
    palpable pyloric o.
    pyloric o.
    o.-shaped
    o.-tip catheter
    o.-tipped bougie

Olympus
    O. adapter
    O. Aloka Gf-EU-series endoscope
    O. CHF-P-series choledochoscope
    O. CV-series endoscope
    O. DES-series endoscope
    O. EF-series esophagoscope
    O. EUS-series endoscope
    O. EVIS series endoscope
    O. gastrostomy
    O. GF-UM-series endoscope

Olympus *(continued)*
    O. GIF-HM-series endo-
      scope
    O. GIF-J-series endoscope
    O. GIF-Q-series endoscope
    O. GIF-T-series endoscope
    O. GIF-XP-series endoscope
    O. JF-T-series endoscope
    O. JF-TV-series endoscope
    O. JF-V-series endoscope
    O. PFJ-series pediatric en-
      doscope
    O. P-series endoscope
    O. TJF-series endoscope
    O. UM-series endoscope
    O. V-series endoscope
    O. XCV-XK-series endo-
      scope
    O. XP-series endoscope
    O. XQ-series endoscope

Ombrédanne operation

omega-shaped incision

omenta *(plural of* omentum)

omental
    o. adhesion
    o. appendices
    o. band
    o. bursa
    o. bursitis
    o. cysts
    o. eminence of body of
      pancreas
    o. enterocleisis
    o. foramen
    o. grafts
    o. hernia
    o. infarction
    o. J-pexy
    o. patch
    o. pedicle
    o. pedicle flap graft
    o. sac
    o. studding
    o. tuber of body of pan-
      creas
    o. tuber of liver
    o. vein

omentalis
    taenia o.
    tenia o.

omentectomy

omentitis

omentofixation

omentopexy

omentoplasty

omentorrhaphy

omentotomy

omentovolvulus

omentum *pl.* omenta
    colic o.
    gastric o.
    gastrocolic o.
    gastrohepatic o.
    gastrosplenic o.
    greater o.
    incarcerated o.
    lesser o.
    o. majus
    o. minus
    pancreaticosplenic o.
    splenogastric o.

omentumectomy

omeprazole
    o.-amoxicillin
    o.-clarithromycin-amoxicil-
      lin therapy

Omnipaque

Omnipen
    O.-N

omphalodiverticular
    o. band

omphalomesaraic

omphalomesenteric

oncocytoma
    renal o.

oncogene-induced carcinogene-
    sis

One-Step gastric button

onionskin lesion

onset of pain

oozing blood

O&P
    ova and parasites

opacification

opacify

opaque meal

open
    o. biopsy
    o. drainage
    o. electrocautery snare
    o.-end flo-thru radiopaque
      tip
    o.-end ostomy pouch
    o. hemorrhoidectomy
    o. hydronephrosis
    o. injury
    o. pyelolithotomy
    o. pyelotomy
    o. retroperitoneal high liga-
      tion
    o. ulcer
    o. wound

opening
    anterior o. of stomach
    appendiceal o.
    o. of bladder
    cardiac o.
    cutaneous o. of male ure-
      thra
    duodenal o. of stomach
    ileocecal o.
    o. to lesser sac of perito-
      neum
    pyloric o.
    o. of vermiform appendix
    vesicourethral o.

operation
    Abbe o.
    Amussat o.
    antireflux o.

operation *(continued)*
    bariatric o.
    Bassini o.
    Battle o.
    Belsey Mark IV o.
    Belsey Mark IV antireflux o.
    Bevan o.
    Bigelow o.
    Billroth o.
    Bricker o.
    Browne o.
    Brunschwig o.
    Cecil o.
    Collis antireflux o.
    Cooper ligament o.
    Delorme rectal prolapse o.
    Denis Browne o.
    Dittel o.
    Duhamel o.
    Duhamel colon o.
    Duplay o.
    Finney o.
    Franco o.
    Frank o.
    Fredet-Ramstedt o.
    Freyer o.
    Fuller o.
    fundic patch o.
    Gauderer-Ponsky PEG o.
    Grondahl-Finney o.
    Halsted o.
    Hartmann o.
    Heineke-Mikulicz o.
    Heller o.
    Hill antireflux o.
    Hochenegg o.
    Hofmeister o.
    Huggins o.
    Kader o.
    Kasai o.
    Kelly o.
    Kocher o.
    Kraske o.
    Lane o.
    Lester Martin modification
      of Duhamel o.
    Lowsley o.
    McBurney o.
    Macewen o.

operation *(continued)*
  Macewen hernia o.
  McGill o.
  McVay o.
  Marshall-Marchetti-Krantz o.
  Maydl o.
  Mayo o.
  Mikulicz o.
  Miles o.
  Millin-Read o.
  Moschcowitz o.
  Nissen o.
  Nissen antireflux o.
  Ombrédanne o.
  Pereyra o.
  Polya o.
  pull-through o.
  Ramstedt o.
  Ripstein rectal prolapse o.
  Roux-en-Y o.
  second-look o.
  Soave o.
  Ssabanejew-Frank o.
  staging o.
  State o.
  Swenson o.
  Tanner o.
  Thiersch anal incontinence o.
  Torek o.
  Toupet o.
  Trendelenburg o.
  Turnbull multiple ostomy o.
  van Hook o.
  Weber-Ramstedt o.
  Whipple o.
  White o.
  Whitehead o.
  Witzel o.
  Wölfler o.
  Young o.

operative
  o. cholangiogram
  o. choledochoscopy
  o. decompression
  o. morbidity
  o. staging

opiate antagonist

opioid
  o. antidiarrheal
  endogenous o.
  o.-mediated pruritus

opisthorchiasis

opportunistic
  o. complication
  o. fungus
  o. infection

Op-Site dressing

opsiuria

opsonic activity

optical esophagoscope

Optiview obturator

Oragrafin contrast medium

oral
  o. barium suspension
  o. bile acid (OBA)
  o. cholecystogram
  o. disease
  o. glucose
  o. intubation
  o. iron
  o. lavage
  o. leukoplakia
  o. preparation
  o. suction catheter
  o. thermometer
  o. thrush
  o. tolerance
  o. transmission
  o. ulcer

orange-colored tonsil

OraSure salivary collection device

orbital
  o. depression
  o. exenteration gastroscopic access technique

orchectomy

orchialgia

orchichorea

orchidalgia

orchidectomy
    radical o.

orchidic

orchiditis

orchidoepididymectomy

orchidometer

orchidoncus

orchidopathy

orchidopexy

orchidoplasty

orchidoptosis

orchidorrhaphy

orchidotomy

orchiectomy
    radical inguinal o.

orchiepididymitis

orchilytic

orchioblastoma

orchiocatabasis

orchiocele

orchiodynia

orchioncus

orchioneuralgia

orchiopathy

orchiopexy
    Bevan o.

orchioplasty

orchiorrhaphy

orchioscheocele

orchioscirrhus

orchiotomy

orchis

orchitic

orchitis
    spermatogenic granuloma-
        tous o.
    traumatic o.

orchitolytic

organ
    artificial o.
    digestive o's
    o. donation
    external genital o's
    genital o's
    o. of Giraldés
    internal genital o's
    male genital o's
    male reproductive o's
    O. Procurement Program
    reproductive o's
    o. transplantation
    urinary o's
    Weber o.

organic impotence

organization
    genomic o.

organoaxial gastric volvulus

organogenesis

organomegaly

organoscopy

organum *pl.* organa
    organa genitalia
    organa genitalia masculina
        externa
    organa genitalia masculina
        interna
    organa urinaria
    organa uropoëtica

Oriental
    O. cholangiohepatitis
    O. cholangitis
    O. schistosomiasis

orifice
  appendiceal o.
  bell-shaped o.
  cardiac o.
  duodenal o. of stomach
  epiploic o.
  external o. of urethra
  external urethral o.
  fistulous o.
  ileal o.
  o. of ileal papilla
  internal o. of urethra
  internal urethral o.
  myopectineal o.
  myopectineal o. of Fru-
    chaud
  sharp-edged o.
  o. of ureter
  ureteral o.
  vesicourethral o.

orificium *pl.* orificia
  o. ureteris
  o. urethrae externum mu-
    liebris
  o. urethrae externum virilis
  o. urethrae internum

O-rings

Ormond disease

orocecal transit time

oroesophageal overtube

orogastric Ewald tube

oropharyngeal
  o. carcinoma
  o. damage
  o. dysphagia
  o. tube

oro-respiratory tract

orosomucoid

orotracheal intubation

Orr
  O. gall duct forceps
  O.-Loygue transabdominal
    proctopexy

orthoglycemic
  o. glycosuria

orthostatic change

orthotopic
  o. appendicocystostomy
  o. bladder
  o. colonic reservoir
  o. continent reservoir
  o. liver transplant
  o. remodeled ileocolonic
    reservoir
  o. transplantation
  o. voiding

orthuria

Os-Cal

oscheal

oscheitis

oscheocele

oscheohydrocele

oscheolith

oscheoma

oscheoncus

oscheoplasty

Osler-Weber-Rendu
  O.-W.-R. disease
  O.-W.-R. syndrome
  O.-W.-R. telangiectasia

osmolality

osmolarity

Osmolite HN enteral feeding

osmotic
  o. diarrhea
  o. diuresis
  o. diuretic
  o. laxative
  o. nephrosis

osseous metaplasia

osteocele

osteoclast-like giant cell

osteodystrophy
　　hepatic o.
　　renal o.

osteogenic
　　o. differentiation
　　o. sarcoma

osteomalacia
　　renal tubular o.

osteopenia

osteophyte
　　esophageal o.

osteoporosis

osteosarcoma

osteotomy
　　anterior innominate o.
　　pelvic o.

ostia (*plural of* ostium)

ostial atherosclerotic plaque

ostiomeatal

ostium *pl.* ostia
　　o. appendicis vermiformis
　　o. cardiacum
　　o. ileale
　　o. ileocaecale
　　o. ileocecale
　　o. pyloricum
　　o. ureteris
　　o. urethrae externum femi-
　　　ninae
　　o. urethrae externum mas-
　　　culinae
　　o. urethrae internum
　　o. valvae ilealis

ostomate

ostomy
　　o. appliance
　　o. bag
　　closed-end o. pouch
　　Coloplast o. irrigation set
　　ConvaTec Durahesive Wa-
　　　ter o.

ostomy (*continued*)
　　Dansac o. irrigation set
　　o. loop
　　loop o. bridge
　　o. skin

O'Sullivan
　　O'S. scoring system
　　O'S.-O'Connor abdominal
　　　retractor

otolaryngologic manifestation

outer
　　o. medulla of kidney
　　o. stripe
　　o. zone of renal medulla

outflow
　　hepatic o. tract
　　hepatic venous o.
　　mean venous o.
　　pulmonary o.
　　o. tract

outlet
　　bladder o.
　　o. dysfunction
　　gastric o.
　　o. obstruction
　　o. obstruction constipation
　　pyloric o.

outline
　　gastric o.

outpatient endoscopy

output
　　intake and o.
　　urinary o.

ova and parasites (O&P)

oval
　　o. esophagoscope
　　o. snare

oval-form colonic groove

oval-open esophagoscope

ovarian
　　o. cancer
　　o. carcinoma
　　o. dermoid cyst

ovarian *(continued)*
    o. disease
    o. endometrioma
    o. enlargement
    o. fibroma
    o. hyperstimulation syndrome
    o. remnant syndrome
    o. vein syndrome

ovarium *pl.* ovaria
    o. masculinum

over-and-over suture

overdistention

overdose
    acetaminophen o.

overflow
    o. fecal incontinence
    o. incontinence

overgrowth
    bacterial o.
    gastric bacterial o.
    small intestine bacterial o.
    tube o.

overload
    hepatic copper o.

overload *(continued)*
    nitrogen o.
    volume o.

overt nephropathy

overtube
    oroesophageal o.

owl eye cells

oxacillin
    o.-associated anicteric hepatitis

oxalate
    calcium o.
    o. calculus
    o. crystal

oxalic acid

oxalosis

oxaluria

oxidosis

oxyntic
    o. cells
    o. glands

oxyosis

pacemaker
    gastric p.

pachycholia

pachychymia

pachyperitonitis

pachyvaginalitis

pack
    gauze p.
    laparotomy p.
    Mikulicz p.

packing
    Adaptic p.
    p. forceps
    p. fraction

pad
    abdominal p.
    abdominal fat p.
    abdominal laparotomy p.
    Active Living incontinen-
      ce p.
    antimesenteric p.
    antimesenteric fat p.
    p. cover
    esophagogastric fat p.
    fat p.
    ileocecal fat p.
    laparotomy p.
    laparotomy p. cover

Paget
    P. disease
    P. disease of perianal area
    P. extramammary disease
    P. perianal disease

pain
    abdominal p.
    biliary p.
    boring p.
    burning p.
    colicky abdominal p.
    constricting p.
    p. control
    cramping p.

pain *(continued)*
    crampy abdominal p.
    deep p.
    diffuse p.
    drug-induced p.
    dull p.
    epicritic p.
    epigastric p.
    exacerbation of p.
    exquisite p.
    functional p.
    gas p's
    gnawing p.
    griping p.
    gripping p.
    hunger p.
    intermittent p.
    knifelike p.
    localized p.
    loin p.
    nagging p.
    nocturnal p.
    noncardiac chest p.
    onset of p.
    palliation of p.
    parietal p.
    perianal p.
    perirectal p.
    poorly localized p.
    postprandial p.
    posture-dependent p.
    protopathic p.
    radiating p.
    rebound p.
    recurrent p.
    recurring p.
    referred p.
    retrosternal chest p.
    severe p.
    somatic p.
    steady p.
    sudden onset of p.
    tearing p.
    terrifying p.
    unrelenting p.
    unrelieved p.
    unremitting p.
    visceral p.

painful defecation

painless
    p. jaundice
    p. rectal bleeding

painter's colic

palate
    cleft p.
    smoker's p.

palatine pillar

palatopharyngeal fold

pale stool

palliation of pain

palliative therapy

pallor
    mucosal p.

palmar
    p. erythema
    p. grasp

Palmer acid test for peptic ulcer

palpable
    p. adenopathy
    p. cord
    p. gallbladder
    p. mass
    p. pyloric olive
    p. rib diastasis
    p. stool

palpably normal

palpating

palpation tenderness

pampinocele

pancolectomy

pancolitis
    necrotizing amebic p.

pancrealgia

pancreas *pl.* pancreata
    aberrant p.

pancreas *(continued)*
    p. accessorium
    accessory p.
    anlage of p.
    annular p.
    Christmas tree appearance
      of p.
    p. divisum
    ectopic p.
    endoscopic retrograde par-
      enchymography of p.
      (ERPP)
    exocrine p.
    head of p.
    heterotopic p.
    lesser p.
    neck of p.
    tail of p.
    uncinate process of p.
    Willis p.
    Winslow p.

Pancrease

pancreas-kidney
    simultaneous p.-k.
    p.-k. transplant

pancreata

pancreatalgia

pancreatectomy
    distal p.
    en bloc distal p.
    left-to-right subtotal p.
    partial p.
    subtotal p.
    total p.
    Whipple p.

pancreatic
    p. abscess
    accessory p. duct
    p. acinar cell
    p. acinar cell carcinoma
    p. acinus
    p. amylase
    p. apoplexy
    p. ascites
    p. calcification

pancreatic *(continued)*
- p. calculus
- p. cancer
- p. carcinoma
- p. cholera
- p. cholera syndrome
- p. colic
- p. cutaneous fistula
- p. cyst
- p. disease
- p. diverticulum
- dorsal p. artery
- p. duct
- p. ductal hypertension
- p. ductal morphological change
- p. duct disruption
- p. duct manipulation
- p. duct sphincter
- p. duct sphincterotomy
- p. duct stent
- p. duct stone
- p. duct stricture
- p. endoprosthesis
- p. enzyme
- p. fibrosis
- p. fistula
- p. function test
- p. gland
- great p. artery
- p. hamartoma
- p. hematochezia
- inferior p. artery
- p. injury
- p. islet cell
- p. islet cell carcinoma
- p. juice
- p. lesion
- p. lipase
- p. lithiasis
- p. lymphangiectasia
- minor p. duct
- p. mucinous cystadenocarcinoma
- non-alpha, non-beta p. islet cell
- p. notch
- p. oncofetal antigen
- p. phlegmon

pancreatic *(continued)*
- p. polypeptide
- p. pseudocyst
- p. pseudocyst abscess
- p. ranula
- p. rest
- p. sarcoidosis
- p. secretory test
- p. sepsis
- p. steatorrhea
- p. stent
- p. stone
- p. tail resection
- p. transpapillary stenting
- p. trauma
- p. tumor localization
- p. veins

pancreaticobiliary
- p. common channel
- p. disease
- p. ductal junction
- p. endoscopy
- p. junction
- p. malignancy
- p. septum
- p. sphincter
- p. tract

pancreaticoduodenal
- anterior superior p. artery
- inferior p. arteries
- posterior superior p. artery
- p. veins

pancreaticoduodenectomy
- Whipple p.

pancreaticoduodenostomy
- Child p.
- Dennis-Varco p.
- Whipple p.

pancreaticoenterostomy

pancreaticogastric
- left p. fold

pancreaticogastrostomy

pancreaticohepatic
- p. syndrome

pancreaticojejunostomy
   caudal p.
   Duval p.
   lateral p.
   longitudinal p.
   Puestow p.
   retrocolic end-to-end p.
   Roux-en-Y p.
   p. stenosis

pancreaticosplenic
   p. omentum

pancreatitis
   acquired p.
   acute p.
   acute gallstone p.
   acute hemorrhagic p.
   acute recurrent p. (ARP)
   acute relapsing p.
   alcoholic p.
   biliary p.
   calcareous p.
   calcific p.
   calcifying p.
   centrilobar p.
   chronic p.
   chronic alcoholic p.
   chronic calcifying p.
   chronic relapsing p.
   coagulopathy p.
   diffuse p.
   drug-induced p.
   edematous p.
   endoscopic sphinctero-
     tomy-induced p.
   familial p.
   focal p.
   fulminating p.
   gallstone p.
   groove p.
   hemorrhagic p.
   hemorrhagic necrotizing p.
   idiopathic p.
   idiopathic fibrosing p.
   idiopathic recurrent p.
   interstitial p.
   Marseille p. classification
   necrotizing p.

pancreatitis *(continued)*
   nodular p.
   nutritional p.
   obstructive p.
   perilobar p.
   post-ERCP induced p.
   postprocedure p.
   purulent p.
   Ranson acute p. classifica-
     tion
   recurrent p.
   segmentary p.
   tropical calcific p.
   ventral chronic calcific p.

pancreatitis-related
   p.-r. bleeding
   p.-r. hemorrhage

pancreatobiliary
   p. canal
   p. region

pancreatoblastoma

pancreatoduodenectomy

pancreatoduodenostomy

pancreatoenterostomy

pancreatogenic

pancreatogenous
   p. fatty diarrhea

pancreatography
   endoscopic retrograde p.

pancreatolith

pancreatolithectomy

pancreatolithiasis

pancreatolithotomy

pancreatolysis

pancreatolytic

pancreatomy

pancreatopathy

pancreatoscopy
  peroral p.

pancreatotomy

pancreatotropic

pancreatropic

pancreectomy

pancreolithotomy

pancreolysis

pancreolytic

pancreopathy

pancreoprivic

pancreotherapy

pancreotropic

pancystitis

panendography

panendoscope
  flexible forward-viewing p.

panendoscopy
  fiberoptic p.

Paneth cells

panmural
  p. cystitis
  p. fibrosis of the bladder

panniculectomy

panniculitis

panniculus
  hanging p.

pannus

panproctocolectomy

pantaloon hernia

pantothenic acid
  p. a. deficiency–induced
    colitis

panthenol

pantoprazole sodium

pantothenol

pantothenyl alcohol

pants-over-vest herniorrhaphy

pants-over-vest repair

Panzer gallbladder scissors

papilla *pl.* papillae
  bile p.
  duodenal p.
  p. duodeni major
  p. duodeni minor
  p. duodeni [Santorini]
  ileal p.
  p. ilealis
  p. ileocaecalis
  ileocecal p.
  major duodenal p.
  minor duodenal p.
  orifice of ileal p.
  p. renalis
  p. of Santorini
  sloughed p.
  p. of Vater

papillary
  p. adenocarcinoma
  p. adenoma
  p. cystic tumor of pancreas
  p. duct
  p. foramina of kidney
  p. gastric carcinoma
  p. hyperplasia
  p. lesion
  p. necrosis
  p. serous cystadenocarci-
    noma
  p. stenosis
  p. tip
  p. transitional cell carci-
    noma
  p. tuber of liver
  p. tubercle

papillectomy

papilledema

papillitis
  necrotizing p.

papillitis *(continued)*
  necrotizing renal p.

papilloma
  esophageal squamous p.
  hirsutoid p.
  hirsutoid p's of penis
  squamous cell p.

papilloma-carcinoma sequence

papillomavirus
  human p. (HPV)
  human p. 16 (HPV 16)

papillosphincterotomy

papillotome
  Bilisystem wire-guided p.

papillotomy

papule
  pearly penile p's

para-appendicitis

paracecal
  p. appendix

paracentesis
  abdominal p.
  diagnostic p.
  large-volume p.

paracentetic

paracetamol absorption

paracolic
  p. abscess
  p. gutter
  p. recesses
  p. sulci

paracolitis

paracystic

paracystitis

paracystium

paradidymal

paradidymis

paradoxical
  p. contraction

paradoxical *(continued)*
  p. diarrhea
  p. incontinence

paradoxus
  pulsus p.

paraductal adenopathy

paraduodenal
  p. fold
  p. fossa
  p. hernia

paraesophageal
  p. diaphragmatic hernia
  p. hernia
  p. hiatal hernia
  p. varix

paraesophagogastric devascularization

parafrenal
  p. abscess
  p. glands

parahepatic

parahepatitis

parahiatal
  p. hernia

parajejunal
  p. fossa

paralysis *pl.* paralyses
  Brown-Séquard p.

paralytic
  p. bladder
  p. colonic obstruction
  p. ileus
  p. intestinal obstruction

paramedian
  p. incision
  p. planes

paranephric
  p. abscess
  p. body
  p. cyst
  p. fat

paranephritis

paraomphalic

parapancreatic

paraparesis
    spastic p.

paraperitoneal
    p. hernia
    p. nephrectomy

paraphimosis

paraproctitis

paraproctium

paraprostatitis

parapyelitic
    p. cysts

pararectal
    p. abscess
    p. fistula
    p. line

pararectus incision

pararenal
    p. fat
    p. fat body
    p. pseudocyst

parasaccular
    p. hernia

parasagittal plane

parasinusoidal

parasite
    intestinal p.

parasitic
    p. infection

paraspadias

parastomal hernia

parasympathomimetic agent

paratesticular
    p. rhabdomyosarcoma

parathyroid
    p. gland

paratyphlitis

paraumbilical
    p. veins

paraurethra

paraurethral
    p. canals of male urethra
    p. ducts of female urethra
    p. ducts of male urethra
    p. glands
    p. tubules

paraurethritis

paravariceal fibrosis

paravertebral fascia

paravisceral
    p. aorta

paregoric

parenchyma
    allograft p.
    p. glandulare prostatae
    hepatic p.
    liver p.
    p. prostatae
    p. testis
    p. of testis

parenchymal
    p. hematoma
    p. hepatic cells
    p. jaundice
    p. liver cells
    p. liver disease
    p. tissue
    p. tumor

parenchymatous
    p. acute renal failure
    chronic p. nephritis
    p. nephritis

parenteral
    p. alimentation
    p. diarrhea
    p. feeding
    p. hyperalimentation
    p. nutrition

parepididymis

parepigastric

paries *pl.* parietes
p. anterior gastris
p. anterior ventriculi
p. posterior gastris
p. posterior ventriculi

parietal
p. cells
p. fistula
p. hernia
p. layer of pelvic fascia
p. layer of tunica vaginalis
of testis
p. pain
p. part of pelvic fascia
postreceptor signaling of p.
cell

parietes (*plural of* paries)

parietocolic
p. fold

Parker-Kerr enteroenterostomy

Parks
P. ileal reservoir
P. ileoanal anastomosis
P. ileostomy pouch
P. method of anal fistulo-
tomy

parorchidium

parorchis

parotid
p. gland

parovarian
p. mass

pars *pl.* partes
p. abdominalis esophagi
p. abdominalis ureteris
p. analis recti
p. anterior faciei diaphrag-
maticae hepatis
p. ascendens duodeni
p. cardiaca gastris

pars (*continued*)
p. cardiaca ventriculi
p. cervicalis esophagi
p. convoluta lobuli corticalis renis
p. cricopharyngea musculi
constrictoris pharyngis
inferioris
p. descendens duodeni
p. dextra faciei diaphrag-
maticae hepatis
p. exocrina pancreatis
p. horizontalis duodeni
p. inferior duodeni
p. intermedia urethrae
masculinae
p. membranacea urethrae
masculinae
p. pelvica ureteris
p. posterior faciei dia-
phragmaticae hepatis
p. profunda musculi
sphincteris ani externus
p. prostatica urethrae masculinae
p. pylorica gastris
p. pylorica ventriculi
p. quadrata
p. radiata lobuli corticalis
renis
p. recta tubuli renalis
p. spongiosa urethrae masculinae
p. subcutanea musculi
sphincteris ani externus
p. superficialis musculi
sphincteris ani externus
p. superior duodeni
p. superior faciei diaphrag-
maticae hepatis
p. thoracica esophagi

part
abdominal p. of esophagus
cardiac p. of stomach
cardial p. of stomach
cervical p. of esophagus
colic p. of omentum
exocrine p. of pancreas
inferior p. of duodenum

part *(continued)*
    intermediate p. of male urethra
    membranous p. of male urethra
    parietal p. of pelvic fascia
    pyloric p. of stomach
    subphrenic p. of esophagus
    thoracic p. of esophagus
    visceral p. of pelvic fascia

partes *(plural of* pars)

partial
    p. bile outflow obstruction
    p. bowel obstruction
    p. enterocele
    p. gastrectomy
    p. hepatectomy
    p. ileal bypass
    p. pancreatectomy

Partipilo gastrostomy

partitioning
    abdominal p.
    gastric p.

paruria

passage
    biliary p's
    p. of stool

passive incontinence

patch
    aortic p.
    colic p.
    colonic p.
    Gore-Tex soft tissue p.
    p. graft
    mucous p.
    omental p.
    p. technique

patchy
    p. colonic ulceration
    p. necrosis

Patella disease

patency
    biliary stent p.
    p. rate

patent airway

pathfinder

pathogenic bacteria

pathologic reflux

patient
    Child C-minus p.
    cirrhotic p.
    diabetic p.
    gastrectomized p.
    shock p.

pattern
    abdominal wall venous p.
    anhaustral colonic gas p.
    cobblestone p.
    colonic mucosal p.
    echo p.
    fine gastric mucosal p.
    fold p.
    gallstone p.
    gas p.
    haustral p.
    histochemical p.
    mosaic duodenal mucosal p.
    mucosal p.
    nodule-in-nodule p.
    nonspecific gas p.
    rugal p.
    sonographic p.
    vascular p.
    venous p.

patulous
    p. anus
    p. cardia
    p. gastroesophageal junction
    p. hiatus
    p. pylorus

pauci-immune
    p. crescentic glomerulonephritis
    p. rapidly progressive glomerulonephritis

paucity
    bile duct p.

Paul-Mixter tube

Pauly point

Payr
    P. clamp
    P. disease

PBC
    primary biliary cirrhosis
        PBC-associated anti-
            body

P cell

peak pressure

pearly penile papules

pea soup stool

peau d'orange

pecten *pl.* pectines
    p. of anal canal
    p. analis

pectenitis

pectenosis

pectenotomy

pectinate line

pectineal
    p. hernia
    p. muscle

pectines (*plural of* pecten)

pectus excavatum

pedal edema

Pedialyte RS electrolyte solu-
    tion

pediatric
    p. colonoscopy
    p. endoscope
    p. endoscopy

Pediazole

pedicellate

pedicellated

pedicellation

pedicle
    cone p.
    p. of lung
    omental p.
    p. of vertebral arch

pedicled

pediculate

pediculation

peduncular

pedunculated
    p. polyp

Pee Wee low profile gastros-
    tomy tube

PEG
    percutaneous endoscopic
    gastrostomy
        PEG-assisted decom-
            pression
        Bard PEG
        Bard PEG tube
        Bower PEG tube
        Dobbhoff PEG tube
        Gauderer-Ponsky PEG
        PEG lavage
        Moss PEG kit
        Ponsky-Gauderer type
            PEG
        Sacks-Vine PEG system
        Sandoz Caluso PEG
            gastrostomy tube

peliosis
    bacillary p.
    p. hepatis
    p. of liver

pelletlike stool

pelvic
    p. abscess
    p. adhesion
    anterior p. exenteration
    p. appendicitis
    p. brim
    p. colon
    p. diaphragm

pelvic *(continued)*
p. exenteration
p. kidney
p. mesocolon
narrow p. plane
p. osteotomy
p. peritonitis
p. plane
p. plane of outlet
posterior p. artery
posterior p. exenteration
p. prolapse
total p. exenteration
transverse p. ligament
visceral p. fascia
wide p. plane

pelvicaliceal
p. stasis
p. system

pelviectasis

pelvifixation

pelvilithotomy

pelviolithotomy

pelvioperitonitis

pelvioplasty

pelvioprostatic capsule

pelvioscopy

pelviostomy

pelviotomy

pelviperitonitis

pelviprostatic
basal p. ligament
p. capsular ligament
p. fascia

pelvirectal
p. abscess
p. achalasia

pelvis *pl.* pelves
extrarenal p.
obstructed p.
pseudospider p.

pelvis *(continued)*
p. renalis
spider p.
p. of ureter

pelviureteral

pelvoscopy

pemphigoid
benign mucous membrane p.

Peña
abdomino-P. pull-through procedure

pencil-thin stool

pendular movement

pendulous abdomen

penectomy

penetration
splenic p.

penial

penile

penis
clubbed p.
concealed p.
double p.
p. palmatus
p. plastica
webbed p.

penischisis

penitis

penoscrotal

Penrose
P. drain
P. sump drain

pentagastrin
p.-stimulated analysis

Pentasa

Pentax
P. EC-series video endoscope

Pentax *(continued)*
P. EG-series video endo-
scope
P. FD-series vide endo-
scope
P. FG-series video endo-
scope

peotomy

Pepcid AC

peppermint oil

pepsic

pepsin
p. secretion

pepsinia

pepsiniferous

Peptamen liquid nutrition

peptic
bleeding p. ulcer
p. cells
chronic p. esophagitis
p. esophageal stricture
p. esophagitis
p. glands
p. reflux
p. stricture
p. ulcer
p. ulcer disease (PUD)

peptide
antral p.
atrial natriuretic p. (ANP)
cellular p.
chemotactic p.
gastric inhibitory p.
gastrin-releasing p.
intestinal p.
vasoactive intestinal p.
(VIP)

Pepto-Bismol

peptogenic

peptogenous

Percival gastric balloon

percussion
dullness to p.
p. tenderness

percutaneous
p. abscess drainage
p. antegrade biliary drainage
p. balloon dilation
p. biliary drainage
p. biopsy
p. cholangiography
p. drainage
dual p. endoscopic gastrostomy
p. endoscopic gastrostomy
p. endoscopic removal
fine-needle p. cholangiogram
p. fine-needle pancreatic biopsy
p. liver biopsy
p. native renal biopsy
p. nephrolithotomy
p. pancreas biopsy
Russell p. endoscopic gastrostomy
p. stone removal
thin-needle p. cholangio-
gram
p. transhepatic biliary
drainage
p. transhepatic cholangiogram
p. transhepatic cholangiography
p. transhepatic decompression
p. transhepatic drainage
p. transhepatic obliteration
p. transluminal renal angioplasty
Surgitek One-Step p. endoscopic gastrostomy
ultrasound-assisted p. endoscopic gastrostomy

Pereyra operation

perforated
p. appendicitis
p. appendix
p. carcinoma

perforated *(continued)*
    p. cholecystitis
    p. diverticulum
    p. peptic ulcer
    p. viscus
perforating
    p. aneurysm
    p. appendicitis
perforation
    appendiceal p.
    bowel p.
    p. of colon
    colonic p.
    ductal system p.
    duodenal p.
    eosinophilic ileal p.
    esophageal p.
    p. of gallbladder
    gastric p.
    intestinal p.
    intraperitoneal p.
    Niemeier gallbladder p.
    peritoneal p.
    prepyloric p.
    retroduodenal p.
    retroperitoneal p.
perforative
    p. appendicitis
    p. peritonitis
perfusate
    p. bag
    esophageal p.
    hyperosmolar p.
perfusion
    allogeneic liver p.
    allogenic liver p.
    intestinal p.
periampullary
    p. carcinoma
    p. duodenal diverticulum
    p. mass
    p. neoplasm
perianal
    p. abscess
    p. edema
    p. fistula

perianal *(continued)*
    p. hematoma
    p. infection
    p. lesion
    p. pain
    p. skin tag
    p. soak
    p. space
    p. wart
periangiocholitis
periappendicitis
periappendicular
pericaliceal
pericalyceal
pericapillary diffusion
pericapsular
pericecal
    p. abscess
pericecitis
pericholangitis
pericholecystic
    p. abscess
    p. edema
pericholecystitis
    gaseous p.
perichromatin granules
Peri-Colace
pericolic
    p. abscess
    p. membrane
    p. membrane syndrome
pericolitis
    p. dextra
    membranous p.
    p. sinistra
pericolonic
    p. abscess
    p. fat
pericolonitis
pericostal suture

pericystitis

perideferentitis

perididymis

perididymitis

peridiverticular

peridiverticulitis

periductal fibrosis

periduodenitis

perienteric

perienteritis

periesophageal

periesophagitis

perigastric

perigastritis

periglandular

perihepatic
   p. adhesion

perihepatitis
   p. chronica hyperplastica
   gonococcal p.

perihernial

perihilar

perijejunitis

periligamentous

perilobar
   p. pancreatitis

perilobular fibrosis

perineal
   p. artery
   deep p. fascia
   p. fistula
   p. flexure of rectum
   p. hernia
   p. hypospadias
   p. incision
   p. infection

perineal *(continued)*
   p. ligament of Carcassone
   p. lithotomy
   p. membrane
   middle p. fascia
   p. muscles
   p. polyp
   p. prostatectomy
   p. section
   p. skin tag
   superficial p. fascia
   transverse p. ligament

perineocele

perineoplasty

perineotomy

perineoscrotal

perinephrial

perinephric
   p. abscess
   p. capsule
   p. fat
   p. sheath

perinephritic

perinephritis

perinephrium

perineum

perinodal

period
   reaction p.

periodic vomiting

periomphalic

perioperative
   p. antibiotic
   p. nutrition
   p. vomiting

periorchitis
   p. adhaesiva
   p. purulenta

periorchium

peripancreatic
   p. fibrosis

peripancreatitis

peripelvic
   p. extravasation

peripenial

peripheral
   p. adrenergic agent
   p. blood mononuclear cell
   p. cholangiocarcinoma
   p. edema
   p. hyperalimentation
   p. intravenous alimentation
   p. necrosis
   p. T cell
   p. venous thrombosis

periphery
   hypoechoic p.

periportal
   p. cirrhosis
   p. fibrosis
   p. hepatocyte

periproctic

periproctitis

periprostatic

periprostatitis

peripyloric

perirectal
   p. mass
   p. pain

perirectitis

perirenal
   p. arteries
   p. abscess
   p. fasciitis
   p. fat
   p. fat capsule
   p. hematoma

perisigmoiditis

perisinusoidal
   p. spaces

perispermatitis
   p. serosa

perisplanchnic

peristalsis
   absent p.
   decreased p.
   esophageal p.
   mass p.
   retrograde p.
   reversed p.
   visible p.

peristaltic
   p. contraction
   p. reflex
   p. unrest

peristomal
   p. infection
   p. skin
   p. varix

peritomist

peritomy

peritoneal
   p. abscess
   p. access
   p. adenocarcinoma
   p. adhesion
   p. anatomy
   p. autoplasty
   p. band
   p. button
   p. biopsy
   p. carcinomatosis
   p. cavity
   p. cavity abscess
   chronic ambulatory p. dialysis
   continuous ambulatory p. dialysis
   continuous cycling p. dialysis
   p. dialysis

peritoneal *(continued)*
    p. fungal infection
    greater p. cavity
    intermittent p. dialysis
    lesser p. cavity
    p. lavage
    p. malignancy
    p. mouse
    p. nodule
    p. perforation
    p. reflection
    p. sclerosis
    p. soilage
    p. space
    p. studding
    p. tap
    p. tuberculosis
    p. window

peritonealgia

peritonealize

peritoneocentesis

peritoneoclysis

peritoneointestinal
    p. reflex

peritoneomuscular

peritoneopathy

peritoneoperineal
    p. fascia

peritoneoplasty

peritoneoscope

peritoneoscopy

peritoneotome

peritoneotomy

peritoneum
    abdominal p.
    intestinal p.
    opening to lesser sac of p.
    p. urogenitale
    p. viscerale

peritonitis
    adhesive p.

peritonitis *(continued)*
    bacterial p.
    barium p.
    benign paroxysmal p.
    bile p.
    biliary p.
    Candida p.
    chemical p.
    p. chronica fibrosa encap-
      sulans
    circumscribed p.
    p. deformans
    diaphragmatic p.
    diffuse p.
    p. encapsulans
    encysted p.
    exudative p.
    fecal p.
    fibrocaseous p.
    fungal p.
    gas p.
    general p.
    granulomatous p.
    hemorrhagic p.
    localized p.
    meconium p.
    pelvic p.
    perforative p.
    purulent p.
    sclerosing p.
    sclerosing encapsulating p.
    secondary bacterial p.
    septic p.
    serous p.
    silent p.
    spontaneous bacterial p.
    sterile p.
    terminal p.
    traumatic p.
    tuberculous p.

peritonization

peritonize

perityphlic

perityphlitis
    p. actinomycotica

periumbilical

periureteral
p. abscess

periureteric
p. fibrosis

periureteritis

periurethral
p. cellulitis
p. phlegmon

periurethritis

perivesical
p. fat

perivesicular

perivesiculitis

perivisceral

Perlman syndrome

permanent
p. end colostomy
p. loop ileostomy
p. section
p. stoma

permeability

permeation
vascular p. of tumor cell

permselectivity

pernasal cholangiogram

pernicious
p. anemia
p. malaria
p. vomiting
p. vomiting of pregnancy

peroral
p. approach
p. cholangioscopy
p. endoprosthesis
p. endoscopy
p. esophageal dilation
p. gastroscope
p. maneuver
p. pancreatoscopy

per rectum
bleeding p. r.

Perry bag

persimmon bezoar

persistent
chronic p. hepatitis
p. chronic hepatitis
p. hematuria
p. müllerian duct
p. viral hepatitis
p. vomiting

persisting
chronic p. hepatitis

personality
ulcer-prone p.

pertussis

petechia pl. petechiae
gastric p.

petechial
p. angioma

Petersen bag

Petit hernia

Peutz
P.-Jeghers hamartoma
P.-Jeghers syndrome

Peyer
aggregated lymphatic follicles of P.
insulae of P.

Peyronie disease

Pezzer catheter

Pfannenstiel incision

Pfuhl sign

phagedenic balanitis

phagocytic stellate cell

pharyngeal
p. anesthesia
p. diverticulum
p. exudate
p. pouch
p. wall

pharyngitis
    exudative p.
    herpes p.

pharyngoesophageal
    p. diverticulectomy
    p. diverticulum
    p. function
    p. junction
    p. sphincter
    p. tear

pharynx

phase
    four p's of swallowing
    p. II marrow transplant re-
        cipient

Phazyme

phencyclidine
    p. abuse

Phenergan

phenoltetrachlorophthalein test

phenyl ethyl alcohol agar

phenomenon *pl.* phenomena
    common cavity p.
    Goldblatt p.

pheochromocytoma
    familial p.
    familial medullary thyroid
        carcinoma-p. syndrome
    malignant p.

Phillips
    P. LaxCaps
    P. Milk of Magnesia

phimosis

phimotic

phlegmon
    pancreatic p.
    periurethral p.

phlegmonous
    p. abscess
    p. alcoholic fatty liver

phlegmonous *(continued)*
    p. change
    p. enteritis
    p. gastritis
    p. mass

pH-metry

phorbol myristate acetate
    (PMA)

PhosLo

phosphate
    stellar p.
    triple p. calculus

Phospho-Soda
    P. enema
    Fleet P.

photogastroscope

photuria

phrenic
    p. ampulla
    p.-pressure point

phrenicocolic
    p. ligament

phrenicohepatic recesses

phrenicolienal ligament

phrenicosplenic ligament

phrenocolic
    p. ligament

phrenogastric

phrenoglottic

phrenohepatic

phrenosplenic

phyllolith

Physick pouches

physiology
    anorectal p.

physiological trophic effect

phytobezoar

phytotrichobezoar

Pick
  P. cell
  P. testicular adenoma
  P. tubular adenoma

picket fence appearance

piecemeal necrosis

Piersol point

pigment
  bile p.
  p. cirrhosis
  p. gallstone
  gastric p.
  hepatogenous p.

pigmentary cirrhosis

pigmented
  p. gallstone
  p. liver

pigtail
  p. biliary stent
  p. catheter
  p. endoprosthesis
  p. stent

Pilcher bag

pile
  prostatic p.
  sentinel p.

piles

pilimictio

pilimiction

pill
  p. esophagitis
  radio p.

pillar
  palatine p.

pillow
  Sand-Eze EGD p.

pilonidal perirectal abscess

pilobezoar

pineal
  p. gland

piperazine citrate

pipestem
  p. cirrhosis
  p. fibrosis
  p. stool

pit
  anal p.
  gastric p's
  postanal p.
  p. of the stomach

pitting
  anal p.
  colonic p.
  p. edema
  gastric p.

pituitary
  p. gigantism
  p. gland

placebo effect

placement
  graft p.

plain film of abdomen

plane
  Addison p's
  Addison clinical p's
  axial p.
  coronal p's
  Hodge p's
  horizontal p.
  ischiorectal fossa p.
  longitudinal p.
  Ludwig p.
  median p.
  midpelvic p.
  midsagittal p.
  narrow pelvic p.
  paramedian p's
  parasagittal p.
  pelvic p.
  pelvic p. of outlet
  transpyloric p.
  transverse p's

plane *(continued)*
  umbilical p.
  vertical p.
  wide pelvic p.

planimetric measurement

planum *pl. plana*
  plana coronalia
  plana frontalia
  plana horizontalia
  p. medianum
  plana paramediana
  plana sagittalia
  p. transpyloricum
  plana transversalia

planuria

plaque
  ostial atherosclerotic p.
  Randall p's

plaquelike
  p. thickening

plaquelike lesion

plasma
  p. bile acid measurement
  p. cell hepatitis
  p. renin activity (PRA)
  seminal p.

plasminogen activator (PA)
  tissue p. a. (TPA)
  tissue-type p. a. (t-PA)
  urokinase p. a.
  vascular p. a. (v-PA)

plastic
  p. induration
  p. vaginalitis

plate
  anal p.
  bowel p.

pleating of small bowel

pleomorphic destructive cholangitis

pleural mass

pleurobiliary fistula

pleuroesophageal

pleuroesophageus

pleurohepatitis

pleurovisceral

plexus *pl.* plexus, plexuses
  Auerbach mesenteric p.
  Auerbach and Meissner p.
  biliary p.
  celiac p.
  celiac p. reflex
  esophageal p.
  gastric p.
  gastroesophageal variceal p.
  hemorrhoidal p.
  ileocolic p.
  rectal p.

plica *pl.* plicae
  plicae caecales
  p. caecalis vascularis
  plicae cecales
  p. cecalis vascularis
  plicae circulares
  plicae circulares [kerckringi]
  plicae conniventes
  p. duodenalis inferior
  p. duodenalis superior
  p. duodenojejunalis
  p. duodenomesocolica
  plicae gastricae
  p. gastropancreatica
  p. hepatopancreatica
  p. ileocaecalis
  p. ileocecalis
  p. interureterica
  p. longitudinalis duodeni
  plicae mucosae vesicae biliaris
  plicae mucosae vesicae felleae
  p. paraduodenalis
  p. pubovesicalis
  plicae recti
  plicae semilunares coli
  plicae sigmoideae coli

plica *(continued)*
    p. spiralis
    plicae transversae recti
    plicae transversales recti
    p. umbilicalis lateralis
    p. umbilicalis media
    p. umbilicalis medialis
    p. umbilicalis mediana
    p. urachi
    p. ureterica
    p. vesicalis transversa
    plicae villosae gastris
    plicae villosae ventriculi

plicate

plicated appendicocystostomy

plication
    Child-Phillips bowel p.
    fundal p.
    Noble bowel p.

plug
    bile p.
    Imlach fat p.
    meconium p.

Plummer bag

plurivisceral

PMA
    phorbol myristate acetate

PMN
    polymorphonuclear
        PMN cell

pneumatic
    p. bag
    p. dilator
    p. esophageal dilation

pneumatinuria

pneumatosis
    p. coli
    p. cystoides intestinalis
    p. cystoides intestinorum
    intestinal p.
    p. intestinalis

pneumaturia

pneumobilia

pneumocholecystitis

pneumococcal infection

pneumococcus nephritis

pneumocolon

pneumogastric

pneumokidney

pneumoperitoneum
    benign p.

pneumoperitonitis

pneumothorax
    iatrogenic p.

pneumouria

pocket cell

pocketed calculus

podocyte

point
    Addison p.
    bleeding p.
    Boas p.
    Brewer p.
    Desjardins p.
    dorsal p.
    Hartmann p.
    Lanz p.
    McBurney p.
    Mackenzie p.
    Pauly p.
    phrenic-pressure p.
    Piersol p.
    Ramond p.
    Robson p.
    p. tenderness
    Voillemier p.

poisoning
    ackee fruit p.
    acute lead p.
    acute mercury p.
    bacterial food p.
    chronic lead p.
    salmonella food p.

pokeweed

Polaroid XS-70 with ACMI adapter

pole
> inferior p. of kidney
> inferior p. of testis
> upper p. of kidney
> upper p. of testis

polkissen

pollakisuria

pollakiuria

Polya operation

polyacrylonitrile

polycholia

polychylia

polyclonal
> p. gammopathy

polycystic
> p. chronic esophagitis
> p. disease of kidneys
> p. disease of liver
> p. kidneys
> p. kidney disease
> p. liver
> p. liver disease
> p. renal disease

polyembryoma

polyglycolic acid

polygonal hepatocyte

polylobar liver

polymicrobial bacterascites

polymorphonuclear cell

polyneuropathy
> uremic p.

polyorchidism

polyorchis

polyorchism

polyp
> adenomatous p. (AP)

polyp *(continued)*
> adenomatous p.–cancer sequence
> adenomatous p. of the colon
> adenomatous colorectal p.
> adenomatous gastric p.
> adenomatous p. of the stomach
> antral p.
> benign adenomatous p.
> bleeding p.
> broad-based p.
> cervical p.
> cholesterol p.
> colonic p.
> colorectal p.
> diminutive adenomatous p.
> diminutive colonic p.
> diminutive hyperplastic p.
> duodenal p.
> elusive p.
> eroded p.
> esophageal p.
> fibroid p.
> filiform p.
> fundic gland p.
> gastric p.
> gastric antral sessile p.
> gastric hyperplastic p.
> hamartomatous p.
> hamartomatous gastric p.
> hyperplastic p.
> hyperplastic adenomatous p.
> hyperplastic epithelial gastric p.
> hyperplastic gastric p.
> inflammatory p.
> invasive colorectal p.
> juvenile p's
> lymphoid p's
> malignant p.
> metaplastic p.
> mucosal p.
> multiple p's
> neoplastic p.
> pedunculated p.
> perineal p.

polyp *(continued)*
    polypoid p.
    postinflammatory p.
    prepyloric p.
    rectal p.
    regenerative p.
    p. relocation
    retention p's
    sentinel hyperplastic p.
    sessile p.
    p. stalk
    synchronous p.
    tuberculosis p.
    tubulovillous p.
    villous p.

polypectomized

polypectomy
    colonoscopic p.
    gastric p.

polypeptide
    gastric inhibitory p. (GIP)
    glucose-dependent insuli-
      notropic p.
    pancreatic p.
    vasoactive intestinal p.
      (VIP)

polyphagia

polypoid
    p. dysplasia
    p. lesion
    p. lymphoma
    p. mass
    p. polyp

polyposis
    adenomatous p.
    adenomatous p. coli (APC)
    p. coli
    familial p.
    familial adenomatous p.
    familial p. coli (FPC)
    familial colorectal p.
    familial gastrointestinal p.
    familial hamartomatous p.
    familial intestinal p.
    familial juvenile p.

polyposis *(continued)*
    familial p. syndrome
    filiform p.
    gastric p.
    gastrointestinal p.
    hamartomatous p.
    hyperplastic p.
    intestinal p.
    juvenile p.
    juvenile intestinal p.
    multiple familial p.
    nonfamilial gastrointesti-
      nal p.

polypotome

polypotrite

polypous
    p. gastritis

polypropylene mesh

polyserositis
    familial recurrent p.

polyspermia

polyspermism

polyvinyl alcohol

Ponka
    P. herniorrhaphy
    P. technique for local anes-
      thesia

pons *pl.* pontes
    p. hepatis

Ponsky-Gauderer type PEG

pontoon

pool
    abdominal p.
    bile acid p.
    gastric p.

pooled saliva

poorly differentiated adenoma

poorly localized pain

popliteal tenderness

porcelain gallbladder

pore
    biliary p.
    Galen p.
    slit p's

pork tapeworm

porotomy

porphyria
    acute p.
    acute intermittent p. (AIP)

port
    subcostal p.

porta *pl.* portae
    p. hepatis
    p. omenti
    p. of omentum
    p. renis

portacaval shunt

Portagen
    P. diet
    P. feeding
    P. formula

portal
    p. canal
    p. circulation
    p. cirrhosis
    p. fissure
    hepatic p.
    p. hypertension
    p. hypertensive gastropa-
      thy
    p. lobulation
    p. lobule
    p. pressure
    p.-systemic anastomosis
    p.-systemic encephalopa-
      thy
    p.-to-p. fibrosis
    p. tract fibrosis
    p. triads
    p. triaditis
    p. vascular bed
    p. vein of liver
    p. venous pressure

portoenterostomy

portojejunostomy

portosystemic
    p. anastomosis
    p. shunt

portoumbilical circulation

porus *pl.* pori
    p. galeni

position
    antero-oblique p.
    body p.
    Buie p.
    cervical p.
    curved flank p.
    decubitus p.
    doral p.
    dorsal lithotomy p.
    dorsosacral p.
    Elliot p.
    final p.
    flank p.
    Fowler p.
    greater curve p.
    jackknife p.
    knee-chest p.
    knee-elbow p.
    kneeling-squatting p.
    lateral decubitus p.
    left decubitus p.
    left lateral decubitus p.
    lithotomy p.
    Mayo-Robson p.
    Noble p.
    prone p.
    reverse Trendelenburg p.
    right antro-oblique p.
    Robson p.
    semioblique p.
    Sims p.
    ski p.
    supine p.
    Trendelenburg p.
    Valentine p.

positive
    p. bowel sounds
    p. nitrogen balance

postanal
  p. dimpling
  p. pit
  p. repair

postbiopsy fistula

postcaval
  p. shunt
  p. ureter

postcholecystectomy
  p. flatulent dyspepsia
  p. syndrome

postcholecystitis
  p. adhesion

postdysenteric

postendoscopic
  p. cholangitis

post-ERCP induced pancreatitis

posterior
  p. abdominal wall
  p. crus of anterior inguinal
    ring
  p. gastric artery
  p. gastric wall
  p. inguinal ligament
  p. margin of testis
  p. mediastinal arteries
  p. mediastinal cavity
  p. nephrectomy
  p. pelvic artery
  p. pelvic exenteration
  p. renal fascia
  p. segment
  p. segmental artery of kidney
  p. segmental artery of liver
  p. superior pancreatico-
    duodenal artery
  p. surface of body of pancreas
  p. surface of kidney
  p. surface of stomach
  p. urethra
  p. urethral valve
  p. vesicourethral angle

posterior *(continued)*
  p. wall of stomach

posterolateral

postfundoplication syndrome

postgastrectomy
  p. bleed
  p. dysfunction
  p. gastritis
  p. hemorrhage
  p. stasis
  p. syndrome

postglomerular
  p. arteriole

posthepatitic
  p. cirrhosis

posthepatitis
  p. aplastic anemia

posthetomy

posthioplasty

posthitis

postholith

postictal

postinfectious glomerulonephritis

postinflammatory
  p. polyp

postischemic
  p. acute renal failure
  p. tubular necrosis

postmenopausal

postmesenteric

postmortem intussusception

postmyotomy reflux

postnasal drip

postnecrotic
  p. cirrhosis
  p. scarring

postobstructive diuresis

postoperative
  p. abscess
  p. adhesion
  p. antibiotic
  p. biliary leakage
  p. fistula
  p. gastritis
  p. hydrocele
  p. ileus
  p. irrigation-suction drainage
  p. reflux
  p. stricture
  p. urinary retention
  p. vomiting

postpartum constipation

postperfusion

postpolypectomy
  p. bleed
  p. hemorrhage

postprandial
  p. distention
  p. nausea
  p. pain
  p. vomiting

postprocedure pancreatitis

postpyloric feeding tube

postreceptor signaling of parietal cell

postrenal
  p. anuria
  p. azotemia

postsinusoidal

postsphincterotomy
  p. ERCP cannulation

postsplenectomy infection

poststreptococcal glomerulonephritis

postsurgical
  p. change
  p. endoscopy

postsurgical *(continued)*
  p. gastric stasis

posttransfusion hepatitis

posttransplant
  p. renal dysfunction

posttraumatic
  p. autotransplantation
  p. pancreatic-cutaneous fistula

posttussive vomiting

postural regurgitation

posture
  Drosin p's
  p.-dependent pain

postvagotomy
  p. diarrhea
  p. dysphagia
  p. gastroparesis

potassemia

potassium
  p. acetate
  p. acid phosphate
  p. acid tartrate
  p. balance
  p. bicarbonate
  p. bitartrate
  canrenoate p.
  p. canrenoate antagonist
  p. citrate
  p. dihydrogen phosphate
  docusate p.
  p.-losing nephritis
  p.-losing nephropathy
  monobasic p. phosphate
  p. sodium tartrate

potato liver

potency

potential
  malignant p.
  neoplastic p.

potentiation of drug hepatotoxicity

Potter
P. facies
P. treatment

pouch
anal p.
Benchekroun p.
p. biopsy
blind upper esophageal p.
Bricker p.
Camey urinary p.
closed-end ostomy p.
Coloplast Flange p.
Coloplast mini p.
continent ileal p.
ConvaTec colostomy p.
ConvaTec Little One Sur-
Fit p.
ConvaTec Sur-Fit two-
piece p.
Dansac Karaya Seal one-
piece drainage p.
dartos p. procedure
Douglas p.
endorectal ileal p.
Foxy P. cover
gastric p.
Hartmann p.
haustral p.
ileal p.
ileal J-p.
ileal S-p.
ileal W-p.
p. ileitis
ileoanal p.
ileocecal p.
intraluminal p.
J p.
Kock p.
open-end ostomy p.
Parks ileostomy p.
pharyngeal p.
Physick p's
rectal p.
rectovaginal p.
rectovesical p.
S p.
Sur-Fit P. cover
terminal ileal p.

pouch (continued)
Willis p.
Zenker p.

pouched ileostomy

pouchitis

pouchogram

Poupart
P. ligament
P. pyelogram

PP-immunoreactive cell

PRA
plasma renin activity

pramoxine hydrochloride

prebladder

precancerous lesion

precipitant urination

precipitated calcium carbonate

precirrhotic hemochromatosis

Precision Isotonic powdered
feeding

precursor
benign neoplastic p.

predigested protein formula

prediverticular

prednisolone
p. enema

Pregestimil formula

preglomerular arteriole

pregnancy
abdominal ectopic p.
ectopic p.
p. gland
pernicious vomiting of p.
toxemia of p.

prehepatic

Prehn sign

prehyoid gland

preileal
    p. appendix

preoperative
    p. antibiotic
    p. lesion

prep
    Colonlite bowel p.
    Dulcolax bowel p.
    Emulsoil bowel p.
    Evac-Q-Kit bowel p.
    Evac-Q-Kwik bowel p.
    Fleet bowel p.
    GoLYTELY bowel p.
    inadequate bowel p.
    OCL bowel p.

prepancreatic
    p. anlagen
    p. artery

preparation
    bowel p.
    bowel p. complication
    oral p.

prepared calcium carbonate

preperitoneal
    p. anesthesia
    p. fat
    p. space

prepuce
    p. of penis

preputial
    p. calculus
    p. concretion
    p. glands
    p. space

preputiotomy

preputium
    p. penis

prepyloric
    p. antrum
    p. atresia
    erosive p. change
    p. gastric ulcer
    p. perforation

prepyloric *(continued)*
    p. polyp
    p. sphincter
    p. ulcer

prerectal lithotomy

prerenal
    p. anuria
    p. azotemia

presbyesophagus

preservation
    cadaver renal p.

presinusoidal

pressure
    abdominal p.
    anal p.
    anal sphincter squeeze p.
    basal p.
    basal anal canal p.
    basal anal sphincter p.
    bile duct p.
    biliary tract p.
    blood p.
    central venous p.
    choledochal basal p.
    closing p.
    p. diverticulum
    p. dressing
    dynamic closure p.
    end-expiratory intragastric p.
    esophageal peristaltic p.
    free hepatic venous p.
    hepatic vein wedge p.
    hepatic venous p.
    hepatic wedge p.
    hydrostatic p.
    interesophageal variceal p.
    intra-abdominal p.
    intra-anal p.
    intracholedochal p.
    intraductal p.
    intraesophageal peristaltic p.
    intragastric p.

pressure *(continued)*
    intraluminal p.
    intraluminal esophageal p.
    leak p.
    lower esophageal sphinc-
        ter p.
    mean arterial p.
    p. measurement
    p. necrosis
    peak p.
    portal p.
    portal venous p.
    proximal p.
    resting anal sphincter p.
    p. sore
    sphincter of Oddi p.
    squeeze p.
    static closure p.
    systemic arterial p.
    urethral p.
    variceal p.
    wedge p.
    wedged hepatic venous p.

prestomal ileitis

Preston salt

preurethral ligament of Wal-
    deyer

prevalence
    cholelithiasis p.

prevascular hernia

prevention
    acute pancreatitis p.

preventriculus

prevertebral fascia

prevesical

priapism
    secondary p.

priapitis

priapus

Prilosec

primary
    p. anastomosis

primary *(continued)*
    p. B cell lymphoma
    p. biliary cirrhosis
    p. diagnostic endoscopy
    p. hematuria
    p. hyperoxaluria
    p. impotence
    p. intention healing
    p. megaloureter
    p. renal calculus
    p. reninism
    p. sclerosing cholangitis
    p. ureteral atony

primed cell

principal cells

principle
    Heineke-Mikulicz p.
    Mitrofanoff p.

privilege
    bathroom p's

probe
    ambulatory p.
    Barr fistula p.
    BICAP P.
    BICAP Silver ACE
        Hemostasis P.
    biliary balloon p.
    blunt p.
    Buie fistula p.
    8-channel cross-sectional
        anal sphincter p.
    Desjardins gallbladder p.
    Desjardins gallstone p.
    Earle rectal p.
    end-fire transrectal p.
    Fenger gallbladder p.
    fistula p.
    gallstone p.
    heater p.
    Larry rectal p.
    Mayo common duct p.
    Moynihan bile duct p.
    Moynihan gallstone p.
    Ochsner flexible spiral
        gallstone p.
    Ochsner gallbladder p.
    rectal p.

problem
  benign pneumatic p.

procedure
  abdominal p.
  abdomino-Peña pull-
    through p.
  antegrade continuous ene-
    ma p. (ACE)
  antireflux p.
  bowel refashioning p.
  Camey p.
  cecal imbrication p.
  Cohen antireflux p.
  dartos pouch p.
  endorectal pull-through p.
  endoscopy p.
  Fowler-Stephens p.
  Hanley rectal bladder p.
  Hartmann p.
  Hofmeister p.
  ileoanal pull-through p.
  Kock p.
  Ladd p.
  MAGPI p.
  Mitrofanoff p.
  Roux-en-Y p. with vagot-
    omy
  Rovsing p.
  Schoemaker p.
  Sugiura p.
  Thal p.
  Whipple p.
  Womack p.
  Young-Dees-Leadbetter p.

process
  caudate p.
  funicular p.
  Todd p.
  transverse p.
  uncinate p. of pancreas
  vermiform p.

processus *pl.* processus
  p. caudatus hepatis
  p. Ferreini lobuli corticalis
    renis
  p. papillaris hepatis
  p. uncinatus pancreatis

processus *(continued)*
  p. vaginalis peritonei
  p. vermiformis

prochlorperazine

procidentia
  anal p.
  internal p.
  rectal p.

proctalgia
  p. fugax

proctatresia

proctectasia

proctectomy

proctencleisis

procteurynter

procteurysis

proctitis
  acute p.
  allergic p.
  chronic ulcerative p.
  diversion p.
  epidemic gangrenous p.
  factitial p.
  gonococcal p.
  gonorrheal p.
  idiopathic p.
  nonspecific ulcerative p.
  radiation p.
  traumatic p.
  ulcerative p.

proctoclysis

proctococcypexy

proctocolectomy
  restorative p.

proctocolitis
  aphthoid p.
  idiopathic p.
  radiation p.
  venereal p.

proctocolonoscopy

ProctoCream-HC

proctocystoplasty

proctocystotomy

proctodynia

Proctofoam-HC

proctogenic

proctogenous
  p. constipation

proctogram
  balloon p.

proctologic

proctologist

proctology

proctoparalysis

proctoperineoplasty

proctoperineorrhaphy

proctopexy
  Orr-Loygue transabdomi-
    nal p.

proctoplasty

proctoplegia

proctoptosis

proctorrhagia

proctorrhaphy

proctorrhea

proctoscope
  Tuttle p.

proctoscopy
  rigid p.

proctosigmoid

proctosigmoidectomy

proctosigmoiditis

proctosigmoidoscope

proctosigmoidoscopy
  rigid p.

proctospasm

proctostasis

proctostenosis

proctostomy

proctotome

proctotomy
  external p.
  internal p.

productive nephritis

profile
  liver function p.
  urethral pressure p.

profilometry
  urethral pressure p.

profound acid reduction

profuse vomiting

progenital

progestational agent

progesterone-associated colitis

prognathic dilatation

prognathion dilatation

program
  Organ Procurement P.

progressing toxicity

progressive
  chronic p. hepatitis
  p. diet
  p. dysphagia
  p. familial cirrhosis
  p. nonsuppurative cholan-
    gitis
  p. renal insufficiency
  p. suppurative cholangitis
  p. systemic sclerosis

projectile vomiting

prokinetic
  p. agent
  p. drug

prokinetic *(continued)*
p. effect

prolapse
anal p.
p. of anus
bladder p.
gastric mucosal p.
p. gastropathy
genitourinary p.
hemorrhoidal p.
intestinal p.
pelvic p.
rectal p.
p. of rectum
stomal p.
valve p.

prolapsed
p. bowel
p. hemorrhoids
p. rectum
p. stoma

prolapsing internal hemorrhoids

prolapsus
p. ani
p. recti

proliferating cell

proliferation
bile duct p.
cell p.
cellular p.
intraluminal p.
neoplastic cell p.

proliferative
p. hypertrophic gastritis

proper
p. hepatic artery

properitoneal
p. fat
p. flank strip
p. hernia

prophylactic
p. antibiotic
p. cholecystectomy

prophylactic *(continued)*
p. urethritis

prophylaxis
antibiotic p.
stricture p.

Propulsid

propulsive waves

Proscar

Prosobee
P. formula
P. liquid formula

prostata
parenchyma prostatae

prostatalgia

prostatauxe

prostate
ductal adenocarcinoma of
the p.
ductal carcinoma of the p.
p. gland
p.-specific antigen
p.-specific membrane antigen

prostatectomy
perineal p.
radical p.
radical retropubic p.
retropubic prevesical p.
suprapubic transvesical p.
transurethral p.

prostatelcosis

prostatic
p. adenocarcinoma
p. calculus
p. adenoma
p. catheter
p. concretions
p. ducts
p. intraepithelial neoplasia
p. mesonephric remnant
p. neoplasm
p. nodule
p. pile

prostatic *(continued)*
  p. sinus
  p. tractor
  p. urethra
  p. utricle
  p. vesicle

prostaticovesical

prostaticovesiculectomy

prostatism
  vesical p.

prostatisme
  p. sans prostate

prostatitic

prostatitis
  allergic p.
  chemical p.
  eosinophilic p.
  granulomatous p.
  nonspecific granuloma-
    tous p.

prostatocystitis

prostatocystotomy

prostatodynia

prostatolith

prostatolithotomy

prostatomegaly

prostatometer

prostatomy

prostatorrhea

prostatotomy

prostatovesiculectomy

prostatovesiculitis

prosthesis *pl.* prostheses
  Angelchik p.
  Angelchik antireflux p.
  Angelchik ring p.
  antireflux p.
  biliary p.
  bilioduodenal p.

prosthesis *(continued)*
  esophageal p.
  Neville tracheal reconstruc-
    tion p.
  penile p.

protection
  gastroduodenal mucosal p.

protective appendicitis

protein
  A-4 p.
  adenovirus-12 viral p.
  ascitic fluid total p.
  p.-calorie malnutrition
  folding of p's
  high p. diet
  p.-losing enteropathy
  R p.
  Tamm-Horsfall p.

proteinaceous cast material

protein serine/threonine kinase
  activity

protoduodenum

proton
  p. flux
  p. pump
  p. pump blocker
  p. pump inhibitor

Protonix

protopathic
  p. pain

Protozoa

protozoal
  p. dysentery

protozoan
  p. enteritis

protruding fat

protrusion
  anal p.

protuberant abdomen

proximal
  p. convoluted tubule

proximal *(continued)*
  p. gastrectomy
  p. gastric vagotomy
  p. pressure
  p. renal tubular acidosis
  p. straight tubule

pruritus
  p. ani
  opioid-mediated p.
  p. scroti
  uremic p.

pseudoachalasia

pseudoalcoholic
  p. hepatitis
  p. liver disease

pseudoaneurysm
  p. formation

pseudoappendicitis
  p. zooparasitica

pseudobile
  p. canaliculus

pseudocapsule

pseudocast

pseudochylous ascites

pseudocirrhosis
  cholangiodysplastic p.

pseudocolitis

pseudocylindroid

pseudocyst
  endosonography-guided
    drainage of pancreatic p.
  infected p.
  pancreatic p.
  pararenal p.

pseudocystobiliary fistula

pseudodiverticulum

pseudodysentery

pseudoesophageal colic

pseudogonorrhea

pseudohaustration

pseudohematuria

pseudohydronephrosis

pseudoileus

pseudolithiasis

pseudomegacolon

pseudomelanosis

pseudomembranous
  p. colitis
  p. enteritis
  p. enterocolitis
  p. gastritis

pseudomyiasis

pseudo-obstruction
  bowel p.
  chronic idiopathic intesti-
    nal p.
  colonic p.
  familial intestinal p.
  idiopathic intestinal p.
  intestinal p.
  nonfamilial intestinal p.

pseudopolyp
  chili bean p.

pseudopolyposis

pseudoptyalism

pseudopyloric
  p. metaplasia

pseudorickets

pseudospider pelvis

pseudotumor
  helminthic p.

pseudovaginal hypospadias

pseudovomiting

psoas
  p. abscess
  p. hitch
  obliteration of the p.
    shadow
  p. sign

psorenteritis

psychogenic
    p. constipation
    p. vomiting

psychologic jaundice

psychrophore

psyllium

ptyocrinous cell

P-type amylase

pubic
    p. artery
    p. region

pubicoperitoneal
    p. muscle

pubococcygeal
    p. muscle

puboischiadic
    p. ligament of prostate
    gland

puboprostatic
    p. ligament
    p. muscle

puborectal
    p. ligament
    p. muscle

pubovaginal
    p. muscle

pubovesical
    p. ligament
    p. muscle

pucker

PUD
    peptic ulcer disease

pudding
    Sustacal p.

puddling
    p. on barium enema
    p. sign

pudendal
    deep external p. artery
    p. hernia
    internal p. artery
    p. nerve function
    superficial external p. ar-
    tery

Puestow pancreaticojejunostomy

pull-through
    Duhamel p.-t.
    endorectal p.-t.
    endorectal ileal p.-t.
    ileal p.-t.
    ileoanal p.-t.
    ileoanal endorectal p.-t.
    p.-t. operation
    rapid p.-t.
    sacroabominoperineal p.-t.
    p.-t. technique

pulmonary
    p. edema
    p. embolism
    p. embolus
    p. outflow

pulpar cell

pulsatile
    p. mass
    p. hematoma

pulse
    abdominal p.
    abrupt p.

pulsion diverticulum

pulsus
    p. abdominalis
    p. paradoxus

pump
    Abbott LifeCare p.
    acid p.
    Companion feeding p.
    Compat feeding p.
    Endolav lavage p.
    Frenta Mat feeding p.

pump *(continued)*
    Frenta System II feeding p.
    Harvard p.
    hepatic artery infusion p.
    infusion p.
    Nutromat Pad S feeding p.
    proton p.
    stomach p.
    suction p.

punch
    aortic p.
    biopsy p.
    p. biopsy
    kidney p.
    Murphy kidney p.

purgation

purge

purging
    self-induced p.

purohepatitis

purpura
    allergic p.
    anaphylactoid p.
    Henoch p.
    Henoch-Schönlein p.
    p. nervosa
    Schönlein-Henoch p.

pursestring
    p. ligature
    p. suture

Purshiana bark

purulent
    p. appendicitis
    p. debris
    p. discharge
    p. material
    p. pancreatitis
    p. peritonitis

pus
    anchovy sauce p.
    p. cast
    p. collection
    frank p.

putrefactive diarrhea

putty kidney

pyelectasia

pyelectasis

pyelic

pyelitic

pyelitis
    calculous p.
    p. cystica
    defloration p.
    encrusted p.
    p. glandularis
    p. granulosa
    p. gravidarum
    hematogenous p.
    hemorrhagic p.
    suppurative p.
    urogenous p.

pyelocaliectasis

pyelocystitis

pyelofluoroscopy

pyelogenic renal cyst

pyelogram
    Poupart p.

pyeloileocutaneous
    p. anastomosis

pyelointerstitial

pyelolithotomy
    open p.

pyelometry

pyelonephritis
    acute p.
    chronic p.
    emphysematous p.
    p. of pregnancy
    xanthogranulomatous p.

pyelonephrosis

pyelopathy

pyelophlebitis

pyeloplasty

pyelostomy

pyelotomy
    open p.

pyeloureterectasis

pyeloureterolysis

pyeloureteroplasty

pyelovenous
    p. backflow

pyemesis

pyloralgia

pylorectomy

pyloric
    p. antrum
    p. artery
    p. atresia
    p. autotransplantation
    p. canal
    p. cap
    p. channel
    p. diaphragm
    p. dilatation
    p. dilation
    p. glands
    hypertrophic p. stenosis
    p. insufficiency
    p. membrane
    p. obstruction
    p. olive
    p. opening
    p. outlet
    p. outlet obstruction
    p. part of stomach
    p. sphincter
    p. sphincter muscle
    p. stenosis
    p. stricture
    p. valve
    p. vein
    p. web

pyloristenosis

pyloritis

pylorodiosis

pyloroduodenal obstruction

pyloroduodenitis

pylorogastrectomy

pyloromyotomy

pyloroplasty
    double p.
    Finney p.
    Heineke-Mikulicz p.
    Jaboulay p.
    Mikulicz p.
    reconstructive p.

pyloroscopy

pylorospasm
    reflex p.

pylorostenosis

pylorostomy

pylorotomy

pylorus
    patulous p.

pyocalix

pyochezia

pyocystis

pyofecia

pyogenic
    p. abscess
    p. bacteria
    p. cholangitis
    p. liver
    recurrent p. cholangiohe-
        patitis
    recurrent p. cholangitis

pyohydronephrosis

pyonephritis

pyonephrolithiasis

pyonephrosis

recess *(continued)*
    subhepatic r's
    subphrenic r's

recessus *pl.* recessus
    r. duodenalis inferior
    r. duodenalis superior
    r. duodenojejunalis
    r. hepatorenalis
    r. ileocaecalis inferior
    r. ileocaecalis superior
    r. ileocecalis inferior
    r. ileocecalis superior
    r. inferior bursae omentalis
    r. intersigmoideus
    r. lienalis
    r. paracolici
    r. paraduodenalis
    r. phrenicohepatici
    r. retrocaecalis
    r. retrocecalis
    r. retroduodenalis
    r. splenicus
    r. subhepatici
    r. subphrenici
    r. superior bursae omentalis

recipient
    r. hepatectomy
    marrow transplant r.
    phase II marrow transplant r.
    renal transplant r.

recirculation

recoil
    elastic r.

recombinant
    r. human alpha interferon
    r. interferon alfa-2a

Recombivax HB

recommended daily allowance (RDA)

reconstruction
    anal sphincter r.
    Billroth I r.
    Billroth II r.

reconstruction *(continued)*
    Roux-en-Y r.
    sphincter r.
    r. technique

reconstructive pyloroplasty

recreational drug

recrudescence

rectal
    r. abscess
    r. alimentation
    r. ampulla
    r. amyloidosis
    r. balloon
    r. biopsy
    r. bleeding
    r. cancer
    r. carcinoma
    r. coil MRI
    r. columns
    r. compliance
    r. cream
    r. dilatation
    r. dilation
    r. dilator
    r. distention
    r. emptying
    r. epithelial cell
    r. evacuation
    r. examination
    r. fascia
    r. fistula
    r. folds
    r. foreign body
    r. gluten challenge
    r. gonorrhea
    r. hypotonia
    r. impaction
    r. incontinence
    inferior r. artery
    inferior r. veins
    r. injury
    r. laceration
    r. lithotomy
    r. mass
    middle r. artery
    middle r. veins
    r. mucosa

rectal *(continued)*
  r. mucosectomy
  r. plexus
  r. polyp
  r. pouch
  r. probe
  r. procidentia
  r. prolapse
  r. reflex
  r. sensation
  r. shelf
  r. sinuses
  r. snare
  r. speculum
  r. sphincter
  r. stenosis
  r. stricture
  r. stump
  superior r. artery
  superior r. vein
  r. suppository
  r. tenderness
  r. tenesmus
  r. thermometer
  r. touch
  r. trauma
  r. tube
  r. ulcer
  r. varix
  r. vault
  r. villous adenoma

rectalgia

rectectomy

rectitis

rectoabdominal

rectoanal
  r. dyssynergia
  r. function
  r. inhibitor
  r. inhibitory reflex

rectocele

rectococcygeal
  r. muscle

rectococcypexy

rectocolitis

rectocutaneous

rectocystotomy

rectolabial fistula

rectopexy
  abdominal r.
  anterior r.
  Marlex mesh abdominal r.

rectoplasty

rectoromanoscope

rectoromanoscopy

rectorrhagia

rectorrhaphy

rectoscope

rectoscopy

rectosigmoid
  r. anastomosis
  r. colon
  r. function
  r. junction
  r. manometry
  r. radiation
  r. varix

rectosigmoidectomy

rectostenosis

rectostomy

rectotome

rectotomy

rectourethral
  r. fistula
  r. muscle

rectourinary fistula

rectouterine
  r. muscle

rectovaginal
  r. fistula

reflex *(continued)*
- anocutaneous r.
- anorectal inhibitory r.
- bladder r.
- r. bladder
- celiac plexus r.
- defecation r.
- diminished gag r.
- r. dyspepsia
- enterogastric r.
- esophagosalivary r.
- gag r.
- gastrocolic r.
- gastroileal r.
- gastropancreatic r.
- ileogastric r.
- intestinointestinal r.
- micturition r.
- myenteric r.
- peristaltic r.
- peritoneointestinal r.
- r. pylorospasm
- rectal r.
- rectoanal inhibitory r.
- renointestinal r.
- renorenal r.
- Roger r.
- urinary r.
- vasovagal r.
- vesical r.
- vesicointestinal r.
- visceromotor r.
- vomiting r.
- von Mering r.

reflux
- acid r.
- acid r. test
- bile r.
- r. bile gastritis
- cholangiovenous r.
- contralateral r.
- r. disease
- duodenal r.
- duodenobiliary r.
- duodenogastric r.
- duodenogastroesopha-
  geal r.
- duodenopancreatic r.
- esophageal r.

reflux *(continued)*
- r. esophagitis
- free r.
- r. gastritis
- gastroesophageal r.
- gastroesophageal r. disease
- gastroesophageal r. scan
- gastrointestinal r.
- hepatojugular r.
- intrarenal r.
- r. megaloureter
- nasopharyngeal r.
- r. nephropathy
- nocturnal acid r.
- nocturnal gastric r.
- nondilating r.
- pathologic r.
- peptic r.
- postmyotomy r.
- postoperative r.
- Roux gastric r.
- scintigraphic r.
- vesicoureteral r.
- vesicoureteric r.

reflux-related stricture

refractory
- r. ascites
- r. duodenal ulcer
- r. esophagitis
- r. sprue
- r. variceal hemorrhage

regenerative
- r. cirrhotic nodule
- large r. nodule
- monoacinar r. nodule
- multiacinar r. nodule
- r. nodule
- r. polyp

regimen
- antireflux r.
- dietetic r.
- immunosuppressive r.
- multidrug r.
- three-drug r.

regio
- regiones abdominales
- r. inguinalis

regio *(continued)*
 r. lateralis
 r. perinealis
 r. pubica
 r. umbilicalis
 r. urogenitalis

region
 abdominal r's
 anal r.
 centrilobular r. of liver
 choledochal r.
 framework r's
 genitourinary r.
 hepatic hilar r.
 hypochondriac r.
 hypogastric r.
 ileocecal r.
 pancreatobiliary r.
 pubic r.
 retroperitoneal r.
 umbilical r.
 urogenital r.

regional
 r. colitis
 r. enteritis
 r. enterocolitis
 r. ileitis

Reglan

regression analysis

regular diet

regurgitant
 r. fraction

regurgitation
 acid r.
 chronic r.
 r. jaundice
 nocturnal r.
 postural r.
 vesicoureteral r.

Rehberg test

Rehfuss stomach tube

Reichmann syndrome

reimplantation
 aortorenal r.

reimplantation *(continued)*
 end-to-side r.

Reinke
 crystalloids of R.
 crystals of R.

rejection
 accelerated transplant r.
 acute cellular r.
 acute r. of liver transplant
 acute vac r.
 acute vascular r.
 allograft r.
 chronic transplant r.
 delayed hyperacute transplant r.
 hyperacute r.
 interstitial r.
 no r.
 renal allograft r.
 transplant r.
 vascular r.

relapsing
 r. appendicitis
 chronic r. pancreatitis

relative dehydration

relaxation
 esophageal sphincter r.

relaxing incision

releasing factor

relocation
 polyp r.

remnant
 cloacal r.
 gastric r.
 mesonephric r.
 prostatic mesonephric r.

removal
 colonoscopic r.
 endoscopic r.
 forceps r.
 foreign body r.
 gastric coin r.
 percutaneous endoscop-
  ic r.

removal *(continued)*
    percutaneous stone r.
    radical en bloc r.
    small polyp r.
    through-the-scope bal-
      loon r.
    tube r.
    ureteral stoma r.

ren *pl.* renes
    r. mobilis
    r. unguliformis

renal
    r. abscess
    acute r. failure
    r. adenocarcinoma
    r. allograft
    r. allograft rejection
    r. amyloidosis
    r. aneurysm
    r. angiography
    r. anuria
    r. apoplexy
    r. arteriolar sclerosis
    r. artery
    r. artery aneurysm
    r. artery stenosis
    r. axis
    r. azotemia
    r. ballottement
    r. biopsy
    r. blockade
    r. calculus
    r. calices
    r. capsule
    r. capsulectomy
    r. capsulotomy
    r. carbuncle
    r. cast
    r. cell carcinoma
    chronic r. failure
    r. clearance
    r. colic
    r. collecting tubule
    r. columns of Bertin
    continuous r. replacement
      therapy
    r. corpuscles
    r. cortex

renal *(continued)*
    r. cortical abscess
    r. cortical adenoma
    r. counterbalance
    r. decapsulation
    r. diabetes
    distal r. tubular acidosis
    r. duct
    r. dwarf
    r. dwarfism
    r. dysplasia
    r. dyspnea
    r. ectopia
    r. edema
    effective r. blood flow
    effective r. plasma flow
    r. failure
    r. fascia
    r. function test
    generalized distal r. tubular
      acidosis
    r. glomeruli
    r. glycosuria
    greater r. calices
    r. hematoma
    r. hematuria
    r. hemorrhage
    r. hyperchloremia acidosis
    r. hypertension
    r. impression of liver
    r. infantilism
    r. insufficiency
    r. leiomyosarcoma
    r. lipomatosis
    r. lobation
    r. lobes
    major r. calices
    r. malacoplakia
    r. medulla
    r. messenger ribonucleo-
      protein acid
    minor r. calices
    multiple recurrent r. colic
    necrosis of r. papillae
    r. oncocytoma
    r. osteodystrophy
    r. papillary necrosis
    r. plasma flow
    primary r. calculus

renal *(continued)*
    proximal r. tubular acidosis
    r. pyramids
    r. replacement therapy
    r. reserve
    r.-retinal dysplasia
    r. rickets
    secondary r. calculus
    r. segments
    r. sinus
    r. threshold
    r. threshold for glucose
    r. toxicity
    r. transplant recipient
    r. tuberculosis
    r. tubular acidosis (types
        1–4)
    r. tubular osteomalacia
    r. tubules
    r. veins

renes *(plural of* ren)

renin
    active r.
    r.-aldosterone axis
    r.-angiotensin axis
    r.-angiotensin system
    r.-angiotensin-aldosterone
        system

reninism
    primary r.

reninoma

renipelvic

renocortical

renocutaneous

renogastric
    r. fistula

renointestinal
    r. reflex

renomedullary
    r. interstitial cell tumor

renopathy

renoprival

renorenal
    r. reflex

renotrophic

renotropic

renovascular
    r. hypertension

Renu enteral feeding

renule

repair
    anal sphincter r.
    Bassini inguinal hernia r.
    Belsey Mark IV r.
    Canadian r.
    Collis r.
    Cooper ligament r.
    esophageal stricture r.
    Halsted-Bassini hernia r.
    Hill r.
    Hill hiatus hernia r.
    Lichtenstein r.
    Lichtenstein hernial r.
    McVay r.
    Marlex hernial r.
    Nissen r.
    pants-over-vest r.
    postanal r.
    Rodney Smith biliary stric-
        ture r.
    Shouldice r.
    slipped Nissen r.
    tight Nissen r.
    transabdominal r.
    two-stage r.
    vest-over-pants r.

Replete liquid nutrition

reprocessor
    American Endoscopy auto-
        matic r.

reproductive
    r. organs

reptilase acid

resection
    abdominal-perineal r.

resection *(continued)*
    abdominoperineal r. (APR)
    anterior r.
    bowel r.
    colon r.
    colosigmoid r.
    curative r.
    en bloc r.
    esophageal r.
    gastric r.
    hepatic r.
    ileal r.
    ileocolic r.
    liver r.
    Miles abdominoperineal r.
    pancreatic tail r.
    segmental colonic r.
    terminal ileal r.
    transanal endoscopic microsurgical r.
    transthoracic r. of esophageal carcinoma
    transurethral r. of bladder tumor
    transurethral r. of the prostate
    transurethral prostatic r.
    transverse r.
    Whipple r.

resective colostomy

resectoscope
    Foroblique r.

resectoscopy

reserve
    renal r.

reservoir
    continent ileal r.
    detubularized right colon r.
    double-barrel r.
    double J-shaped r.
    double-stapled ileal r.
    fecal r.
    ileal r.
    ileoanal r.
    ileocecal r.
    ileocecal continent urinary r.

reservoir *(continued)*
    intra-abdominal ileal r.
    isoperistaltic ileal r.
    J-shaped r.
    J-Vac suction r.
    lateral internal pelvic r.
    Le Bag pouch r.
    r. mucosal absorption
    orthotopic colonic r.
    orthotopic continent r.
    orthotopic remodeled ileo-colonic r.
    Parks ileal r.
    S-shaped r.

residual
    r. barium
    r. stool
    r. urine

residue
    fecal r.
    low r. diet

residuum *pl.* residua
    gastric r.

resin
    anion exchange r.
    bile salt–binding r.

resistance
    basal renal vascular r.
    drug r.

resistant ascites

resonant abdomen

resorption
    tubular r.

Resource enteral feeding

respiratory acidosis

respiratory-esophageal fistula

response
    cell-mediated immunohistological r.
    cellular immune r.
    gag r.
    immune r.

rest
 adrenal r.
 bowel r.
 gut r.
 pancreatic r.
 total bowel r.

restaging of cancer

resting anal sphincter pressure

restorative proctocolectomy

retained
 r. antrum
 r. barium
 r. feces
 r. gallstone

retch

retching

rete *pl.* retia
 r. of Haller
 r. Halleri
 r. testis
 r. testis [halleri]

retention
 r. band
 barium r.
 r. cyst
 r. enema
 r. esophagitis
 gastric r.
 r. jaundice
 r. meal
 r. polyps
 postoperative urinary r.
 sodium r.
 stool r.
 r. suture
 urinary r.
 r. of urine
 r. vomiting

retia (*plural of* rete)

reticulum *pl.* reticula
 Ebner r.

retracted stoma

retractile
 r. mesenteritis
 r. testis

retractor
 Balfour r.
 Balfour abdominal r.
 Balfour self-retaining r.
 Barr rectal r.
 Beardsley esophageal r.
 Berens esophageal r.
 Christie gallbladder r.
 Crile angle r.
 Denis Browne abdominal r.
 Doyen r.
 Doyen abdominal r.
 fan-type laparoscopic r.
 Finochietto r.
 Foss bifid gallbladder r.
 Foss biliary duct r.
 Franz abdominal r.
 Harrington Deaver r.
 Hill-Ferguson rectal r.
 Hill rectal r.
 Kirschner abdominal r.
 Mayo abdominal r.
 Mayo-Adams appendectomy r.
 McBurney r.
 Mikulicz r.
 Murphy gallbladder r.
 O'Sullivan-O'Connor abdominal r.
 Robin-Masse abdominal r.
 Roux r.

retransplantation

retrocaval
 r. ureter

retrocecal
 r. abscess
 r. appendicitis
 r. appendix
 r. fossa
 r. hernia

retrocolic
 r. end-to-end pancreaticojejunostomy

retrocolic *(continued)*
    r. end-to-side choledocho-
      jejunostomy

retroduodenal
    r. arteries
    r. fossa
    r. perforation

retrograde
    r. cannulation
    r. cholangiography
    endoscopic r. cannulation
    endoscopic r. cholangio-
      gram
    endoscopic r. cholangiogra-
      phy
    endoscopic r. cholangio-
      pancreatography (ERCP)
    endoscopic r. cholecys-
      toendoprosthesis
    r. fashion
    r. flow on barium enema
    r. hernia
    r. intussusception
    r. migration
    r. peristalsis

retrohepatic vena cava

retroileal
    r. appendicitis
    r. appendix

retroiliac
    r. ureter

retropancreatic tunnel

retroperitoneal
    r. approach
    r. cavity
    r. fibrosis
    r. fistula
    r. hernia
    r.-iliopsoas abscess
    r. lymphadenectomy
    r. neoplasm
    r. perforation
    r. region
    r. space
    r. tumor

retroperitoneum

retropubic
    r. prevesical prostatectomy

retrostalsis

retrosymphysial

retrourethral
    r. catheterization

retrovascular
    r. hernia

retrovesical

retrovirus infection

Retzius
    R. cavity
    space of R.

revenge
    Montezuma's r.

reversal
    r. of gradient

reverse
    r. filtration

reversed
    r. reimplanted appendico-
      cystostomy
    r. peristalsis

rhabdoid
    r. tumor of the kidney

rhabdomyosarcoma
    paratesticular r.
    r. of prostate

rhabdosphincter
    intrinsic r.

rhacoma

Rhamnus

Rheum
    R. officinale

rheumatoid
    r. factor

rhubarb

ribbon
   r. gut
   r. stool

ribonucleic acid (RNA)

Richter hernia

ricinus oil

rickets
   celiac r.
   renal r.

ridge
   interureteric r.

Riedel lobe

Rieux hernia

right
   r.-angled end-to-side anas-
     tomosis
   r. colectomy
   r. colic artery
   r. colic vein
   r. colon
   r. colonic flexure
   r. epiploic vein
   r. flexure of colon
   r. gastric artery
   r. gastric vein
   r. gastroepiploic artery
   r. gastroepiploic vein
   r. gastro-omental artery
   r. gastro-omental vein
   r. gastropancreatic fold
   r. hemicolectomy
   r. hepatic duct
   r. hepatic radicle
   r. inferior gastric artery
   r. lobe of liver
   r. mesocolon
   r. suprarenal vein
   r. triangular ligament of liver

rigid
   r. abdomen
   r. endoscope

rigid *(continued)*
   r. proctoscopy
   r. proctosigmoidoscopy
   r. sigmoidoscope

rigidity
   abdominal r.
   boardlike r.
   boardlike r. of abdomen
   involuntary reflex r.
   nuchal r.

Rigiflex
   R. achalasia balloon
   R. achalasia dilator
   R. TTS balloon

RigiScan measurement

rigor mortis

ring
   A r.
   A r. of esophagus
   abdominal r.
   anorectal r.
   apex of external r.
   biofragmentable anasto-
     motic r.
   crural r.
   deep abdominal r.
   deep inguinal r.
   distal esophageal r.
   esophageal r.
   esophageal A r.
   esophageal B r.
   esophageal contractile r.
   esophageal mucosal r.
   esophageal muscular r.
   external r.
   external abdominal r.
   external inguinal r.
   femoral r.
   ilioinguinal r.
   iliopsoas r.
   inguinal r.
   internal abdominal r.
   internal inguinal r.
   Ochsner r.
   Schatzki r.
   superficial abdominal r.

ring *(continued)*
    superficial inguinal r.

Ringer solution
    iced lactated R. s.
    lactated R. s.

Riolan muscle

Riopan Plus

Ripstein rectal prolapse operation

RNA
    ribonucleic acid

Roberts
    R. esophagoscope
    R.-Jesberg esophagoscope

Robin-Masse abdominal retractor

Robson
    R. point
    R. position

Rochelle salt

Rocher sign

Rockey-Davis incision

rod
    colostomy r.
    gram-negative r.
    r's of Heidenhain

Rodney Smith biliary stricture repair

Roger
    R. reflex
    R. syndrome

Rokitansky
    R. disease
    R. diverticulum
    R. hernia
    R.-Aschoff ducts
    R.-Aschoff sinuses
    R.-Cushing ulcers

Rolaids

roll
    iliac r.

rolling hernia

romanoscope

rosacic acid

rose bengal test

Rose-Bradford kidney

rosebud stoma

Rosenbach sign

Rossbach disease

Rossetti modification of Nissen fundoplication

rot
    liver r.

rotation
    external r.

rotavirus
    r. diarrhea
    r. gastroenteritis
    r. infection

Rotazyme test

Roth
    vas aberrans of R.

Rotor syndrome

rotund abdomen

roughage
    high r. diet
    low r. diet

round ulcer

Roux
    R. gastric reflux
    R. limb
    R.-limb stasis
    R. retractor
    R. stasis syndrome

Roux-en-Y
    R.-en-Y anastomosis
    R.-en-Y biliary bypass with antrectomy
    R.-en-Y choledochojejunostomy

Roux-en-Y *(continued)*
    R.-en-Y distal jejunoileos-
      tomy
    R.-en-Y esophagojejunos-
      tomy
    R.-en-Y gastric bypass
    R.-en-Y gastroenterostomy
    R.-en-Y gastrojejunostomy
    R.-en-Y hepaticojejunos-
      tomy
    R.-en-Y jejunal limb
    R.-en-Y limb enteroscopy
    R.-en-Y loop
    R.-en-Y operation
    R.-en-Y pancreaticojejunos-
      tomy
    R.-en-Y procedure with va-
      gotomy
    R.-en-Y reanastomosis
    R.-en-Y reconstruction

Rovighi sign

Rovsing
    R. procedure
    R. sign
    R. syndrome

Rowasa enema

R protein

rubber band ligation
    r. b. l. of hemorrhoid

rubor
    dependent r.

ructus

Rudd-Clinic hemorrhoidal for-
    ceps

rudiment
    r. of vaginal process

rudimentary testis syndrome

rudimentum *pl.* rudimenta
    r. processus vaginalis

ruga *pl.* rugae
    rugae gastricae
    rugae of stomach
    rugae vesicae biliaris

rugal
    r. fold
    r. hypertrophy
    r. pattern

rugitus

rule
    Goodsall r.

rumbling bowel sounds

rumination

runny stool

"runs"

rupture
    acute hepatic r.
    duodenopancreaticocho-
      ledochal r.
    esophageal r.
    hepatic r.
    Mallory-Weiss mucosal r.
    splenic r.

ruptured
    r. aneurysm
    r. appendix
    r. sigmoid diverticulum

rush

Russell percutaneous endo-
    scopic gastrostomy

Ruysch
    R. disease
    R. glomeruli

Ryle tube

sac
   epiploic s.
   fluid-filled s.
   greater peritoneal s.
   greater s. of peritoneum
   hernial s.
   lesser peritoneal s.
   lesser s. of peritoneal cav-
      ity
   omental s.
   splenic s.

sacciform
   s. kidney

saccular
   s. aneurysm
   s. colon

sacculated
   s. bladder

sacculation
   s's of colon

sacculus *pl.* sacculi
   sacculi of Beale

Sacks-Vine
   S.-V. feeding gastrostomy
      tube
   S.-V. PEG system

sacral
   s. edema
   s. flexure of rectum
   lateral s. arteries
   lateral s. veins
   median s. artery
   median s. vein

sacred bark

sacroabominoperineal pull-
   through

sacrococcygeal artery

sagittal
   s. fissure of liver

sago
   s.-grain stool

sago *(continued)*
   s. liver

Sahli-Nencki test

Saint triad

sal
   s. ammoniac
   s. diureticum

salicylate abuse

saline
   s. cathartic
   s. cleansing enema
   s.-filled cholangiocatheter
   s. laxative
   normal s. solution
   warm s. solution

saliva
   s. bicarbonate
   pooled s.
   s. substitute

salivary
   s. amylase
   s. glands
   s. mass
   s. tenderness

salivation

Salmonella
   S. colitis
   S. enteritidis
   S. food poisoning
   S. typhimurium enterocoli-
      tis

salmonella
   s. colitis
   s. food poisoning
   nontyphoidal s.

salmonellosis
   nontyphoidal s.

salol test

salpingitis

salpinx

salt
  bile s's
  bismuth s.
  Carlsbad s.
  diuretic s.
  Glauber s.
  s.-losing nephritis
  Preston s.
  Rochelle s.
  Seignette s.

salt-and-pepper duodenal erosion

sample
  random stool s.
  stool s.

sampling
  tissue s.

Sam Roberts esophagoscope

sanded nucleus

Sand-Eze EGD pillow

Sandifer syndrome

Sandoz Caluso PEG gastrostomy tube

sandpaper gallbladder

Sandström's gland

sanguirenal

Santorini
  accessory duct of S.
  S. canal
  circular S. muscles
  duct of S.
  papilla of S.

saphenous
  accessory s. vein
  great s. vein
  s. loop fistula
  small s. vein

Sappey
  accessory portal system
    of S.

Sappey *(continued)*
  veins of S.

sarcocele

sarcohydrocele

sarcoidosis
  hepatic s.
  pancreatic s.

sarcoma *pl.* sarcomas, sarcomata
  clear cell s. of kidney
  embryonal s.
  Ewing s.
  gastric s.
  gastric Kaposi s.
  gastrointestinal Kaposi s.
  intracolonic Kaposi s.
  Kaposi s.
  Kupffer cell s.
  osteogenic s.

satellite lesion

satiety
  early s.

saturnine colic

saucerized biopsy

saw palmetto

sawtooth irregularity of bowel
  contour

SBFT
  small-bowel follow-through

SBO
  small-bowel obstruction

scale
  Goldberg Anorectic Attitude s.
  Graham s. for drug-induced
    gastric damage

scalpel
  s. blade

scan
  s.-directed biopsy

scan *(continued)*
  gallbladder s.
  gastroesophageal reflux s.
  hepatic blood pool s.
  hepatobiliary s.
  intercostal s.
  liver s.

scaphoid abdomen

scapus *pl.* scapi
  s. penis

Scardino-Prince ureteropelvioplasty

scarlatinal nephritis

Scarpa
  S. fascia
  S. sheath

scarring
  gastrostomy s.
  local s.
  postnecrotic s.

scatologic

scatoma

SCFA
  short-chain fatty acid

Schachowa spiral tubes

Schatzki ring

Schiff biliary cycle

Schindler esophagoscope

schistocystis

schistosomal
  s. bladder cancer
  s. bladder carcinoma
  s. dysentery
  s. liver disease

schistosomiasis
  Asiatic s.
  hepatic s.
  intestinal s.
  Japanese s.

schistosomiasis *(continued)*
  Manson s.
  Oriental s.

Schnidt gall duct forceps

Schoemaker
  S. anastomosis
  S. gastroenterostomy
  S. procedure

Schoenberg intestinal forceps

Schönlein
  S.-Henoch purpura
  S.-Henoch syndrome

Schüller
  S. ducts
  S. glands

Schwann cell

schwannian spindle cell

sciatic hernia

scintigraphic reflux

scintigraphy
  adrenal s.
  gastroesophageal s.
  hepatobiliary s.
  quantitative hepatitis B s.

scintiscan
  biliary s.
  gastroesophageal s.

scirrhous adenocarcinoma

scissors
  Buie rectal s.
  Doyen abdominal s.
  Mayo s.
  Panzer gallbladder s.

sclera
  anicteric s.
  icteric s.
  nonicteric s.

scleroderma
  s. bowel disease
  esophageal s.
  s. of esophagus

sclerosant
absolute alcohol s.

sclerosing
s. adenosis
s. agent
s. cholangitis
s. encapsulating peritonitis
s. hepatic carcinoma
intrahepatic s. cholangitis
s. peritonitis
primary s. cholangitis

sclerosis
alcohol s.
biliary s.
endoscopic s.
esophageal variceal s.
focal glomerular s.
gastric s.
glomerular s.
hepatic s.
hepatoportal s.
injection s.
multiple s.
peritoneal s.
progressive systemic s.
renal arteriolar s.
tuberous s.
variceal s.

sclerotherapy
esophageal variceal s.
fiberoptic injection s.
hemorrhoidal s.
variceal s. in esophagus

sclerotic stomach

scoliosis

scoop
Desjardins gallbladder s.
Ferguson gallstone s.
gallbladder s.
Mayo common duct s.
Mayo gallstone s.
Moynihan gallstone s.

scoparius

Scopinaro pancreaticobiliary
bypass

scorbutic
s. dysentery

score
Gleason s.

Scott jejunoileal bypass

"scotty dog" graft

screening
cancer s.
colon cancer s.
colonoscopy s.
s. colonoscopy

Scribner shunt

scrotal
s. hematocele
s. hernia
s. hydrocele
s. mass
s. raphe
s. septum

scrotectomy

scrotitis

scrotocele

scrotoplasty

scrotum
acute s.
s. lapillosum
watering-can s.

scybala (*plural of* scybalum)

scybalous

scybalum *pl.* scybala

sea anemone ulcer

searcher

second
s. convoluted tubule

secondary
s. achalasia
s. amyloidosis
s. bacterial peritonitis
s. biliary cirrhosis

secondary *(continued)*
    s. biliary fibrosis
    s. cholangitis
    s. closure
    s. contraction
    s. diaphragm
    s. impotence
    s. incontinence
    s. jejunal ulcer
    s. metastatic carcinoma
    s. peristaltic wave
    s. priapism
    s. pseudo-obstruction syndrome
    s. renal calculus
    s. surgery
    s. volvulus

second-look
    s.-l. laparotomy
    s.-l. operation

secretin
    s. test

secretion
    biliary cholesterol s.
    gastric acid s.
    gastrin s.
    idiopathic gastric acid s.
    mucoid s.
    pepsin s.

secretory
    s. diarrhea

section
    abdominal s.
    perineal s.
    permanent s.

sedation
    benzodiazepine conscious s.

seed

seeding
    malignant s.

segment
    aganglionic s. of colon
    anterior inferior s.
    anterior superior s.

segment *(continued)*
    ileocecal s.
    inferior s.
    s's of kidney
    posterior s.
    renal s's
    superior s.
    thin s.

segmental
    anterior s. artery of liver
    anterior inferior s. artery of kidney
    anterior superior s. artery of kidney
    s. appendicitis
    s. change
    s. colitis
    s. colonic adenomatous polyposis syndrome
    s. colonic resection
    s. colonic tuberculosis
    s. enteritis
    s. glomerulonephritis
    inferior s. artery of kidney
    s. ischemic colitis
    lateral s. artery of liver
    s. liver graft
    medial s. artery of liver
    posterior s. artery of kidney
    posterior s. artery of liver
    superior s. artery of kidney

segmentary pancreatitis

segmentation
    s. contraction
    haustral s.
    s. movement

segmentectomy of liver

segmented intestine

segmentum *pl.* segmenta
    segmenta renalia

segregator

Seignette salt

Seldinger cystic duct catheterization

selective
- s. cannulation
- s. ductal cannulation
- s. mesenteric angiography
- s. proximal vagotomy

self-induced
- s.-i. purging
- s.-i. vomiting

self-retaining catheter

semen

semenologist

semenology

semiflexible endoscope

semiformed stool

semilunar
- s. folds of colon
- s. fold of transversalis fascia
- s. valves of colon
- s. valves of Morgagni

seminal
- s. canal
- s. cells
- s. crest
- s. cyst
- s. ducts
- s. fluid
- s. gland
- s. granules
- s. hillock
- s. plasma
- s. vesicle

seminiferous
- convoluted s. tubules
- s. epithelium
- straight s. tubules
- s. tubules

seminologist

seminology

seminoma
- anaplastic s.
- classic s.

seminoma *(continued)*
- spermatocytic s.

seminuria

semi-open hemorrhoidectomy

semipedunculated lesion

semirigid endoscope

semisolid stool

senescent cell

Sengstaken
- S.-Blakemore esophageal balloon
- S.-Blakemore tube

senile nephrosclerosis

Senior-Loken syndrome

senna
- s. fluidextract
- s. syrup

sennoside

Senokot

Senokot-S

Sensa
- Hemoccult S.

sensation
- rectal s.

sensitivity
- anaphylactoid food s.

sensor
- FiberOptic s.

sensorium change

sensory
- s. finding
- s. paralytic bladder

sentinel
- s. clot
- s. fold
- s. gland
- s. hyperplastic polyp
- s. loop
- s. node

sentinel *(continued)*
    s. pile
    s. tag

separation
    cell s. technique

separator
    Benson pylorus s.

sepsis
    anorectal s.
    biliary s.
    gram-negative s.
    gram-positive s.
    intra-abdominal s.
    pancreatic s.

septal
    s. hematoma

septic
    s. cholangitis
    s. peritonitis
    s. shock
    s. wound

septicemia

septulum *pl.* septula
    septula testis

septum *pl.* septa
    s. bulbi urethrae
    s. glandis penis
    s. of glans penis
    pancreaticobiliary s.
    s. pectiniforme
    s. penis
    rectovesical s.
    s. rectovesicale
    s. renis
    scrotal s.
    s. scrotale
    s. scroti
    septa of testis

sequela *pl.* sequelae

sequence
    adenoma-carcinoma s.
    esophageal manometric s.
    metaplasia-dysplasia-carci-
      noma s.

sequencing analysis

sequential motility

sequestration of fluid

Serafini hernia

serangitis

serial cholangiogram

series
    Gastrografin GI s.
    GI s.

serocolitis

seroenteritis

seromuscular
    s. intestinal patch graft

serosa
    cecal s.
    gastric s.

serosal
    s. tear

serosanguineous drainage

serotonin
    s. antagonist
    s. cell

serous
    s. diarrhea
    s. hepatosis
    s. peritonitis

serpiginous

Sertoli
    S. cells
    S.-cell–only syndrome
    S. cell tumor
    column of S.
    S.-Leydig cell

serum
    s. amylase
    s. bile acid measurement
    s. bilirubin
    s. cholinesterase activity
    familial nephritis s.

serum *(continued)*
    s. ferritin
    s. haptoglobin
    s. hepatitis
    s. uric acid
    s. virus antibody

sessile
    s. adenoma
    s. hydatid
    s. lesion
    s. nodular carcinoma
    s. polyp

set
    Coloplast ostomy irrigation s.
    Dansac ostomy irrigation s.
    Eliminator nasal biliary catheter s.
    first s.
    French introducer s.

severe
    s. erosive esophagitis
    s. gastritis
    s. pain
    s. reflux esophagitis

sexual function

shadow
    obliteration of the psoas s.

shaft
    s. of penis

sham feeding
    s. f. test

sharp dissection

sharp-edged
    s.-e. orifice
    s.-e. tip

shave biopsy

sheath
    anterior rectus s.
    common s. of testis and spermatic cord
    fascial s. of prostate
    masculine s.

sheath *(continued)*
    perinephric s.
    rectus s.
    Scarpa s.

sheathing canal

shelf
    Blumer rectal s.
    mesocolic s.
    rectal s.

shellac calculus

shield
    Active Living incontinence s.
    Fuller rectal s.

shift
    fluid s.
    mediastinal s.

shifting dullness

Shiner tube

shock
    hypovolemic s.
    s. liver
    s. patient
    septic s.
    testicular s.

Shohl solution

Shouldice
    S. inguinal herniorrhaphy
    S. repair

short
    s.-bowel syndrome
    s.-chain fatty acid (SCFA)
    s. circuit
    s. gastric arteries
    s. gastric veins
    s.-gut syndrome
    s.-incubation hepatitis
    s.-segment lesion

shrunken liver

shotty lymph node

Shouldice inguinal herniorrhaphy

shrapnel-induced
  s.-i. biliary obstruction
  s.-i. obstructive jaundice

shrunken liver

shunt
  angiographic portacaval s.
  arteriovenous s.
  AV (arteriovenous) s.
  biliopancreatic s.
  Buselmeier s.
  Cimino s.
  congenital portacaval s.
  Denver s.
  Denver peritoneovenous s.
  distal splenorenal s.
  end-to-side portacaval s.
  esophageal s.
  extrahepatic s.
  gastric venacaval s.
  gastrorenal s.
  intrahepatic s.
  jejunoileal s.
  LeVeen ascites s.
  LeVeen peritoneal s.
  Linton s.
  mesocaval s.
  portacaval s.
  portosystemic s.
  postcaval s.
  Quinton-Scribner s.
  Ramirez s.
  Scribner s.
  side-to-side s.
  small-bowel s.
  splenorenal s.
  Thomas s.
  transhepatic portacaval s.
  transjugular intrahepatic
    portosystemic s. (TIPS)
  ventriculoperitoneal s.
  Warren s.

sialogastrone

sickle cell
  s. c. anemia
  s. c. nephropathy

sickness
  Jamaican vomiting s.

sideropenic dysphagia

siderosis
  hepatic s.
  urinary s.

side-to-side
  s.-t.-s. anastomosis
  s.-t.-s. shunt

side-viewing endoscope

Siffert method

sigmoid
  s. arteries
  s. colectomy
  s. colon
  s. colon volvulus
  s. curve
  s. cystoplasty
  s. disease
  s. diverticulitis
  s. diverticulum
  s.-end colostomy
  s. enterocystoplasty
  s. flexure
  s. fold
  s. folds of colon
  s. kidney
  s. loop
  s. loop reduction
  s.-loop rod colostomy
  s. rectum pouch
  s. ulcer
  s. valves of colon
  s. veins
  s. volvulus

sigmoidectomy

sigmoiditis

sigmoidopexy

sigmoidoproctostomy

sigmoidorectostomy

sigmoidoscope
  adult s.

sigmoidoscope *(continued)*
    American ACMI (S3565, TX-915) flexible fiberoptic s.
    fiberoptic s.
    flexible s.
    Lloyd-Davis s.
    rigid s.

sigmoidoscopy
    fiberoptic s.

sigmoidosigmoidostomy

sigmoidostomy

sigmoidotomy

sigmoidovesical

sign
    Aaron s.
    Blumberg s.
    Boas s.
    Boyce s.
    Brodie s.
    Christmas tree s.
    colon cutoff s.
    Cope s.
    Courvoisier s.
    Cullen s.
    double-bubble duodenal s.
    Federici s.
    flush-tank s.
    Gilbert s.
    Grey Turner s.
    Guyon s.
    Hennings s.
    Horn s.
    Howship-Romberg s.
    iliopsoas s.
    Kelly s.
    Lennhoff s.
    Lloyd s.
    McBurney s.
    Meltzer s.
    Murphy s.
    obturator s.
    Pfuhl s.
    Prehn s.
    psoas s.
    puddling s.

sign *(continued)*
    rebound s.
    Rocher s.
    Rosenbach s.
    Rovighi s.
    Rovsing s.
    string s.
    tethered-bowel s.
    Thornton s.
    Trimadeau s.
    Turner s.

signaling
    postreceptor s. of parietal cell

signet cell
    Dukes A, B, C s. c.

signet-ring cell

Silastic
    S. collar
    S. silo reduction of gastroschisis
    S. sling

silent
    s. abdomen
    s. aspiration
    s. gallstone
    s. peritonitis
    s. stone
    s. thrombosis

silicone elastomer ring vertical gastroplasty

Silon tent for gastroschisis

Silvestrini-Corda syndrome

simple mechanical obstruction

simple urethritis

Sims test

simultaneous pancreas-kidney

single-contrast barium enema

sinus *pl.* sinus, sinuses
    anal s's
    s. anales
    s. epididymidis

sinus *(continued)*
    s. of epididymis
    Guérin s.
    s. of kidney
    s. of Morgagni
    mucous s's of male urethra
    s. pocularis
    prostatic s.
    s. prostaticus
    rectal s's
    s. rectales
    renal s.
    s. renalis
    Rokitansky-Aschoff s's
    s. tenderness

sinusoid
    s.-lining cell

sinusoidal
    s. fibrosis

Sippy
    S. diet
    S. esophageal dilator

siqua

site
    bleeding s.
    stoma s.

situs
    abdominal s. inversus
    s. inversus

sitz bath
    HydraClense s. b.

Sitz Marker

Skene
    S. ducts
    S. glands
    S. tubules

skenitis

skenoscope

skin
    anicteric s.
    s. atrophy
    s. bleeding time
    s. crease

skin *(continued)*
    s. dimpling
    dry s.
    icteric s.
    jaundiced s.
    s. knife
    nonicteric s.
    ostomy s.
    peristomal s.
    s. staple
    s. tag
    s. turgor
    s. xanthoma

skinny-needle biopsy

skip
    s. appendicitis
    s. lesion

sleeve
    ileal s.

slide
    Hemoccult Sensa s.

sliding
    s. esophageal hiatal hernia
    s. hernia
    s. hiatal hernia

sling
    fascial s.
    rectus fascial s.
    intestinal s.
    Silastic s.
    suburethral s.
    vaginal wall s.

slip hernia

slipped
    s. hernia
    s. Nissen fundoplication
    s. Nissen repair

slit
    filtration s's
    s. membrane
    s. pores

slotted anoscope

sloughed papilla

sloughing of mucosa

slow
  s. colonic transit
  S. Fe
  s. transit constipation

sludge
  biliary s.
  gallbladder s.

slurry of stool

small
  s. bowel
  s.-droplet fatty liver
  s. iliac artery
  s. intestinal infarction
  s. intestinal stenosis
  s. intestinal villi
  s. intestine
  s. intestine bacterial over-
    growth
  s. intestine mesentery
  s. noncleaved-cell lym-
    phoma
  s. polyp removal
  s. saphenous vein

small-bowel
  s.-b. biopsy
  s.-b. enema
  s.-b. follow-through (SBFT)
  s.-b. infarct
  s.-b. obstruction (SBO)
  s.-b. shunt
  s.-b. tube
  video s.-b. enteroscopy

smiling incision

smoker
  s's palate
  s's tongue

smooth
  s. diet
  s. muscle isoform actin

snap-frozen biopsy

snare
  colorectal s.
  Douglas rectal s.
  Frankfeldt rectal s.

snare *(continued)*
  s. loop biopsy
  Norwood rectal s.
  open electrocautery s.
  oval s.
  rectal s.

soak
  perianal s.

soap colitis

soapsuds enema

Soave
  S. endorectal pull-through
  S. operation

soda
  baking s.
  bicarbonate of s.

sodium
  s. acetate
  s. acid phosphate
  s. balance
  s. benzoate
  s. bicarbonate
  s. biphosphate
  s. chloride irrigation
  s. chloride solution
  s. citrate
  dibasic s. phosphate
  docusate s.
  s. hyposulfite
  low s. diet
  monobasic s. phosphate
  s. phosphate
  s. phosphate and biphos-
    phate enema
  s. phosphates enema
  s. phosphates rectal solu-
    tion
  potassium s. tartrate
  s. retention
  s. sulfate
  s. thiosulfate

soft
  s. abdomen
  s. bland diet
  s. diet
  s. food dysphagia

soft *(continued)*
    s. stool
    s. tissue
    s. tissue mass

softener
    stool softener

softening
    s. of the stomach

soilage
    peritoneal s.

soiling
    colostomy s.

solid
    s. bolus challenge
    s.-cystic tumor of pancreas
    s. emptying
    s. food
    s. food digestion
    s. food dysphagia
    s. pseudopapillary tumor of
      pancreas
    s. tumor

solid-state esophageal manom-
    etry catheter

soluble liver antigen

solution
    Albright s.
    amino acid–based dialy-
      sate s.
    balanced electrolyte s.
    Balance lavage s.
    Belzer s.
    Belzer UW liver preserva-
      tion s.
    bile acid–EDTA s.
    buffer s.
    colonic lavage s.
    electrolyte flush s.
    Gastrolyte oral s.
    GoLYTELY s.
    iced lactated Ringer s.
    lactated Ringer s.
    lactulose s.
    lavage s.
    magnesium citrate oral s.

solution *(continued)*
    normal saline s.
    Pedialyte RS electrolyte s.
    Shohl s.
    sodium chloride s.
    sodium phosphates rec-
      tal s.
    warm saline s.

somatic pain

somatostatin (SS)
    antral s.
    s. cell

somatostatinoma

Somogyi unit

Sonne dysentery

sonographic pattern

sonography
    colonic transabdominal s.
      (CTAS)

sonoguided biopsy

sorbitol

sordes
    s. gastricae

sore
    canker s.
    pressure s.

sorter
    fluorescence-activated
      cell s. (FACS)

sorting
    fluorescence-activated
      cell s. (FACS)

sound
    absent bowel s's
    active bowel s's
    apical s.
    auscultation of bowel s's
    auscultatory s.
    bowel s's
    common duct s.
    diminished bowel s's
    esophageal s.

sound *(continued)*
    gurgling bowel s's
    high-pitched bowel s's
    hyperactive bowel s's
    hypoactive bowel s's
    Le Fort s.
    low-pitched bowel s's
    musical bowel s's
    normoactive bowel s's
    positive bowel s's
    quiet bowel s's
    rumbling bowel s's
    tinkling bowel s's
    urethral s.

source
    active s. of bleeding

sour stomach

Southern blot analysis

soya-induced enteropathy

Soyalac formula

soy-based formula

space
    anorectal s.
    Bowman s.
    capsular s.
    chyle s's
    dead s.
    deep postanal anorectal s.
    s's of Disse
    extraperitoneal s.
    extravascular s.
    intercostal s.
    intercostal supraclavicu-
      lar s.
    intersphincteric s.
    intersphincteric anorec-
      tal s.
    ischiorectal s.
    ischiorectal anorectal s.
    Kiernan s's
    Lesshaft s.
    s.-occupying lesion
    perianal s.
    perisinusoidal s's
    peritoneal s.
    preperitoneal s.

space *(continued)*
    preputial s.
    retroperitoneal s.
    s. of Retzius
    subhepatic s.
    subperitoneal appendicitis
    subphrenic s.
    subumbilical s.
    suprahepatic s.
    supraomental s.

span
    hepatic s.
    levator s.
    liver s.

Spanish collar

spasm
    acid-provoked s.
    cricopharyngeal s.
    diffuse esophageal s.
    esophageal s.

spasmodic stricture

spastic
    s. bladder
    s. bowel syndrome
    s. colon
    s. constipation
    s. dysuria
    s. esophagus
    s. gait
    s. ileus
    s. paraparesis

spatial change

spatium *pl.* spatia
    s. extraperitoneale

spatula
    Haberer abdominal s.

spatulation
    graft s.

specific
    s. activity
    s. gangrenous and ulcera-
      tive balanoposthitis
    s. gastritis

spectral analysis

spectrophotometric analysis

speculum *pl.* specula
Barr rectal s.
Barr-Shuford rectal s.
Brinkerhoff s.
Brinkerhoff rectal s.
Cook s.
Hinkle-James rectal s.
Hirschmann s.
Kelly s.
Martin s.
Martin and Davy s.
Mathews s.
rectal s.

Spencer disease

sperma

spermacrasia

spermagglutination

spermatemphraxis

spermatic
s. abscess
s. calculus
s. canal
s. cord
s. duct
external s. fascia
false s. vesicle
s. fistula
internal s. fascia

spermatism

spermatitis

spermatocele

spermatocelectomy

spermatocyst

spermatocystectomy

spermatocystitis

spermatocystotomy

spermatocytoma

spermatogenic

spermatogenous

spermatology

spermatopathia

spermatopathy

spermatopoietic

spermatorrhea

spermatoschesis

spermaturia

spermectomy

spermiation

spermiduct

spermocytoma

spermolith

spermoneuralgia

spermophlebectasia

spherospermia

sphincter
anal s.
s. ani
anorectal s.
artificial s.
s. atony
biliary s.
s. of Boyden
cardiac s.
cardioesophageal s.
choledochal s.
cricopharyngeal s.
s. dysfunction
esophageal s.
external anal s.
external s. muscle of anus
external rectal s.
s. function
gastroesophageal s.
Giordano s.
Glisson s.
Henle s.
s. of hepatopancreatic ampulla

sphincter *(continued)*
  Hyrtl s.
  ileocecal s.
  incompetent s.
  inguinal s.
  internal s.
  internal anal s.
  internal s. muscle of anus
  lower esophageal s.
  Lütkens s.
  s. muscle of bile duct
  s. muscle of hepatopan-
    creatic ampulla
  s. muscle of membranous
    urethra
  s. muscle of pylorus
  s. muscle of urethra
  s. muscle of urinary blad-
    der
  Nélaton s.
  neo-anal s.
  O'Beirne s.
  s. of Oddi
  s. of Oddi manometry
  s. of Oddi pressure
  pancreatic duct s.
  pancreaticobiliary s.
  pharyngoesophageal s.
  prepyloric s.
  pyloric s.
  s. reconstruction
  rectal s.
  s. tone
  upper esophageal s.
  s. urethrae
  s. vesicae
sphincteral
  s. achalasia
sphincterectomy
sphincteric
  s. mechanism
sphincterismus
sphincteritis
sphincterometry
sphincteroplasty

sphincteroscope
  Kelly s.
sphincterotome
sphincterotomy
  biliary s.
  external s.
  internal s.
  pancreatic duct s.
spider
  s. angioma
  colonic arterial s.
  s. nevus
  s. pelvis
  s. telangiectasia
spigelian
  s. hernia
  s. lobe
spike-burst electrical activity
spiking fever
spillage
  fecal s.
  s. of tumor cells
spinach stool
spinal
  s. cord necrosis
  s. fluid finding
spindle
  s. colonic groove
  urine s's
spindle cell
  schwannian s. c.
spinous tenderness
spiral
  s. bacteria
  s. cast
  s. fold
  s. fold of cystic duct
  s. tubule
  s. valve of cystic duct
  s. valve of Heister
spirillar dysentery

splanchnic

splanchnolith

splanchnopathy

splanchnotribe

spleen
    s. tip

splenalgia

splenectomy
    incidental s.

splenic
    s. abscess
    s. angiogram
    s. anlage
    s. arterial embolization
    s. artery
    s. atrophy
    s. AV fistula
    s. avulsion
    s. capillary hemangiomato-
    sis
    s. dullness
    s. flexure
    s. flexure carcinoma
    s. flexure of colon
    s. flexure colonoscopy
    s. flexure syndrome
    s. fossa of omental sac
    s. function
    s. hilum
    s. penetration
    s. rupture
    s. sac
    s. tissue
    s. trauma
    s. vein
    s. vein thrombosis

splenocolic
    s. ligament

splenodynia

splenogastric
    s. ligament
    s. omentum

splenomegalia

splenomegaly
    congenital s.
    congestive s.
    Egyptian s.
    Gaucher s.
    hemolytic s.
    infectious s.
    infective s.
    tropical s.

splenonephric

splenopancreatic

splenopathy

splenophrenic
    s. ligament

splenoportal
    s. hypertension

splenorenal
    s. angle
    s. bypass
    distal s. shunt
    s. ligament
    s. recess
    s. shunt
    s. venous anastomosis

splint
    Toronto s.

splinting of abdomen

split
    s. ileostomy
    s.-liver transplant
    s.-thickness skin graft

sponge
    absorbable s.
    absorbable gelatin s.

spongeitis

sponge kidney

spongiitis

spongiose urethra

spongiositis

spongy
s. body of male urethra
s. body of penis
s. urethra

spontaneous bacterial peritonitis

spoon
gall duct s.
Mayo common duct s.
Volkmann s. for pancreatic
calculus

sporadic dysentery

spore
fungal s.

spot
epigastric s.
hot s.
milk s's
tendinous s's

S pouch

spout
ileal s.

spread
hematogenous s. of infection

spreading factor

Sprinz
S.-Dubin syndrome
S.-Nelson syndrome

sprue
celiac s.
collagenous s.
hypogammaglobulinemic s.
nontropical s.
refractory s.
subclinical s.
tropical s.
unclassified s.

spurious
s. cast

spurious *(continued)*
s. tube cast

spurting blood

sputum
s. aeroginosum
green s.
icteric s.

squamous cell
esophageal s. c. carcinoma
s. c. papilloma
supraglottic s. c. carcinoma

squeeze pressure

SS
somatostatin

Ssabanejew-Frank operation

S-shaped ileal pouch-anal anastomosis

S-shaped reservoir

stable incision

stab wound drain

stack of coins appearance

staff

stage
anhepatic s. of liver transplantation
Dukes s.
Hoehn and Yahr s.
Tanner s.

staghorn calculus

staging
Ann Arbor cancer s.
s. of cancer
s. laparotomy
neoplasm s.
s. operation
operative s.
TNM system for tumor s.
tumor s.

stagnant
s. bile

stagnant *(continued)*
  s. loop syndrome

stain
  Gram s.
  Gram s. of stool
  hematoxylin s.
  hematoxylin and eosin s.
  Wright s. of stool

stalk
  polyp s.

Stamm
  S. gastroplasty
  S. gastrostomy

Staphylococcus aureus
  methicillin-resistant *S. aureus* (MRSA)

staple
  s. line dehiscence
  skin s.

stapler
  EEA s.
  EEA AutoSure s.
  GIA s.
  intraluminal s.
  LDS s.

stapling
  gastric s.

starch blocker

Starck dilator

stasis *pl.* stases
  antral s.
  bile s.
  biliary s.
  s. cirrhosis
  s. esophagitis
  fecal s.
  s. gallbladder
  gastric s.
  ileal s.
  intestinal s.
  liver s.
  pelvicaliceal s.
  s. syndrome

stasis *(continued)*
  s. ulceration
  urinary s.

State
  S. end-to-end anastomosis
  S. operation

static
  s. closure pressure
  s. compliance

status
  nutritional s.

steady pain

stearrhea

steatocele

steatohepatitis
  nonalcoholic s.

steatorrhea
  biliary s.
  idiopathic s.
  intestinal s.
  pancreatic s.

steatosis
  drug-induced s.
  hepatic s.
  toxic s.

Steinstrasse

stellar phosphate

stellate
  s. cell
  phagocytic s. cell
  s. veins of kidney
  s. venules of kidney

stenosis *pl.* stenoses
  ampullary s.
  anal s.
  anorectal s.
  antral s.
  aortic s.
  aortic valvular s.
  atherosclerotic s.
  benign s.
  benign papillary s.

stenosis *(continued)*
>> choledochoduodenal junctional s.
>> congenital s.
>> congenital hypertrophic pyloric s.
>> congenital pyloric s.
>> distal esophageal s.
>> duodenal s.
>> esophageal s.
>> hypertrophic pyloric s.
>> infantile hypertrophic gastric s.
>> infantile hypertrophic pyloric s.
>> malignant s.
>> pancreaticojejunostomy s.
>> papillary s.
>> pyloric s.
>> radiation s.
>> rectal s.
>> renal artery s.

stenotic
>> s. lesion
>> s. stoma

stent
>> Angiomed blue s.
>> Angiomed Puroflex s.
>> antireflux double-J s.
>> biliary s.
>> Braun s.
>> common bile duct s.
>> Eliminator biliary s.
>> Eliminator pancreatic s.
>> EndoCoil biliary s.
>> EsophaCoil esophageal s.
>> French s.
>> Greenen pancreatic s.
>> mesh s.
>> pancreatic s.
>> pancreatic duct s.
>> pigtail biliary s.
>> pigtail s.

stenting
>> biliary s.
>> endoscopic s.
>> endoscopic pancreatic s.

stenting *(continued)*
>> pancreatic transpapillary s.
>> tumor s.

stepladder incision technique

stercobilin

stercobilinogen

stercolith

stercoraceous
>> s. abscess
>> s. ulcer
>> s. vomiting

stercoral
>> s. abscess
>> s. appendicitis
>> s. colic
>> s. diarrhea
>> s. fistula
>> s. tumor
>> s. ulcer
>> s. ulceration

stercorolith

stercoroma

stercorous

stercus *pl.* stercora

sterile
>> s. dressing
>> s. pancreatic necrosis
>> s. peritonitis

sterility
>> male s.

sterilization

sterilize

sternzellen

steroid
>> anabolic s.
>> s.-dependent Crohn disease

stigmata of recent hemorrhage

stimulant
>> s. cathartic

stimulant *(continued)*
  s. laxative

stimulation
  anocutaneous s.
  hilum s.

stimulus
  external s.

Stokvis-Talma syndrome

stoma *pl.* stomas, stomata
  abdominal s.
  anastomotic s.
  Benchekroun s.
  bowel s.
  concealed umbilical s.
  ConvaTec Active Life s. cap
  diverting s.
  divided-s. colostomy
  dusky s.
  end s.
  end-loop s.
  gastrointestinal s.
  ileostomy s.
  Laws gastroplasty with Si-
    lastic collar–reinforced s.
  loop s.
  maturing of s.
  Mitrofanoff s.
  nippled s.
  permanent s.
  prolapsed s.
  retracted s.
  rosebud s.
  Silastic collar–reinforced s.
  s. site
  stenotic s.
  s. ulcer

stomach
  aberrant umbilical s.
  s. ache
  acid-suppressed s.
  anacidic s.
  anal electrical stimulation
  antrum of s.
  bilocular s.
  s. brush
  s. calculus

stomach *(continued)*
  cardia of s.
  cardiac s.
  cirrhosis of s.
  dilatation of the s.
  distal blind s.
  dumping s.
  functional disorder of
    the s.
  greater curvature of s.
  hourglass s.
  s. lavage
  leather bottle s.
  lesser curvature of s.
  s. neoplasm
  s. pump
  s. reefing
  sclerotic s.
  thoracic s.
  trifid s.
  s. tube
  upside-down s.
  waterfall s.
  watermelon s.

stomachal
  s. vertigo

stomachalgia

stomachic
  s. calculus

stomachodynia

stomal
  s. bag
  s. prolapse
  s. ulcer

stoma-like
  s. channel

stomata *(plural of* stoma)

stomatal

stomatitis *pl.* stomatitides
  aphthous s.
  erythematopultaceous s.
  herpetic s.
  tropical s.
  uremic s.

stone
    ampullary s.
    bile duct s.
    biliary tract s.
    bilirubinate s.
    black pigment s.
    bladder s.
    common bile duct s. (CBD
      stone)
    common duct s.
    gallbladder s.
    s. granuloma
    s. granuloma formation
    impacted s.
    impacted ampullary s.
    s. impaction
    infection s.
    intraluminal s.
    kidney s.
    mulberry s.
    pancreatic s.
    pancreatic duct s.
    s. retrieval balloon
    silent s.

Stone clamp applier

stone-searcher

stool
    acholic s.
    bilious s.
    black tarry s.
    blood in s.
    blood passed with s.
    blood-streaked s.
    blood on surface of s.
    bloody s.
    brown s.
    bulky s.
    butter s.
    clay-colored s.
    Clinitest-negative s.
    Clinitest-positive s.
    Clinitest s. test
    s. color
    continent of s.
    s. culture
    currant jelly s.
    dark s.

stool *(continued)*
    diarrhea s.
    s. evacuation
    fatty s.
    floating s.
    foamy s.
    formed s.
    foul-smelling s.
    frank blood in s.
    frequency of s.
    green s.
    guaiac-negative s.
    guaiac-positive s.
    hard s.
    heme-negative s.
    heme-positive s.
    impacted s.
    s. incontinence
    lienteric s.
    liquid s.
    loose s.
    malodorous s.
    maroon-colored s.
    melenic s.
    mucoid s.
    mucous s.
    mushy s.
    nonbloody s.
    s. for occult blood
    oily s.
    s. osmolality test
    s. osmotic gap
    s. for ova and parasites
    pale s.
    palpable s.
    passage of s.
    pea soup s.
    pelletlike s.
    pencil-thin s.
    pipestem s.
    rabbit s.
    residual s.
    s. retention
    ribbon s.
    runny s.
    sago-grain s.
    s. sample
    semiformed s.
    semisolid s.

stool *(continued)*
    slurry of s.
    soft s.
    s. softener
    spinach s.
    straining at s.
    tarry black s.
    undigested food in s.
    unformed s.
    watery s.
    Wright stain of s.

Storz esophagoscope

straight
    s. arteries of kidney
    s. arterioles of kidney
    s. collecting tubule
    distal s. tubule
    false s. arterioles of kidney
    s. intestine
    s. margin of testis
    proximal s. tubule
    s. seminiferous tubules
    true s. arterioles of kidney
    s. tubule
    s. venules of kidney

straining
    defecatory s.
    s. at stool

stranding
    soft tissue s.

strangulated
    s. bowel
    s. bowel obstruction
    s. hemorrhoid
    s. hernia
    s. viscus

strangulation necrosis

stranguria

strangury

stratum *pl.* strata
    s. circulare gastris
    s. circulare tunicae muscu-
        laris coli
    s. circulare tunicae muscu-
        laris gastris

stratum *(continued)*
    s. circulare tunicae muscu-
        laris intestini tenuis
    s. circulare tunicae muscu-
        laris recti
    s. circulare tunicae muscu-
        laris ventriculi
    s. circulare ventriculi
    s. externum tunicae muscu-
        laris ductus deferentis
    s. externum tunicae muscu-
        laris ureteris
    s. externum tunicae muscu-
        laris vesicae urinariae
    s. longitudinale gastris
    s. longitudinale tunicae
        muscularis coli
    s. longitudinale tunicae
        muscularis gastris
    s. longitudinale tunicae
        muscularis intestini te-
        nuis
    s. longitudinale tunicae
        muscularis recti
    s. longitudinale tunicae
        muscularis ventriculi
    s. longitudinale ventriculi
    s. medium tunicae muscu-
        laris ductus deferentis
    s. medium tunicae muscu-
        laris ureteris
    s. medium tunicae muscu-
        laris vesicae urinariae
    submucous s. of bladder
    submucous s. of colon
    submucous s. of rectum
    submucous s. of small in-
        testine
    submucous s. of stomach

strawberry
    s. gallbladder
    s. hemangioma

straw-colored ascites

strep
    anhemolytic s.
    hemolytic s.

streptococcal
    s. esophagitis

streptococcus
    alpha-hemolytic s.
    s. enteritis

Streptococcus viridans

stress
    s. erosion
    s. gastritis
    s. incontinence
    s.-induced gastric ulcer-
      ation
    s. lesion
    s. ulcer
    s. ulceration
    s. ulcer hemorrhage

Stresstein liquid feeding

stricture
    anal s.
    anastomotic s.
    annular esophageal s.
    antral s.
    benign s.
    benign bile duct s.
    benign biliary s.
    bile duct s.
    biliary s.
    biliary tract s.
    cicatricial s.
    colorectal s.
    contractile s.
    corrosive esophageal s.
    diaphragmlike s.
    distal esophageal s.
    ductal s.
    esophageal s.
    extrahepatic biliary s.
    filiform s.
    hourglass s.
    Hunner s.
    intestinal s.
    intrahepatic biliary s.
    irritable s.
    longitudinal esophageal s.
    malignant s.
    pancreatic duct s.

stricture *(continued)*
    peptic s.
    peptic esophageal s.
    postoperative s.
    s. prophylaxis
    pyloric s.
    rectal s.
    recurrent s.
    reflux-related s.
    spasmodic s.

strictured esophagus

strictureplasty

stricturoplasty

stricturotome

stricturotomy

string
    s. bladder
    s. sign

strip
    s. biopsy
    properitoneal flank s.

stripe
    inner s.
    outer s.

strongyloidiasis
    intestinal s.

struma
    Hashimoto s.

struvite
    s. calculus

studding
    omental s.
    peritoneal s.

study
    antegrade contrast s.
    anti–hepatitis A–IgM im-
      munological s.
    barium s.
    bulb tip retrograde s.
    cinefluorographic s.
    colonic transit s.
    colorectal physiologic s.
    Framingham follow-up s.

study (*continued*)
    hematologic s.

stump
    appendiceal s.
    blind s.
    dehiscence of s.
    duodenal s.
    gastric s.
    s. ligation
    rectal s.

stuttering
    urinary s.
    s. urination

stymatosis

S-type amylase

subabdominal

subabdominoperitoneal

subacute
    s. abscess
    s. atrophy of liver
    s. fatty liver of pregnancy
    s. glomerulonephritis
    s. hepatic necrosis
    s. hepatitis
    s. necrosis
    s. nephritis
    s. nonspecific peritonitis

subanal

subcapsular
    s. hematoma
    s. hemorrhage
    s. hepatic abscess

subcecal
    s. appendix
    s. fossa

subcarinal node

subchronic atrophy of liver

subclinical
    s. hepatitis
    s. sprue

subconjunctival hemorrhage

subcostal
    s. flank incision
    s. incision
    s. port
    s. transperitoneal incision

subcutaneous
    s. fat
    s. fungus
    s. tissue
    s. veins of abdomen

subdiaphragmatic
    s. abscess

subfulminant liver failure

subglottic lesion

subhepatic
    s. abscess
    s. area
    s. recesses
    s. space

subicteric

sublobular
    s. veins

submassive hepatic necrosis

submucosa

submucosal
    s. calculus
    s. gastric hemorrhage
    s. lesion
    s. mass
    s. tattoo
    s. thickening

submucous
    s. cystitis
    s. lamina of stomach
    s. layer of bladder
    s. layer of colon
    s. layer of esophagus
    s. layer of small intestine
    s. layer of stomach
    s. layer of urinary bladder
    s. membrane of stomach
    s. stratum of bladder

submucous *(continued)*
s. stratum of colon
s. stratum of rectum
s. stratum of small intestine
s. stratum of stomach
s. ulcer

subperitoneal
s. abscess
s. appendicitis
s. fascia
s. space

subperitoneoabdominal

subperitoneopelvic

subphrenic
s. abscess
s. part of esophagus
s. recesses
s. space

subpreputial

subpubic

subrectal

subsegmentectomy
hepatic s.

subserous
s. layer of gallbladder
s. layer of liver
s. layer of peritoneum
s. layer of small intestine
s. layer of stomach
s. layer of urinary bladder

subsigmoid
s. fossa

substance
s. abuse
cortical s. of kidney
medullary s. of kidney
s. P

substantia *pl.* substantiae
s. corticalis renis
s. glandularis prostatae

substantia *(continued)*
s. medullaris renis
s. muscularis prostatae

substitute
olestra fat s.
saliva s.

subsymphyseal epispadias

subtotal
s. colectomy
s. gastrectomy
s. pancreatectomy

subtraction angiography

subumbilical
s. space

suburethral
s. sling

succus *pl.* succi
s. entericus
s. gastricus
s. pancreaticus
s. prostaticus

suction
s. biopsy
s. drainage
Gomco s.
lavage and s.
s. lipectomy
low intermittent s.
nasogastric (NG) s.
s. pump
s. tip
s. tube
Wangensteen s.

suctioning
intermittent s.

sudden onset of pain

Sudeck atrophy

sugar
fasting blood s. (FBS)
s.-icing liver
s. indigestion

Sugiura procedure

suite
    endoscopy s.

sulcus *pl.* sulci
    angular s.
    s. intermedius gastricus
    paracolic sulci
    sulci paracolici
    s. for vena cava
    s. venae cavae

sulfacytine

sulfaethidole

sulfaguanidine

sulfalene

sulfamethizole

sulfamethoxazole

sulfamethoxypyridazine

sulfamethylthiadiazole

sulfanuria

sulfasalazine

sulfate
    ferrous s.

sulfisomidine

sulfobromophthalein
    s. excretion test
    s. sodium

sulfolithocholylglycine

sulfolithocholyltaurine

sulfuric acid

summer
    s. cholera
    s. diarrhea

summit
    s. of bladder

sump
    s. drain
    s. nasogastric tube

sump *(continued)*
    s.-Penrose drain
    s. ulcer

superficial
    s. abdominal ring
    chronic s. gastritis
    s. epigastric artery
    s. epigastric vein
    s. esophageal carcinoma
    s. external pudendal artery
    s. fascia of perineum
    s. gastric carcinoma
    s. gastritis
    s. inguinal ring
    s. layer of fascia of peri-
        neum
    s. layer of triangular liga-
        ment
    s. perineal fascia
    s. tumor

superimposed alcoholic hepati-
    tis

superinfection
    delta hepatitis s.
    hepatitis D s.

superior
    s. aberrant ductule
    s. angle of duodenum
    s. border of body of pan-
        creas
    s. border of pancreas
    s. duodenal fold
    s. duodenal fossa
    s. epigastric artery
    s. epigastric veins
    s. flexure of duodenum
    s. fossa of omental sac
    s. hemorrhoidal artery
    s. ileocecal fossa
    s. layer of pelvic dia-
        phragm
    s. ligament of epididymis
    s. lip of ileocecal valve
    s. margin of pancreas
    s. mediastinal cavity
    s. mesenteric angiography
    s. mesenteric artery

superior *(continued)*
    s. mesenteric artery syndrome
    s. mesenteric vein
    s. mesenterorenal bypass
    s. rectal artery
    s. rectal vein
    s. segment
    s. segmental artery of kidney
    s. suprarenal arteries
    s. thoracic aperture
    s. vesical arteries

supernumerary kidney

superselective vagotomy

support
    artificial hepatic s.
    nutritional s.
    s. parenteral nutrition

suppository
    rectal s.
    vaginal s.

suppression
    acid s.
    cell-mediated s.

suppressive anuria

suppurative
    acute s. cholangitis
    acute s. nephritis
    acute obstructive s. cholangitis
    s. appendicitis
    s. appendix
    s. cholangitis
    chronic s. nephritis
    s. nephritis
    progressive s. cholangitis
    s. pyelitis

suppressor T cell

supra-anal

supraceliac aorta

supradiaphragmatic
    s. diverticulum

supraduodenal
    s. artery

supraglottic squamous cell carcinoma

suprahepatic
    s. abscess
    s. space

suprainguinal

supraintestinal

supralevator
    s. abscess
    s. pelvic exenteration
    s. perirectal abscess

supraomental
    s. space

suprapelvic

suprapubic
    s. cystostomy
    s. cystotomy
    s. lithotomy
    s. transvesical prostatectomy

suprarenal
    aortic s. artery
    s. gland
    s. impression of liver
    inferior s. artery
    left s. vein
    middle s. artery
    right s. vein
    superior s. arteries

supraumbilical

supravesical

surface
    anterior s. of kidney
    anterior s. of pancreas
    anterior s. of stomach
    anteroinferior s. of body of pancreas
    anterosuperior s. of body of pancreas
    cut s. of liver
    diaphragmatic s. of liver

surface *(continued)*
    s. nodularity
    s. nodule
    posterior s. of body of pancreas
    posterior s. of kidney
    posterior s. of stomach
    ventral s.

Surfak

surgery
    abdominal s.
    anorectal s.
    antireflux s.
    bariatric s.
    colorectal s.
    intestinal s.
    radical s.
    rectovaginal s.
    secondary s.

surgical
    s. abdomen
    complete s. exploration
    s. extirpation
    s. flap
    s. gut
    s. incision
    s. kidney
    s. triangle
    s. vagotomy

Surgitek One-Step percutaneous endoscopic gastrostomy

Surgiwip suture ligature

surreptitious vomiting

survival
    graft s.

suspension
    barium s.
    charcoal s.
    oral barium s.

suspensorius

suspensory
    s. ligament of bladder
    s. ligament of liver
    s. ligament of penis

suspensory *(continued)*
    s. ligament of spleen
    s. muscle of duodenum

Sustacal
    S. HC liquid feeding
    S. pudding

Sustagen liquid feeding

sustentacular

sustentaculum *pl.* sustentacula
    s. lienis

suture
    absorbable s.
    Albert s.
    anastomotic s.
    anchoring s.
    Appolito s.
    Connell s.
    Cushing s.
    Czerny s.
    Czerny-Lembert s.
    Dupuytren s.
    furrier s.
    Gély s.
    glover s.
    s. granuloma
    Gussenbauer s.
    Halsted s.
    heavy silk s.
    hemostatic s.
    Horsley s.
    inverting s.
    Lembert s.
    s. ligature
    s. line dehiscence
    lock-stitch s.
    loop s.
    s. material
    over-and-over s.
    pericostal s.
    pursestring s.
    retention s.
    traction s.

suture applier
    Advanced surgical s. a.

sutureless bowel anastomosis

swallow
  barium s.
  dry s.
  Gastrografin s.
  Hypaque s.
  ice-water s.
  modified barium s.
  water-soluble contrast eso-
    phageal s.

swallowing
  four phases of s.
  s. mechanism

sweep
  duodenal s.

swelling
  cell s.
  external s.

swollen tongue

Swenson operation

sychnuria

Sydney
  S. classification of gastritis
  S. system gastritis classifi-
    cation

sylvian fistula

Symmers fibrosis

sympathetic
  s. nervous system activity

symphyseal bar

symptom
  gastrointestinal s.
  incarceration s.

symptomatic gallstone

symptomatology
  chronic functional s.

Syms tractor

synanthrin

syncholia

synchondroseotomy

synchronous
  s. adenomas
  s. lesion
  s. polyp

syncope
  defecation s.

syncytial giant-cell hepatitis

syndrome
  abdominal muscle deficien-
    cy s.
  acquired immunodeficien-
    cy s. (AIDS)
  acute flank pain s.
  adult respiratory distress s.
  acute nephritic s.
  Addison s.
  adrenogenital s.
  adult respiratory distress s.
    (ARDS)
  afferent loop s.
  anorexia-cachexia s.
  anterior abdominal wall s.
  anterior cord s.
  apple-peel bowel s.
  argentaffinoma s.
  autoimmune deficiency s.
  bacterial overgrowth s.
  Barrett s.
  Bartter s.
  Bearn-Kunkel s.
  Bearn-Kunkel-Slater s.
  Behçet s.
  blind loop s.
  Boerhaave s.
  BOR s.
  Bouveret s.
  bowel bypass s.
  branchio-oto-renal s.
  brown bowel s. (BBS)
  Budd-Chiari s.
  Bywaters s.
  Canada-Cronkhite s.
  carcinoid s.
  celiac s.
  cerebrohepatorenal s.

syndrome *(continued)*
  Charcot s.
  Chiari s.
  Chilaiditi s.
  cholestatic s.
  chronic intestinal ischemic s.
  compression s.
  constipation-predominant irritable bowel s.
  Courvoisier-Terrier s.
  Crigler-Najjar s.
  Cronkhite-Canada s.
  crush s.
  Cruveilhier-Baumgarten s.
  del Castillo s.
  de Toni-Fanconi s.
  dialysis dysequilibrium s.
  diarrheogenic s.
  Dubin-Johnson s.
  Dubin-Sprinz s.
  dumping s.
  Eagle-Barrett s.
  embryonic testicular regression s.
  Epstein s.
  familial medullary thyroid carcinoma-pheochromocytoma s.
  Fanconi s.
  Fitz-Hugh–Curtis s.
  flulike s.
  fragile X s.
  Fraser s.
  functional bowel s.
  functional prepubertal castrate s.
  gas-bloat s.
  Gasser s.
  gastrointestinal immunodeficiency s.
  gastrojejunal loop obstruction s.
  Gee-Herter-Heubner s.
  Gilbert s.
  Gitelman s.
  glioma-polyposis s.
  Goodpasture s.
  HELLP s.

syndrome *(continued)*
  hematuria-dysuria s.
  hemolytic uremic s.
  Henoch-Schönlein s.
  hepatorenal s.
  Hinman s.
  hypotonic s's
  iatrogenic immunodeficiency s.
  ileocecal s.
  inflammatory bowel s. (IBS)
  inspissated bile s.
  irritable bowel s. (IBS)
  irritable colon s.
  jejunal s.
  juvenile polyposis s.
  Kimmelstiel-Wilson s.
  König s.
  Kunkel s.
  late dumping s.
  Laubry-Soulle s.
  levator s.
  Liddle s.
  Lightwood s.
  Lignac s.
  Lignac-Fanconi s.
  liver-kidney s.
  Mallory-Weiss s.
  megacystis-megaureter s.
  megacystis-microcolon–intestinal hypoperistalsis s. (MMIHS)
  minimal change nephrotic s.
  nephrotic s.
  obesity hypoventilation s.
  Ogilvie s.
  Oldfield s.
  ovarian hyperstimulation s.
  ovarian remnant s.
  ovarian vein s.
  pancreatic cholera s.
  pancreaticohepatic s.
  pericolic membrane s.
  Perlman s.
  Peutz-Jeghers s.
  postcholecystectomy s.
  postfundoplication s.
  postgastrectomy s.

syndrome *(continued)*
>   s. of primary biliary cirrho-
>   sis
>   Reichmann s.
>   Roger s.
>   Rotor s.
>   Roux stasis s.
>   Rovsing s.
>   rudimentary testis s.
>   Sandifer s.
>   Schönlein-Henoch s.
>   secondary pseudo-obstruc-
>   tion s.
>   segmental colonic adenom-
>   atous polyposis s.
>   Senior-Loken s.
>   Sertoli-cell–only s.
>   short-bowel s.
>   short-gut s.
>   Silvestrini-Corda s.
>   spastic bowel s.
>   splenic flexure s.
>   Sprinz-Dubin s.
>   Sprinz-Nelson s.
>   stagnant loop s.
>   stasis s.
>   Stokvis-Talma s.
>   superior mesenteric ar-
>   tery s.
>   Thorn s.
>   toxic shock s.
>   Turcot s.
>   urethral s.
>   vanishing testes s.
>   Verner-Morrison s.
>   WDHA s.
>   WDHH s.
>   Young s.
>   Zollinger-Ellison s.

synechtenterotomy

syngeneic transplantation

syngenesioplastic transplantation

synorchidism

synorchism

synoscheos

synthase
>   citrate s.

synthetic
>   s. mesh
>   s. vascular graft

syphilitic
>   s. cirrhosis
>   s. gastritis
>   s. nephritis

syrup
>   ipecac s.
>   lactulose s.
>   senna s.

system
>   Abbott Lifeshield needle-
>   less s.
>   accessory portal s. of Sap-
>   pey
>   AJCC/UICC staging s.
>   alimentary s.
>   anomalous arrangement of
>   pancreaticobiliary duc-
>   tal s. (AAPBDS)
>   Atkinson scoring s. for dys-
>   phagia
>   automated endoscopic s.
>   for optimal positioning
>   (AESOP)
>   BICAP Hemorrhoid S.
>   BICAP Hemostatic S.
>   Cell Soft S.
>   digestive s.
>   ductal s.
>   Dukes staging s.
>   Edmondson grading s. for
>   hepatocellular carcinoma
>   gastrointestinal s.
>   genitourinary s.
>   glucose transport s.
>   Hopkins rod-lens s. for
>   rigid choledochoscope
>   mechanical assist s.
>   O'Sullivan scoring s.
>   pelvicaliceal s.
>   Ranson grading s.

system *(continued)*
  renin-angiotensin s.
  renin-angiotensin-aldoster-
    one s.
  Sacks-Vine PEG s.
  Sydney s. gastritis classifi-
    cation
  TNM s. for tumor staging
  urinary s.
  urogenital s.

systema
  s. digestorium
  s. urogenitale

systematic sextant biopsy

systemic
  s. arterial pressure
  s. effect
  s. fungus

T_m

tabetic bladder

tache
    t. blanche

tachyalimentation

tachygastria

tactoid

tadpole-like appearance

taenia *pl.* taeniae
    taeniae coli
    t. libera
    t. mesocolica
    t. omentalis
    taeniae pylori
    taeniae of Valsalva

taenial

tag
    edematous t.
    external skin t.
    hemorrhoidal t.
    perianal skin t.
    perineal skin t.
    sentinel t.
    skin t.

Tagamet
    T. HB

tail
    t. of epididymis
    t. of pancreas

takedown
    colostomy t.
    t. of colostomy

taking down of adhesions

talc embolus

Tamm
    T.-Horsfall mucoprotein
    T.-Horsfall protein

tamponade
    balloon t.

tamponade *(continued)*
    esophageal balloon t.
    esophagogastric t.

tamponage

tamponing

tampon tube

tandem colonoscopy

tangential
    t. biopsy
    t. colonic submucosal in-
        jection

tangle of hemorrhoidal veins

Tanner
    T. operation
    T. stage

tannic acid

tap
    abdominal t.
    peritoneal t.
    t. water enema

tape
    adhesive t.
    appendectomy t.
    laparotomy t.

tapeworm
    beef t.
    Cestoda t.
    fish t.
    pork t.

target
    t. gland
    t. lesion

target cell
    non–antigen-expressing
        t. c.

tarry black stool

tartar
    cream of t.

tattoo
    colonoscopic t.

tattoo *(continued)*
    endoscopic t.
    submucosal t.

tattooing
    four-quadrant t.

taurine

taurochenodeoxycholic acid

taurocholaneresis

taurocholanopoiesis

taurocholate

taurocholic acid

Taylor gastric balloon

T cell
    T c. adhesion
    effector T c. function
    T c. function
    T c. growth factor
    HBV-specific T c.
    T c. lymphoma
    peripheral T c.
    suppressor T c.

tear
    capsular t.
    diastatic serosal t.
    esophageal t.
    gastric t.
    Mallory-Weiss t.
    mesenteric t.
    mucosal t.
    pharyngoesophageal t.
    serosal t.

tearing
    t. pain
    t. trough

TEC
    transpapillary endoscopic
      cholecystectomy

technique
    abdominal pressure t.
    Belt t.
    blind t.
    Brackin t.

technique *(continued)*
    cell separation t.
    Farr t.
    fiberoptic instrument t.
    Hartmann reconstruction t.
    Hofmeister t.
    hot biopsy t.
    lateral window t.
    LeDuc t.
    Lich t.
    Marlex plug t.
    Mitrofanoff t.
    orbital exenteration gastro-
      scopic access t.
    patch t.
    pull-through t.
    reconstruction t.

T effector cell

Teflon
    T. ERCP cannula
    T. nasobiliary drain
    T. tube

Tegaderm dressing

tela *pl.* telae
    t. submucosa esophagi
    t. submucosa gastris
    t. submucosa intestini
      crassi
    t. submucosa intestini te-
      nuis
    t. submucosa oesophagi
    t. submucosa recti
    t. submucosa ventriculi
    t. submucosa vesicae uri-
      nariae
    t. subserosa gastris
    t. subserosa hepatis
    t. subserosa intestini crassi
    t. subserosa intestini tenuis
    t. subserosa peritonei
    t. subserosa ventriculi
    t. subserosa vesicae biliaris
    t. subserosa vesicae felleae
    t. subserosa vesicae urina-
      riae

telangiectasia
    duodenal t.

telangiectasia *(continued)*
    gastrointestinal t.
    hepatic t.
    hereditary hemorrhagic t.
    Osler-Weber-Rendu t.
    radiation t.
    spider t.

telangiectatic
    t. angioma
    t. vessel

telar

telemetering capsule

telescope
    forward-viewing t.

Telfa dressing

telotism

temp end colostomy

temporary
    t. end colostomy
    t. loop ileostomy

Tenckhoff
    T. catheter
    T. peritoneal catheter

tender
    t. liver
    t. thyroid

tenderness
    adnexal t.
    ballottement t.
    bony t.
    cervical motion t.
    costochondral t.
    costovertebral angle t.
    diffuse t.
    exquisite t.
    focal t.
    frontal t.
    localizing t.
    palpation t.
    percussion t.
    point t.
    popliteal t.
    rebound t.
    rectal t.

tenderness *(continued)*
    salivary t.
    sinus t.
    spinous t.
    thyroid t.
    uterine t.

tendinous
    t. arch of levator ani muscle
    t. spots

tendo *pl.* tendines
    t. cricooesophageus

tendon
    cricoesophageal t.

tenesmus
    rectal t.
    vesical t.

tenia *(variant of* taenia*)*
    teniae coli
    tenia libera
    tenia mesocolica
    tenia omentalis
    teniae pylori
    teniae of Valsalva

tenial

teniamyotomy

tense ascites

tension-free
    t.-f. anastomosis
    t.-f. hernioplasty

teratocarcinogenesis

teratocarcinoma

teratoma *pl.* teratomas, teratomata
    benign cystic t.
    malignant t.

teratospermia

terminal
    t. bile duct
    t. colostomy
    t. enteritis
    t. fossa

terminal *(continued)*
    t. ileal pouch
    t. ileal resection
    t. ileitis
    t. ileostomy
    t. ileum
    t. ileus
    t. peritonitis

terminus
    amino t.
    duodenal t.
    intrapapillary t.

terrifying pain

tertiary
    t. contraction
    t. radicle

Tesberg esophagoscope

test
    acid clearance t. (ACT)
    acidemia of stool t.
    acid hemolysis t.
    acid perfusion t.
    acid reflux t.
    alkalinization t.
    angiotensin II infusion t.
    anorectal t.
    augmented histamine t.
    Baermann stool t.
    belt t.
    Bernstein t.
    bile acid breath t.
    bile acid tolerance t.
    bile solubility t.
    bilirubin t.
    Boas t.
    cellobiose/mannitol sugar t.
    chew-and-spit t.
    Chiron RIBA HCV (hepatitis C virus) t.
    citrate t.
    Clinitest stool t.
    colonic transit t.
    diabetes home screening t.
    Einhorn string t.
    esophageal acid infusion t.
    esophageal function t.
    fecal fat t.

test *(continued)*
    fecal occult blood t.
    Fishberg concentration t.
    flocculation t.
    fluorescent treponemal antibody absorption t.
    followup t.
    Frei t.
    fructose tolerance t.
    FTA t.
    FTA-ABS t.
    gastric accommodation t.
    gastric function t.
    Gastroccult t.
    glucagon t.
    glucose tolerance t. (GTT)
    glycyltryptophan t.
    Hamel t.
    Hematest t.
    Hema-Wipe t.
    Hemoccult t.
    Hemoccult II t.
    Hemoccult Sensa t.
    HemoSelect t.
    hepatic function t.
    Histalog t.
    histamine t.
    Huhner t.
    iliopsoas t.
    inulin clearance t.
    irrigation t.
    Jadassohn t.
    Jatrox *Helicobacter pylori* t.
    Javorski t.
    Jaworski t.
    Jones and Cantarow t.
    kidney function t.
    lipase t.
    liver function t. (LFT)
    Lundh t.
    Macdonald t.
    MacLean-de Wesselow t.
    McNemar ascites t.
    t. meal
    MEGX t.
    monoethylglycinexylidide t.
    Moynihan t.
    Neubauer and Fischer t.

test *(continued)*
    obturator t.
    Palmer acid t. for peptic ulcer
    pancreatic function t.
    pancreatic secretory t.
    phenoltetrachlorophthalein t.
    qualitative fecal fat t.
    quantitative fecal fat t.
    Quick t.
    radioisotope renal excretion t.
    Rehberg t.
    renal function t.
    rose bengal t.
    Rotazyme t.
    Sahli-Nencki t.
    salol t.
    secretin t.
    sham feeding t.
    Sims t.
    stool osmolality t.
    sulfobromophthalein excretion t.
    thallium exercise stress t.
    thallium exercise stress t. fundoplasty
    urea breath t.
    urea concentration t.
    Urecholine supersensitivity t.
    water-gurgle t.
    Whipple t.
    Woldman t.

testalgia

testectomy

testes

testicle

testicular
    t. feminization
    t. shock
    t. torsion
    t. tubular adenoma

testiculoma

testiculus *pl.* testiculi

testing
    anorectal physiology t.

testis *pl.* testes
    abdominal t.
    common sheath of t. and spermatic cord
    Cooper irritable t.
    ectopic t.
    inverted t.
    obstructed t.
    parenchyma t.
    parenchyma of t.
    t. redux
    retained t.
    retractile t.
    undescended t.

testitis

test meal
    Ewald t. m.

testopathy

tetany
    gastric t.

tethered-bowel sign

texture
    heterogeneous t.
    homogeneous t.

Thal
    T. esophagogastroscopy
    T. procedure

thallium
    t. exercise stress test
    t. exercise stress test fundoplasty

thamuria

Thaysen disease

Theile glands

theophylline
    t. olamine enema
    t. toxicity

theory
    forbidden clone t.
    germ line t.

therapeutic
    t. angiography
    t. colonoscopy
    t. endoscopy
    t. laparoscopy
    t. upper endoscopy
    t. value

therapy
    acid-suppression t.
    adrenalin injection t.
    alpha interferon t.
    antibiotic t.
    antireflux t.
    bile acid t.
    bismuth-free triple t.
    bubble t.
    chemoradiation t.
    continuous renal replace-
      ment t.
    drug t.
    esophageal photodynam-
      ic t.
    external beam radiation t.
    H_2 antagonist t.
    heater probe t.
    H_2 receptor antagonist t.
    interferon t.
    nutritional t.
    omeprazole-clarithromycin-
      amoxicillin t.
    palliative t.
    radiation t.
    renal replacement t.
    triple t.

thermometer
    Celsius t.
    centigrade t.
    Fahrenheit t.
    oral t.
    rectal t.

thick
    t. adhesion
    t. ascending limb

thick (continued)
    t. bile

thickened gallbladder wall

thickening
    apical t.
    mediastinal t.
    plaquelike t.
    submucosal t.
    wall t.

thickness
    esophageal wall t.
    mucous gel t.

thick-walled gallbladder

Thiersch anal incontinence operation

thigh graft arteriovenous fistula

thin
    t. adhesion
    t. ascending limb
    t. basement membrane ne-
      phropathy
    t. segment
    t. tubule

thin-needle
    t.-n. percutaneous cholan-
      giogram

thin-walled gallbladder

thirst fever

Thomas shunt

thoracal

thoraces

thoracic
    t. aorta
    t. aortorenal bypass
    t. esophagus
    t. fistula
    inferior t. aperture
    t. kidney
    t. part of esophagus
    t. stomach
    superior t. aperture

thoracicoabdominal

thoracoabdominal
    t. aorta
    t. incision

thoracoepigastric
    t. veins

thoracolaparotomy

thoracotomy
    esophagectomy with t.

thorax

Thorn syndrome

Thornton sign

three-drug regimen

threshold
    renal t.
    renal t. for glucose

thrive
    failure to t.

thrombolytic agent

thrombosed
    t. hemorrhoid
    t. internal and external
      hemorrhoid

thrombosis
    bland t.
    hepatic vein t.
    mesenteric arterial t.
    mesenteric venous t.
    nonocclusive mesenteric t.
    peripheral venous t.
    silent t.
    splenic vein t.
    venous t.

thrombus *pl.* thrombi
    bile t.
    mural t.

through
    t. drainage

through-the-scope
    t.-t.-s. balloon
    t.-t.-s. balloon removal

through-the-scope *(continued)*
    t.-t.-s. dilation

thrush
    oral t.

thymus
    t.-derived cell
    t. gland

thyroid
    t. gland
    t. nodule
    tender t.
    t. tenderness

thyroiditis
    Hashimoto t.

tidal drainage

Tigan

tight
    t. abdomen
    t. adhesion
    t. Nissen repair

time
    abdominopelvic orocecal
      transit t.
    activated partial thrombo-
      plastin t.
    activated thromboplastin t.
    bleeding t.
    chromoscopy t.
    colonic transit t.
    dextrinizing t.
    emptying t.
    esophageal transit t.
    gastric bleeding t.
    gastric emptying t.
    gastric transit t.
    orocecal transit t.
    skin bleeding t.
    transit t.

tincture
    belladonna t.
    t. of benzoin
    camphorated opium t.

tinidazole

tinkling bowel sounds

tip
    Buie rectal suction t.
    Buie suction t.
    filiform t.
    open-end flo-thru radio-
        paque t.
    papillary t.
    sharp-edged t.
    spleen t.
    suction t.
    vessel t.

TIPS
    transjugular intrahepatic
        portosystemic shunt
        stenosis of TIPS

tissue
    acinar t.
    adipose t.
    ampullary granulation t.
    cicatricial t.
    connective t.
    t. culture
    extraperitoneal t.
    fatty t.
    fibroadipose t.
    fibroelastic t.
    fibroelastic connective t.
    fibrous t.
    t. forceps
    gut-associated lymphoid t.
        (GALT)
    lipomalike t.
    lipomatous t.
    mucosa-associated lym-
        phoid t. (MALT)
    t. necrosis
    necrotic t.
    neoplastic t.
    nonviable t.
    parenchymal t.
    t. plasminogen activator
        (TPA)
    redundant t.
    t. sampling
    soft t.
    splenic t.
    subcutaneous t.

tissue (continued)
    t.-type plasminogen activa-
        tor (t-PA)

tissue adhesive
    fibrin t. a.

titer
    anti-HSV IgM Ab t.

Titralac Plus

TLA
    transperitoneal laparo-
        scopic adrenalectomy

TNM
    tumor-node-metastasis
        TNM classification of
            carcinoma
        TNM system for tumor
            staging

Todd
    T. cirrhosis
    T. process

tolbutamide
    t.-induced cholestasis

Toldt membrane

tolerance
    oral t.

tolterodine tartrate

tomography
    computed t. (CT)

tone
    anal sphincter t.
    bowel t.
    lower esophageal sphinc-
        ter t.
    sphincter t.

tongue
    bifid t.
    black hairy t.
    t. deviation
    fissured t.
    hairy t.
    t. movement
    mucosal t.

tongue *(continued)*
    smoker's t.
    swollen t.

tongue-shaped villus

tonic
    bitter t.
    t. contraction

tonsil
    orange-colored t.

tooth grasper
    Allis t. g.

topical
    t. anesthesia
    t. anesthetic
    t. antibiotic
    t. oropharyngeal anesthesia

Torek operation

tormina

torminal

Toronto splint

torsion
    adnexal t.
    biliary tract t.
    gallbladder t.
    testicular t.

tortuous
    t. esophagus
    t. venous ectasia

torus *pl.* tori
    t. uretericus

Toshiba video endoscope

total
    t. abdominal colectomy
    t. abdominal evisceration
    t. bilateral vagotomy
    t. bilirubin
    t. bowel rest
    t. colonoscopy
    t. enteral nutrition
    t. gastrectomy
    t. infarction

total *(continued)*
    t. internal reflection
    t. pancreatectomy
    t. parenteral alimentation
    t. parenteral nutrition
      (TPN)
    t. pelvic exenteration

touch
    rectal t.

Touhy-Borst adapter

Toupet
    T. fundoplication
    T. operation

tourniquet occlusion

toxemia
    hepatic t.
    t. of pregnancy

toxic
    t. cirrhosis
    t. colitis
    t. diarrhea
    t. dilation of colon
    t. gastritis
    t. hepatitis
    t. megacolon
    t. nephrosis
    t. shock syndrome
    t. steatosis

toxicity
    acute hepatic t.
    octreotide-induced hepatic t.
    progressing t.
    renal t.
    theophylline t.

toxicosis
    hemorrhagic capillary t.

toxigenic
    t. bacteria
    t. diarrhea

toxin
    cholera t.
    cholera t.–induced diarrhea

toxuria

TPN
  total parenteral nutrition
  (TPN)

trabecula *pl.* trabeculae
  trabeculae corporum cav-
  ernosorum penis
  trabeculae corporis spon-
  giosi penis

trabecular

trace-gas analysis

trachelocystitis

tracheoesophageal
  t. fistula

tract
  alimentary t.
  biliary t.
  digestive t.
  fistulous t.
  gastrointestinal t.
  gastrointestinal t. hemorrhage
  genitourinary t.
  GI t.
  hepatic outflow t.
  ileal inflow t.
  ileal outflow t.
  infected t.
  intestinal t.
  intramural fistulous t.
  oro-respiratory t.
  outflow t.
  pancreaticobiliary t.
  urinary t.

traction
  t. diverticulum
  t. suture

tractor
  prostatic t.
  Syms t.
  urethral t.

tractus *pl.* tractus
  t. iliopubicus

training
  bladder t.
  bowel t.

transabdominal
  t. repair

transanal endoscopic microsur-
  gical resection

trans-blotting cell

transcatheter
  t. arterial embolization
  t. hepatic arterial embolization
  t. splenic arterial embolization
  t. variceal embolization

transcolonic
  t. endoscopy

transcription
  t.-activating factor

transcutaneous biopsy

transducer
  antral pressure t.

transduodenal
  t. drainage
  t. endoscopic decompression

transection
  esophageal t.

transesophageal
  t. endoscopy
  t. ligation of varix

transfer factor

transformation
  neoplastic t.
  nodular t.
  nodular t. of the liver
  t. zone

transfusion
  t.-associated hepatitis
  autologous t.
  t. hepatitis

transfusion *(continued)*
    t. nephritis
    t.-related chronic liver disease

transgastric
    t. fine-needle aspiration biopsy
    t. cholangiogram
    t. drainage
    t. esophageal bougienage
    t. ligation

transgastrostomic enteroscopy

transhepatic
    t. biliary drainage
    t. cholangiogram
    t. cholangiography
    t. embolization
    fine-needle t. cholangiogram
    fine-needle t. cholangiography
    percutaneous t. cholangiogram
    percutaneous t. cholangiography
    percutaneous t. decompression
    percutaneous t. drainage
    t. portacaval shunt

transhiatal
    t. esophagectomy

transient
    t. cholangitis
    t. gastroparesis

transit
    colonic t.
    esophageal t.
    gastrointestinal t.
    mean colonic t.
    slow colonic t.
    t. time

transitional
    t. cell
    t. cell carcinoma
    papillary t. cell carcinoma

transitional *(continued)*
    t. zone biopsy

transjugular
    t. intrahepatic portosystemic shunt (TIPS)
    t. liver biopsy

transmission
    mother-to-infant t. of hepatitis C virus
    oral t.

transmural
    t. approach
    t. colitis
    t. drainage
    t. fibrosis
    t. ileocolitis

transnasal endoscopy

transpapillary
    t. approach
    t. biopsy
    t. cannulation
    t. catheterization
    t. drainage
    endoscopic t. cannulation
    t. endoscopic cholecystectomy (TEC)

transparietal

transperitoneal
    t. laparoscopic adrenalectomy (TLA)

transplant
    allogeneic kidney t.
    allogenic kidney t.
    cadaveric t.
    cadaveric liver t.
    cadaveric renal t.
    chronic t. rejection
    delayed hyperacute t. rejection
    Gallie t.
    heart-kidney t.
    liver t.
    orthotopic liver t.
    pancreas-kidney t.

transplant *(continued)*
    t. rejection
    split-liver t.

transplantation
    allogeneic t.
    allogenic t.
    genetically identical t.
    heterotopic t.
    homotopic t.
    liver t.
    living nonrelated donor t.
    living related donor t.
    living unrelated donor t.
    organ t.
    orthotopic t.
    syngeneic t.
    syngenesioplastic t.
    xenogeneic t.

transport maximum for glucose

transposition
    gastric t.

transpubic
    t. incision

transpyloric
    t. plane

transrectal
    t. ultrasound-guided–sextant biopsy

transsphincteric anal fistula

transthoracic
    t. esophagectomy
    t. hepatotomy
    t. resection of esophageal carcinoma

transudative ascites

transureteroureteral
    t. anastomosis

transureteroureterostomy

transurethral
    t. prostatectomy
    t. prostatic resection
    t. resection of bladder tumor

transurethral *(continued)*
    t. resection of the prostate

transvaterian

transvenous liver biopsy

transversalis fascia

transverse
    t. colectomy
    t. colostomy
    t. colostomy effluent
    t. colon
    t. duodenotomy
    t. fascia
    t. fissure
    t. folds of rectum
    t. incision
    t. ligament of pelvis
    t. loop
    loop t. colostomy
    t.-loop rod colostomy
    t. pelvic ligament
    t. perineal ligament
    t. planes
    t. process
    t. resection
    t. semilunar skin incision
    t. umbilical line
    t. vesical fold
    t. view

transversourethralis

transversus abdominis muscle

transvesical

trauma
    bile duct t.
    blunt t.
    blunt abdominal t.
    blunt liver t.
    blunt pancreatic t.
    colorectal t.
    duodenal t.
    esophageal t.
    external t.
    gallbladder t.
    gastric t.
    hepatic t.
    iatrogenic t.

trauma *(continued)*
    iatrogenic pancreatic t.
    liver t.
    pancreatic t.
    rectal t.
    splenic t.

Trauma-Aid HBC enteral feeding

TraumaCal enteral feeding

traumatic
    t. appendicitis
    t. lesion
    t. orchitis
    t. peritonitis
    t. proctitis

Travasol amino acid

Travasorb
    T. HN powdered feeding
    T. MCT liquid feeding
    T. STD liquid feeding

traveler's diarrhea

treatment
    acorn t.
    alpha interferon t.
    alternate-day t.
    anabolic steroid t.
    anoplasty t.
    anti–*Helicobacter pylori* t.
    t. channel
    cholecystitis t.
    chronic anoplasty t.
    t. failure
    interferon t.
    Potter t.

tree
    biliary t.
    cannulation of biliary t.
    hepatobiliary t.

Treitz
    fossa of T.
    T. hernia
    ligament of T.
    muscle of T.

Trendelenburg operation

Treves fold

triad
    Charcot t.
    Dieulafoy t.
    hepatic t's
    portal t's
    Saint t.
    t. of Schultz

triaditis
    portal t.

triamterine
    hydrochlorothiazide-triamterene (HCTZ-TA)

triangle
    Calot t.
    cardiohepatic t.
    Charcot t.
    cystohepatic t.
    digastric t.
    Grynfeltt t.
    t. of Grynfeltt and Lesshaft
    iliofemoral t.
    inguinal t.
    Lesshaft t.
    Lieutaud t.
    Livingston t.
    mesenteric t.
    surgical t.
    urogenital t.
    vesical t.

triangular
    t. ligament of Colles
    left t. ligament of liver
    right t. ligament of liver
    t. ligament of urethra

trichinelliasis

trichinellosis

trichiniasis

trichinosis

trichobezoar

trichophytobezoar

trifid stomach

trigonal muscle

trigone
    t. of bladder
    urogenital t.
    vesical t.

trigonectomy

trigonitis

trigonum *pl.* trigona
    t. urogenitale
    t. vesicae
    t. vesicae [Lieutaudi]

trilabe

Trimadeau sign

trimipramine
    t. maleate

triorchid

triorchidism

triorchis

triorchism

triple
    t. intussusception
    t. lobe hepatectomy
    t. phosphate calculus
    t. therapy

trisegmentectomy
    left t.

trisplanchnic

trocar
    accessory t.
    gallbladder t.
    Ochsner gallbladder t.

trophic change

tropical
    t. calcific pancreatitis
    t. diarrhea
    t. splenomegaly
    t. sprue
    t. stomatitis

trough
    tearing t.

Trousseau
    T. esophageal bougie
    T.-Lallemand bodies

Tru-Cut
    T.-C. biopsy
    T.-C. needle biopsy

true
    anterior t. ligament of bladder
    t. straight arterioles of kidney

truncal
    t. vagotomy
    t. vagotomy and gastroenterostomy

truss

trypan blue–stained cell

trypanosomiasis
    American t.

T-tube
    T-tube cholangiogram
    T-tube drainage

tubal
    t. ligation
    t. nephritis

tube
    Abbott-Miller t.
    Abbott-Rawson t.
    Abbott -Rawson double-lumen gastrointestinal t.
    Anderson gastric t.
    ascites drainage t.
    Baker intestinal decompression t.
    Baker jejunostomy t.
    Bard gastrostomy feeding t.
    Bard PEG t.
    Bower PEG t.
    Broncho-Cath double-lumen endotracheal t.

tube *(continued)*
 Buie rectal suction t.
 Cantor t.
 t. cast
 Celestin esophageal t.
 Compat feeding t.
 cuffed endotracheal t.
 decompression t.
 t. decompression
 Dennis t.
 Dennis intestinal t.
 digestive t.
 Dobbhoff feeding t.
 Dobbhoff gastric decom-
  pression t.
 Dobbhoff PEG t.
 drainage t.
 endotracheal t.
 esophageal t.
 Ewald t.
 fallopian t.
 feeding t.
 t. feeding
 French T-t.
 gastric aspiration t.
 gastric lavage t.
 gastrostomy t.
 gastrostomy t. migration
 Har-el pharyngeal t.
 Harris t.
 Keofeed feeding t.
 large-bore gastric lavage t.
 Levin t.
 long intestinal t.
 Malecot gastrostomy t.
 Malecot nephrostomy t.
 Miller-Abbott t.
 Moss t.
 Moss gastrostomy t.
 nasobiliary t.
 nasoduodenal feeding t.
 nasoenteric feeding t.
 nasogastric t.
 nasogastric feeding t.
 nasoileal t.
 nasojejunal t.
 nephrostomy t.
 Nuport PEG t.

tube *(continued)*
 orogastric Ewald t.
 oropharyngeal t.
 t. overgrowth
 Paul-Mixter t.
 Pee Wee low profile gas-
  trostomy t.
 postpyloric feeding t.
 rectal t.
 Rehfuss stomach t.
 t. removal
 Ryle t.
 Sacks-Vine feeding gastrostomy t.
 Sandoz Caluso PEG gas-
  trostomy t.
 Schachowa spiral t's
 Sengstaken-Blakemore t.
 Shiner t.
 small-bowel t.
 stomach t.
 suction t.
 T-t.
 tampon t.
 Teflon t.
 Wangensteen t.

tubeless cystostomy

tuber *pl.* tubers, tubera
 omental t. of body of pancreas
 omental t. of liver
 t. omentale corporis pancreatis
 t. omentale hepatis
 papillary t. of liver

tubercle
 caudal t. of liver
 Farre t's
 papillary t.

tuberculate

tuberculated

tuberculocele

tuberculosis
 colonic t.
 duodenal t.

tuberculosis *(continued)*
    esophageal t.
    gastric t.
    ileocecal t.
    intestinal t.
    miliary t.
    peritoneal t.
    t. polyp
    renal t.
    segmental colonic t.

tuberculous
    t. enteritis
    t. esophagitis
    t. gastritis
    t. ileocolitis
    t. infectious esophagitis
    t. nephritis
    t. peritonitis

tuberous sclerosis

tubular
    t. ectasia
    t. epithelial cell
    t. hyposthenuria
    t. iron accumulation
    t. maximum
    t. necrosis
    t. nephritis
    t. resorption

tubularized cecal flap

tubule
    Albarrán t's
    arcuate renal t.
    attenuated t.
    Bellini t.
    biliferous t.
    collecting t.
    connecting t.
    convoluted t.
    convoluted seminiferous t's
    cortical collecting t.
    distal convoluted t.
    distal straight t.
    Ferrein t's
    first convoluted t.
    Henle t.
    junctional t.
    Kobelt t's

tubule *(continued)*
    medullary collecting t.
    metanephric t's
    paraurethral t's
    proximal convoluted t.
    proximal straight t.
    renal t's
    renal collecting t.
    second convoluted t.
    seminiferous t's
    Skene t's
    spiral t.
    straight t.
    straight collecting t.
    straight seminiferous t's
    thin t.
    uriniferous t.
    uriniparous t.

tubulitis

tubulointerstitial
    hereditary t. nephritis
    t. nephritis

tubulopathy

tubulorrhexis

tubulotoxic effect

tubulous

tubulovesicle

tubulovesicular

tubulovillous
    t. adenoma
    t. lesion
    t. polyp

tubulus
    t. attenuatus
    t. biliferus
    t. colligens rectus
    t. contortus distalis
    t. contortus proximalis
    t. rectus distalis
    t. rectus proximalis
    t. renalis
    t. renalis arcuatus
    t. renalis colligens

tubulus *(continued)*
    tubuli seminiferi contorti
    tubuli seminiferi recti

tubus *pl.* tubi
    t. digestorius

Tucks ointment

Tuffier inferior ligament

Tulpius
    valve of T.

tumeur
    t. pileuse

tumor
    abdominal desmoid t.
    t. ablation
    Abrikosov t.
    adenomatoid t.
    adnexal t.
    adrenal rest t.
    ampullary t.
    t. angiogenesis
    benign t.
    bifurcation t.
    biliary tract t.
    bleeding t.
    carcinoid t.
    celiac t.
    t. cell
    duodenal t.
    endodermal sinus t.
    esophageal t.
    fecal t.
    gastrin-secreting non–beta
      islet cell t.
    germ cell t.
    gonadal stromal t.
    Grawitz t.
    hepatic t.
    interstitial cell t.
    juxtaglomerular t.
    juxtaglomerular cell t.
    Klatskin t.
    Leydig cell t.
    mesenchymal t.
    t. necrosis
    t. necrosis factor
    t. of Oddi

tumor *(continued)*
    papillary cystic t. of pan-
      creas
    parenchymal tissue
    renomedullary interstitial
      cell t.
    retroperitoneal t.
    rhabdoid t. of the kidney
    Sertoli cell t.
    solid t.
    solid-cystic t. of pancreas
    solid pseudopapillary t. of
      pancreas
    t. staging
    t. stenting
    stercoral t.
    superficial esophageal car-
      cinoma
    t.-suppressor gene
    testicular t.
    UICC t. classification
    vascular permeation of t.
      cell
    villous t.
    Wilms t.
    yolk sac t.

Tums

tunic
    fibrous t. of liver
    t's of spermatic cord

tunica *pl.* tunicae
    t. adnata testis
    t. adventitia ductus defer-
      entis
    t. adventitia esophagi
    t. adventitia glandulae sem-
      inalis
    t. adventitia glandulae vesi-
      culosae
    t. adventitia oesophagi
    t. adventitia ureteris
    t. adventitia vesiculae sem-
      inalis
    t. albuginea corporis spon-
      giosi
    t. albuginea corporum cav-
      ernosorum
    t. albuginea testis

tunica *(continued)*
    t. dartos
    t. fibrosa hepatis
    t. fibrosa renis
    tunicae funiculi spermatici
    t. mucosa ductus deferen-
        tis
    t. mucosa esophagi
    t. mucosa gastris
    t. mucosa glandulae semin-
        alis
    t. mucosa glandulae vesicu-
        losae
    t. mucosa intestini crassi
    t. mucosa intestini recti
    t. mucosa intestini tenuis
    t. mucosa oesophagi
    t. mucosa recti
    t. mucosa ureteris
    t. mucosa urethrae femini-
        nae
    t. mucosa urethrae mulie-
        bris
    t. mucosa ventriculi
    t. mucosa vesicae biliaris
    t. mucosa vesicae felleae
    t. mucosa vesicae urinariae
    t. mucosa vesiculae semin-
        alis
    t. muscularis coli
    t. muscularis ductus defer-
        entis
    t. muscularis esophagi
    t. muscularis gastris
    t. muscularis glandulae
        seminalis
    t. muscularis glandulae ve-
        siculosae
    t. muscularis intestini te-
        nuis
    t. muscularis oesophagi
    t. muscularis recti
    t. muscularis ureteris
    t. muscularis urethrae femi-
        ninae
    t. muscularis urethrae mu-
        liebris
    t. muscularis ventriculi

tunica *(continued)*
    t. muscularis vesicae bil-
        iaris
    t. muscularis vesicae fel-
        leae
    t. muscularis vesicae uri-
        nariae
    t. muscularis vesiculae
        seminalis
    t. propria tubuli testis
    t. serosa gastris
    t. serosa hepatis
    t. serosa intestini crassi
    t. serosa intestini tenuis
    t. serosa peritonei
    t. serosa testis
    t. serosa ventriculi
    t. serosa vesicae biliaris
    t. serosa vesicae felleae
    t. serosa vesicae urinariae
    t. spongiosa urethrae femi-
        ninae
    t. submucosa urethrae fem-
        ininae
    tunicae testis
    t. vaginalis testis

tunnel
    t. infection
    retropancreatic t.

turbid
    t. bile
    t. peritoneal fluid

Turck zone

Turcot syndrome

Turcotte
    Child-T. classification

turgor
    skin t.

turista

Turnbull
    T. colostomy
    T. end-loop ileostomy

Turnbull *(continued)*
  T. multiple ostomy operation

Turner sign

Tuttle proctoscope

two-channel endoscope

two-layer
  t.-l. anastomosis
  t.-l. enteroenterostomy

two-stage repair

two-way catheter

tympania

tympanism

tympanites
  false t.

tympanitic
  t. abdomen
  t. dullness

tympanous

tympany
  abdominal t.

type
  t. A gastritis
  t. B gastritis
  t. C cirrhosis

typhlectasis

typhlectomy

typhlitis

typhlodicliditis

typhlopexy

typhlostomy

typhlotomy

typhoid
  abdominal t.
  t. fever

tyrosine kinase activity

Tyrrell fascia

Tyson
  crypts of T.
  glands of T.

tysonitis

UC
  ulcerative colitis

UICC
  International Union against
  Cancer
    UICC tumor classifica-
    tion

UGI
  upper gastrointestinal
    UGI angiomata
    UGI endoscope

UGIB
  upper gastrointestinal
  bleeding

ulcer
  acid peptic u.
  active duodenal u.
  anastomotic u.
  anastomotic/stomal u.
  anterior duodenal u.
  anterior wall antral u.
  antral u.
  aphthoid u.
  aphthous u.
  apical duodenal u.
  Barrett u.
  u. base
  bear claw u.
  u. bed
  benign u.
  benign gastric u.
  bulbar peptic u.
  cecal u.
  colonic u.
  colorectal u.
  Crohn duodenal u.
  Cruveilhier u.
  Cushing u.
  Cushing-Rokitansky u's
  Dieulafoy u.
  drug-induced u.
  duodenal u.
  elusive u.
  esophageal u.
  Fenwick-Hunner u.
  flask u.

ulcer *(continued)*
  focal colonic mucosal u.
  gastric u.
  gastroduodenal double u.
  giant peptic u.
  girdle u.
  greater curvature u.
  u. with heaped-up edges
  herpetic u.
  Hunner u.
  idiopathic esophageal u.
  jejunal u.
  kissing u's
  Kocher dilatation u.
  lesser curvature u.
  malignant u.
  marginal u.
  open u.
  oral u.
  peptic u.
  perforated peptic u.
  prepyloric u.
  prepyloric gastric u.
  rectal u.
  recurrent u.
  Rokitansky-Cushing u's
  round u.
  sea anemone u.
  secondary jejunal u.
  stercoraceous u.
  stercoral u.
  stoma u.
  stomal u.
  stress u.
  submucous u.
  sump u.
  visible u. vessel

ulcerating
  u. adenocarcinoma
  u. carcinoma

ulceration
  anal u.
  anastomotic u.
  ASA-induced gastric u.
  CMV-associated u.
  CMV-induced esophageal u.
  collar-button u.

ulceration *(continued)*
    duodenal u.
    esophageal u.
    gastric u.
    necrotic u.
    patchy colonic u.
    radiation-induced u.
    stasis u.
    stercoral u.
    stress u.
    stress-induced gastric u.

ulcerative
    u. colitis (UC)
    u. enteritis
    u. esophagitis
    u. gastritis
    u. lymphoma
    u. proctitis

ulcerlike dyspepsia

ulceroerosive
    u. disease

ulcerogenic
    u. fistula

ulcer-prone personality

ulcus *pl.* ulcera
    u. simplex vesicae
    u. ventriculi

ultrafilter

ultrafiltration

ultrasonographic finding

ultrasonography
    abdominal u.
    intraoperative u. and angi-
      ography

ultrasound
    abdominal u.
    u.-assisted percutaneous
      endoscopic gastrostomy
    Doppler u.
    endorectal u.
    u.-guided biopsy

ultrastructural basket-weave
  change

umbilical
    u. artery
    u. fissure
    u. fistula
    u. granuloma
    u. incisure
    u. notch
    u. plane
    u. region
    u. vein catheterization

umbilicated angioma

umbilicus
    amniotic u.
    decidual u.

unbanded gastroplasty

uncinate process of pancreas

unclassified sprue

unconjugated
    u. bilirubin
    u. hyperbilirubinemia

undersurface of liver

undescended testis

undifferentiated
    u. adenoma
    u. cell

undigested food in stool

unformed stool

unilateral
    u. subcostal incision

unilobular
    u. cirrhosis

uninephrectomy

uninhibited neurogenic bladder

union
    anomalous pancreaticobili-
      ary ductal u. (APBDU)

unit
    amylase u.
    French u.
    Somogyi u.

Universal esophagoscope

unrelenting
    u. diarrhea
    u. pain

unrelieved pain

unremitting pain

unresectable hepatocellular
    carcinoma

unrest
    peristaltic u.

upper
    u. alimentary endoscopy
    u. endoscopy and colonos-
        copy
    u. esophageal sphincter
    u. gastrointestinal (UGI)
    u. gastrointestinal angio-
        mata
    u. gastrointestinal bleeding
        (UGIB)
    u. gastrointestinal endo-
        scope
    u. gastrointestinal endos-
        copy
    u. gastrointestinal hemor-
        rhage
    u. GI endoscope
    u. GI tract foreign body
    u. pole of testis

upside-down stomach

upstream pancreatic duct

uptake
    hepatic u.

urachal
    u. adenocarcinoma
    u. diverticulum
    u. fistula

uracrasia

uracratia

uranyl acetate

urate
    acute u. nephropathy

urate *(continued)*
    u. cast
    chronic u. nephropathy
    u. nephropathy

urea
    u. breath test
    u. clearance
    u. concentration test
    u. kinetics
    u. kinetic modeling

urease
    gastric u. activity

urecchysis

Urecholine supersensitivity test

uredema

urelcosis

uremia

uremic
    u. acidosis
    u. bone disease
    u. cachexia
    u. colitis
    u. encephalopathy
    u. polyneuropathy
    u. pruritus
    u. stomatitis

uremigenic

uresiesthesis

uresis

uretal

ureter
    circumcaval u.
    ectopic u.
    orifice of u.
    postcaval u.
    retrocaval u.
    retroiliac u.

ureteral
    u. orifice
    u. stoma removal

ureteralgia

ureterectasia

ureterectasis

ureterectomy

ureteric
    u. bridge

ureteritis
    u. cystica
    u. glandularis

ureterocele
    ectopic u.

ureterocelectomy

ureterocolonic
    u. anastomosis

ureterocolostomy

ureterocutaneostomy

ureterocystanastomosis

ureterocystoneostomy

ureterocystoscope

ureterocystostomy

ureteroduodenal

ureteroenteric

ureteroenteroanastomosis

ureteroenterostomy

ureteroileal
    u. anastomosis

ureteroileocutaneous
    u. anastomosis

ureteroileostomy
    Bricker u.

ureterointestinal

ureterolith

ureterolithiasis

ureterolithotomy

ureterolysis

ureteromeatotomy

ureteroneocystostomy

ureteroneopyelostomy

ureteronephrectomy

ureteropathy

ureteropelvic
    u. junction
    u. junction obstruction

ureteropelvioneostomy

ureteropelvioplasty
    Culp-DeWeerd u.
    Foley Y-V u.
    Scardino-Prince u.

ureterophlegma

ureteroplasty

ureteroproctostomy

ureteropyelitis

ureteropyeloneostomy

ureteropyelonephritis

ureteropyelonephrostomy

ureteropyeloplasty

ureteropyelostomy

ureteropyosis

ureterorectal

ureterorectoneostomy

ureterorectostomy

ureterorenoscope

ureterorenoscopy

ureterorrhagia

ureterorrhaphy

ureteroscope

ureteroscopy

ureterosigmoid
    u. anastomosis

ureterosigmoidostomy

ureterostenosis

ureterostoma

ureterostomy
cutaneous u.

ureterotomy

ureterotrigonal
u. complex

ureterotrigonoenterostomy

ureterotrigonosigmoidostomy

ureterotubal
u. anastomosis

ureteroureteral
u. anastomosis

ureteroureterostomy

ureterovesical
u. junction

ureterovesicoplasty

ureterovesicostomy

urethra
anterior u.
double u.
u. feminina
u. masculina
membranous u.
u. muliebris
posterior u.
prostatic u.
spongiose u.
spongy u.
u. virilis

urethral
u. abscess
anterior u. valve
u. artery
u. calculus
u. caruncle
u. catheter
u. chill
u. fever
u. glands of female urethra
u. glands of male urethra

urethral *(continued)*
u. hematuria
u. lacunae
u. lacunae of Morgagni
u. obstruction
posterior u. valve
u. pressure
u. pressure profile
u. pressure profilometry
u. sound
u. syndrome
u. tractor
u. utricle

urethralgia

urethratresia

urethrectomy

urethremphraxis

urethreurynter

urethrism

urethritis
u. cystica
u. glandularis
gouty u.
u. granulosa
nongonococcal u.
nonspecific u.
u. orificii externi
u. petrificans
prophylactic u.
simple u.

urethroblennorrhea

urethrobulbar

urethrocecal
u. anastomosis

urethrocystitis

urethrocystopexy

urethrodynia

urethrograph

urethrometer

urethrometry

urethropenile

urethroperineal

urethroperineoscrotal

urethropexy

urethrophraxis

urethrophyma

urethroplasty

urethroprostatic

urethrorectal

urethrorrhagia

urethrorrhaphy

urethrorrhea

urethroscope

urethroscopic

urethroscopy

urethroscrotal

urethrospasm

urethrostaxis

urethrostenosis

urethrostomy

urethrotome
  Maisonneuve u.

urethrotomy
  external u.
  internal u.

urethrotrigonitis

urethrovaginal
  u. fistula

urethrovesical

uretic

URF-P2 choledochoscope

urge incontinence

urgency
  defecatory u.
  u. incontinence

urian

uric

uric acid
  acute u. a. nephropathy
  u. a. calculus
  chronic u. a. nephropathy
  u. a. lithiasis
  u. a. nephropathy

uriesthesis

urinable

urinaccelerator

urinaemia

urinal

urinary
  u. abscess
  u. acidity
  u. amylase
  u. ascites
  u. bladder
  u. calculus
  Camey u. pouch
  u. cast
  u. continence
  u. cylinder
  u. extravasation
  u. fever
  u. fistula
  u. frequency
  u. incontinence
  u. lithiasis
  u. organs
  u. output
  u. reflex
  u. retention
  u. siderosis
  u. stasis
  u. stuttering
  u. system
  u. tract
  u. tract infection

urinate

urination
  precipitant u.

urination *(continued)*
  stuttering u.

urine
  u. bilirubin
  residual u.
  retention of u.

urinemia

uriniferous
  u. tubule

urinific

uriniparous
  u. tubule

urinogenital

urinologist

urinology

urinoma

urinothorax

urinous
  u. infiltration

uroammoniac

urobilin
  u. complex

urobilinogen

Uro-Bond skin adhesive

urocele

urochezia

urochrome

urochromogen

urocinetic

uroclepsia

urocystitis

urodialysis

urodynamic
  u. obstruction

urodynamics

urodynia

uroedema

uroflow

uroflowmeter

urogastrone

urogenital
  u. canals
  u. diaphragm
  u. fistula
  u. region
  u. system
  u. triangle
  u. trigone

urogenous
  u. pyelitis

urohematonephrosis

urokinase plasminogen activator

urokinetic

urokymography

urolith

urolithiasis

urolithic

urolithology

urologic

urological

urologist

urology

urometric

urometry

uromodulin

uroncus

uronephrosis

uronology

urononcometry

uropathogen

uropathy
    obstructive u.

uropenia

uropittin

uroplania

uropoiesis

uropoietic

uroprotection

uroprotective

uropyonephrosis

uropyoureter

uroscheocele

uroschesis

urosepsis

uroseptic

urosis

urostealith
    u. calculus

urothelial

urothelium

urotoxia

urotoxic

urotoxicity

urotoxin

urotoxy

uroureter

ursodeoxycholate

ursodeoxycholic acid

ursodeoxycholylglycine

ursodeoxycholyltaurine

urticaria
    colonic u.

urticarial fever

uterine
    u. colic
    u. fibroid
    u. tenderness

uterus *pl.* uteri
    anteflexed u.
    bicornuate u.
    u. masculinus

utricle
    prostatic u.
    urethral u.

utriculitis

utriculus *pl.* utriculi
    u. masculinus
    u. prostaticus

uvula *pl.* uvulae
    u. of bladder
    Lieutaud u.
    u. vesicae

vaccine
   hepatitis B virus v. (HBVV)

vacuolar nephrosis

Vacutainer bag

vagina *pl.* vaginae
   v. masculina

vaginal
   v. bleeding
   v. cuff cellulitis
   v. fistula
   v. flora
   v. hematocele
   v. lithotomy
   v. wall sling
   v. suppository

vaginalitis
   plastic v.

vaginitis
   v. testis

vagosympathetic balance

vagotomy
   highly selective v.
   laparoscopic v.
   medical v.
   proximal gastric v.
   Roux-en-Y procedure
      with v.
   selective proximal v.
   superselective v.
   surgical v.
   total bilateral v.
   truncal v.

vagus nerve

Valentine position

vallecula *pl.* valleculae
   v. ovata

vallecular
   v. dysphagia

valproic acid

Valsalva maneuver

value
   therapeutic v.

valva *pl.* valvae
   v. ilealis
   v. ileocaecalis

valve
   v. ablation
   anal v's
   anterior urethral v.
   Ball v's
   Bauhin v.
   Benchekroun hydraulic v.
   Benchekroun ileal v.
   blunting of v.
   competent ileocecal v.
   fallopian v.
   Gerlach v.
   Guérin v.
   Heister v.
   Houston v's
   hymenal v. of male urethra
   ileocecal v.
   ileocolic v.
   incompetent v.
   incompetent ileocecal v.
   Kerckring (Kerkring) v's
   Kohlrausch v's
   LeVeen v.
   Lopez enteral v.
   v. of Macalister
   Mercier v.
   Mitrofanoff v.
   Morgagni v's
   v. of navicular fossa
   O'Beirne v.
   v. prolapse
   pyloric v.
   semilunar v's of colon
   semilunar v's of Morgagni
   sigmoid v's of colon
   spiral v. of cystic duct
   spiral v. of Heister
   v. of Tulpius
   ureteral v.
   posterior urethral v.
   v. of Varolius
   v. of vermiform appendix

valvula
    valvulae anales
    valvulae conniventes
    v. fossae navicularis
    v. ileocolica
    v. processus vermiformis
    v. pylori
    v. spiralis [Heisteri]

van Buren
    v. B. disease

van den Bergh
    v. d. B. disease

Van der Waals force

van Hook
    v. H. operation

vanishing testes syndrome

variceal
    v. band ligation
    v. bleeding
    v. decompression
    v. hemorrhage
    v. pressure
    v. sclerosis
    v. sclerotherapy in esopha-
      gus
    v. wall

varicella
    v. zoster
    v. zoster infection

varices (*plural of* varix)

varicocele

varicocelectomy

varicole

varioliform gastritis or gastro-
    pathy

Varolius
    valve of V.

varix *pl.* varices
    actively bleeding v.
    alcoholic v.
    anorectal v.

varix *(continued)*
    bar-type esophageal v.
    colonic v.
    common bile duct varices
    duodenal v.
    ectopic varices
    esophageal v.
    familial colonic varices
    fundal v.
    gallbladder varices
    gastric varices
    idiopathic varices
    ileal v.
    v. ligation
    mesenteric v.
    obliterated varices
    paraesophageal v.
    peristomal v.
    rectal v.
    rectosigmoid v.
    transesophageal ligation
      of v.

vas *pl.* vasa
    v. aberrans
    v. aberrans of Roth
    vasa aberrantis hepatis
    v. afferens glomeruli
    v. deferens
    v. efferens glomeruli
    v. epididymidis
    vasa recta renis

vasa (*plural of* vas)

vascular
    v. abnormality
    v. access
    v. access failure
    v. anastomosis
    cecal v. ectasia
    v. cecal fold
    v. cirrhosis
    v. coat of stomach
    v. ectasia
    v. hemangioma
    v. insufficiency
    v. lamina of stomach
    v. lesion
    v. malformation
    v. nephritis

vascular *(continued)*
    v. pattern
    v. permeation of tumor cell
    v. plasminogen activator
        (v-PA)
    v. rejection
    v. smooth muscle cell

vasculitic
    v. lesion
    v. neuropathy

vasculitis
    allergic v.
    necrotizing bowel v.
    necrotizing v.

vasculopathy
    acute renal transplant v.

vasculum
    v. aberrans

vasectomized

vasectomy

vasitis

vasoactive
    v. intestinal peptide (VIP)
    v. intestinal polypeptide
        (VIP)

vasoepididymostomy

vasoligation

vasomotor nephropathy

vaso-orchidostomy

vasopuncture

vasoresection

vasorrhaphy

vasosection

vasostomy

vasotomy

vasovagal reflex

vasovasostomy

vasovesiculectomy

vasovesiculitis

Vater
    ampulla of V.
    papilla of V.

vault
    rectal v.

Vectastain
    alkaline phosphatase V.
    ABC

vegetarian
    v. diet

veil
    Jackson v.

vein
    aberrant obturator v.
    accessory saphenous v.
    appendicular v.
    arciform v's
    arcuate v's of kidney
    ascending lumbar v.
    central v's of hepatic lob-
        ules
    central v's of liver
    central v. of suprarenal
        gland
    cystic v.
    great saphenous v.
    hepatic v's
    ileal v's
    ileocolic v.
    iliac v.
    inferior epigastric v.
    inferior mesenteric v.
    inferior rectal v's
    interlobar v's of kidney
    interlobular v's of kidney
    intermediate colic v.
    intermediate hepatic v's
    internal pudendal v.
    jejunal v's
    v's of kidney
    lateral sacral v's
    left colic v.
    left epiploic v.
    left gastric v.

vein *(continued)*
    left gastroepiploic v.
    left gastroomental v.
    left hepatic v.
    left suprarenal v.
    lumbar v's
    median sacral v.
    mediastinal v's
    middle colic v.
    middle hepatic v's
    middle rectal v's
    middle sacral v.
    omental v.
    pancreatic v's
    pancreaticoduodenal v's
    paraumbilical v's
    portal v. of liver
    pyloric v.
    Retzius v's
    renal v's
    right colic v.
    right epiploic v.
    right gastric v.
    right gastroepiploic v.
    right gastroomental v.
    right suprarenal v.
    v's of Sappey
    short gastric v's
    sigmoid v's
    small saphenous v.
    splenic v.
    stellate v's of kidney
    subcutaneous v's of abdo-
      men
    sublobular v's
    superficial epigastric v.
    superior epigastric v's
    superior mesenteric v.
    superior rectal v.
    thoracoepigastric v's
    umbilical v.

Velpeau
    V. canal
    V. hernia

vena *pl.* venae
    v. adrenalis dextra
    v. appendicularis

vena *(continued)*
    venae arciformes renis
    venae arcuatae renis
    v. cava inferior
    venae centrales hepatis
    v. colica dextra
    v. colica intermedia
    v. colica media
    v. colica sinistra
    v. cystica
    v. epigastrica inferior
    v. epigastrica superficialis
    venae epigastricae supe-
      riores
    v. epiploica dextra
    v. epiploica sinistra
    venae esophageae
    venae esophageales
    venae gastricae breves
    v. gastrica dextra
    v. gastrica sinistra
    v. gastroepiploica dextra
    v. gastroepiploica sinistra
    v. gastroomentalis dextra
    v. gastroomentalis sinistra
    venae hepaticae
    venae hepaticae dextrae
    venae hepaticae interme-
      diae
    venae hepaticae mediae
    venae hepaticae sinistrae
    venae ileales
    v. ileocolica
    v. iliaca communis
    v. iliaca externa
    v. iliaca interna
    v. iliolumbalis
    venae interlobares renis
    venae interlobulares hepa-
      tis
    venae interlobulares renis
    venae lumbales
    v. lumbalis ascendens
    v. mediana colli
    venae mediastinales
    v. mesenterica inferior
    v. mesenterica superior
    venae pancreaticae

vena *(continued)*
    venae pancreaticoduodenales
    venae paraumbilicales
    v. portae hepatis
    v. prepylorica
    v. portalis hepatis
    venae rectales inferiores
    venae rectales mediae
    v. rectalis superior
    venae renales
    venae renis
    venae sacrales laterales
    v. sacralis media
    v. sacralis mediana
    v. saphena accessoria
    v. saphena magna
    v. saphena parva
    venae sigmoideae
    v. splenica
    venae stellatae renis
    v. suprarenalis dextra
    v. suprarenalis sinistra
    venae thoracoepigastricae

vena cava
    retrohepatic v. c.

venereal
    v. disease
    v. proctocolitis
    v. wart

venogram
    hepatic v.

veno-occlusive disease of the liver

venoperitoneostomy

venous
    v. arches of kidney
    v. ligament of liver
    v. pattern
    v. thrombosis
    v. web

venovenous
    v. access

ventilation
    mechanical v.

venting percutaneous gastrostomy

ventral
    v. celiotomy
    v. chronic calcific pancreatitis
    v. hernia
    v. herniorrhaphy
    v. surface

ventricular
    v. canal

ventriculoperitoneal shunt

ventriculus

ventrocystorrhaphy

ventroptosia

ventroptosis

venula *pl.* venulae
    venulae rectae renis
    venulae stellatae renis

venule
    hepatic v.
    stellate v's of kidney
    straight v's of kidney

verdohemoglobin

Veress cannula

verge
    anal v.

vermicular
    v. appendage
    v. colic
    v. movements

vermiculation

vermiform
    v. appendix
    v. artery
    v. bodies
    v. process

verminous
    v. appendicitis
    v. colic

verminous *(continued)*
   v. ileus

vermix

Vermox

Verner-Morrison syndrome

verotoxin

verrucous
   v. gastritis

vertebrated catheter

vertical
   v. banded gastroplasty
   v. midline incision
   v. plane
   v. ring gastroplasty
   v. Silastic ring gastroplasty

vertigo
   v. ab stomacho laeso
   gastric v.
   objective v.
   stomachal v.

verumontanitis

verumontanum

very late activation (VLA)

vesica *pl.* vesicae
   v. biliaris
   v. fellea
   v. prostatica
   v. urinaria

vesical
   v. calculus
   v. diverticulum
   v. fibrosis
   v. fistula
   v. hematuria
   v. hernia
   inferior v. artery
   v. prostatism
   v. reflex
   superior v. arteries
   v. tenesmus
   transverse v. fold
   v. triangle
   v. trigone

vesicle
   false spermatic v.
   prostatic v.
   seminal v.

vesicoabdominal

vesicocele

vesicoclysis

vesicocolic
   v. fistula

vesicocolonic

vesicocutaneous
   v. fistula

vesicoenteric

vesicofixation

vesicointestinal
   v. reflex

vesicoperineal

vesicoprostatic
   v. calculus

vesicopubic
   v. ligament

vesicorectal

vesicorenal

vesicosigmoid

vesicosigmoidostomy

vesico-sphincter dyssynergia

vesicostomy
   cutaneous v.

vesicotomy

vesicoumbilical

vesicourachal

vesicoureteral
   v. reflux
   v. regurgitation

vesicoureteric
   v. reflux

vesicourethral
    v. anastomosis
    v. angle
    anterior v. angle
    v. opening
    v. orifice
    posterior v. angle

vesicovaginal
    v. fistula
    v. lithotomy

vesicula *pl.* vesiculae
    v. bilis
    v. fellea
    v. prostatica
    v. seminalis

vesicular

vesiculectomy

vesiculitis

vesiculotomy

vessel
    accessory v.
    afferent v. of glomerulus
    bile v's
    efferent v. of glomerulus
    gastroepiploic blood v.
    hemorrhoidal v's
    ileal blood v.
    ileocolic v.
    telangiectatic v.
    v. tip
    visible ulcer v.

vestibule
    v. of omental bursa

vestibulum *pl.* vestibula
    v. bursae omentalis

vestige
    v. of vaginal process

vestigial

vestigium *pl.* vestigia
    v. processus vaginalis

vest-over-pants herniorrhaphy

vest-over-pants repair

viability
    intestinal v.

video
    v. colonoscope
    v. duodenoscope
    v. endoscope
    v. endoscopy
    v. small-bowel enteroscopy

videoendoscope (*variant* video endoscope)
    double-channel v.

videolaparoscopy

view
    longitudinal v.
    transverse v.

vigorous achalasia

villoglandular
    v. adenoma

villose

villous
    v. atrophy
    v. adenoma
    v. coat of small intestine
    v. colorectal adenoma
    v. epithelium
    v. folds of stomach
    v. polyp
    v. tumor

villus *pl.* villi
    colonic v.
    duodenal v.
    fingerlike v.
    villi intestinales
    jejunal v.
    leaflike v.
    small intestinal villi
    villi of small intestine
    tongue-shaped v.

Vim-Silverman technique for liver biopsy

violin-string adhesion

VIP
>   vasoactive intestinal pep-
>   tide
>   vasoactive intestinal poly-
>   peptide

VIPoma

viral
>   v. cholangitis
>   v. colitis
>   v. diarrhea
>   v. dysentery
>   v. enteritis
>   v. esophagitis
>   v. gastritis
>   v. gastroenteritis
>   v. hemorrhagic fever
>   v. hepatitis
>   v. infection

Virchow's gland

viremia
>   hepatitis C v.

virucidal agent

virulent diarrhea

virus
>   adeno-associated v. (AAV)
>   dengue v.
>   v. diarrhea
>   esophageal condyloma v.
>   fowlpox v.
>   Hanta v.
>   hepatitis A v. (HAV)
>   hepatitis B v. (HBV)
>   hepatitis C v. (HCV)
>   hepatitis D v. (HDV)
>   hepatitis delta v. (HDV)
>   hepatitis E v. (HEV)
>   herpes simplex v.
>   human immunodeficien-
>   cy v. (HIV)
>   mother-to-infant transmis-
>   sion of hepatitis C v.

viruslike action (VLA)

viscera (*plural of* viscus)

viscerad

visceral
>   v. cavity
>   v. fascia of pelvis
>   v. ischemia
>   v. layer of pelvic fascia
>   v. layer of tunica vaginalis
>   of testis
>   v. neuropathy
>   v. pain
>   v. part of pelvic fascia
>   v. pelvic fascia

visceromotor
>   v. reflex

visceroperitoneal

viscerotome

viscerotomy

viscid bile

viscoelastic collagen fiber

viscous
>   v. bile
>   v. lidocaine
>   v. Xylocaine gargle

viscus *pl.* viscera
>   abdominal v.
>   hollow v.
>   intra-abdominal v.
>   intraperitoneal v.
>   perforated v.
>   strangulated v.

visible
>   v. abdominal distention
>   v. peristalsis
>   v. ulcer vessel

visibly normal

Visick dysphagia classification

Vistaril

visual laser ablation

vitamin
v. B$_{12}$ malabsorption

Vital feeding

Vitaneed feeding

vividiffusion

vivo
ex v.
in v.

Vivonex TEN feeding

VLA
very late activation
viruslike action

voiding
orthotopic v.

Voillemier point

Volkmann spoon for pancreatic calculus

voltage-gated channel

volume
liver v.
v. overload

voluntary
v. dehydration
v. guarding

volvulate

volvulus
cecal v.
colonic v.
gastric v.
idiopathic v.
intestinal v.
mesenteroaxial gastric v.
v. neonatorum
organoaxial gastric v.
v. reduction
secondary v.
sigmoid v.
sigmoid colon v.

vomit
Barcoo v.

vomit *(continued)*
bilious v.
black v.
coffee-ground v.

vomiting
bilious v.
v. center
chemotherapy-induced v.
concealed v.
cyclic v.
dry v.
epidemic v.
episodic v.
erotic v.
fecal v.
hysterical v.
intractable v.
ipecac-induced v.
nausea and v.
nervous v.
periodic v.
perioperative v.
pernicious v.
pernicious v. of pregnancy
persistent v.
postoperative v.
postprandial v.
posttussive v.
profuse v.
projectile v.
psychogenic v.
recurrent v.
recurrent bouts of v.
v. reflex
retention v.
self-induced v.
stercoraceous v.
surreptitious v.

vomiturition

vomitus
Barcoo v.
bile-stained v.
black v.
bloody v.
bright red v.
v. cruentus
feculent v.
v. matutinus

vomitus *(continued)*
  nonbilious v.

von Haberer gastroenterostomy

von Hansemann
  v. H. cells

von Kupffer
  v. K. cells

von Mering
  v. M. reflex

von Recklinghausen
  v. R. gastric neurofibroma
  v. R. neurofibromatosis

vulvovaginal anus

W

Waldeyer
  W. fascia
  W. fossa
  preurethral ligament of W.

wall
  abdominal w.
  anterior abdominal w.
  anterior gastric w.
  anterior w. of stomach
  bowel w.
  capillary w.
  colonic w.
  esophageal w.
  gallbladder w.
  gallbladder w. abscess
  midabdominal w.
  pharyngeal w.
  posterior abdominal w.
  posterior gastric w.
  posterior w. of stomach
  thickened gallbladder w.
  w. thickening
  variceal w.

wandering
  w. gallbladder
  w. kidney
  w. liver

Wangensteen
  W. apparatus
  W. drainage
  W. suction
  W. tube

warm saline solution

Warren shunt

wart
  anal w.
  cervical w.
  exophytic w.
  genital w.
  intra-anal w.
  perianal w.
  venereal w.

water
  w. brash

water (continued)
  w.-gurgle test
  w. intoxication
  w.-jet
  w.-jet dissector

water-soluble
  w.-s. bilirubin
  w.-s. contrast enema
  w.-s. contrast esophageal
    swallow

waterfall stomach

watermelon
  w. cecum
  w. rectum
  w. stomach

watery
  w. diarrhea
  w. stool

Watson capsule biopsy

wave
  abdominal fluid w.
  propulsive w's
  secondary peristaltic w.

wax-tipped bougie

waxy
  w. cast
  w. kidney
  w. liver

WDHA
  watery diarrhea, hypokale-
    mia, achlorhydria
      WDHA syndrome

WDHH
  watery diarrhea, hypokale-
    mia, hypochlorhydria
      WDHH syndrome

web
  antral w.
  duodenal w.
  esophageal w.
  hepatic w.
  intestinal w.
  mucosal w.

web *(continued)*
    pyloric w.
    venous w.

Weber
    W. corpuscle
    W. organ
    W.-Ramstedt operation

weddellite
    w. calculus

wedged hepatic venous pressure

wedge
    w. hepatic biopsy
    w. pressure

wedge pressure

Wegener granulomatosis

weight
    ideal body w. (IBW)

Weight Watchers
    W. W. diet

Welch Allyn video endoscope

well-differentiated adenoma

Wernicke encephalopathy

Western blot analysis

wet colostomy

W hernia

whewellite
    w. calculus

whip bougie

Whipple
    W. disease
    W. operation
    W. pancreatectomy
    W. pancreaticoduodenectomy
    W. pancreaticoduodenostomy
    W. procedure
    W. resection
    W. test

whipworm
    w. infection

whistle-tip catheter

white
    w. bile
    w. diarrhea
    w. line of pelvis
    w. spot disease

White operation

Whitehead
    modified W. hemorrhoidectomy
    W. operation

whitlockite
    w. calculus

Whitmore bag

WHO gastric carcinoma classification

wide albumin gradient ascites

Willis
    W. pancreas
    W. pouch

Wilms tumor

Wilson
    W. muscle
    W.-Cook dilating balloon
    W.-Cook esophageal balloon
    W.-Cook gastric balloon

window
    gastric w.
    mesenteric w.
    peritoneal w.

windowed esophageal balloon

winged catheter

Winslow
    foramen of W.
    hiatus of W.
    W. pancreas

winter acidosis

wire
    bypass w.

wiring
    jaw w.

Wirsung
    canal of W.
    duct of W.

Witzel
    W. duodenostomy
    W. gastrostomy
    W. operation

Woldman test

Wölfler
    W. gastroenterostomy
    W's gland
    W's operation

Womack procedure

wooden belly

Woodward esophagogastros-
    copy

worm colic

wound
    anal w.
    w. dehiscence
    w. drainage
    w. infection
    open w.
    septic w.

wrapping
    fundic w.

Wright stain of stool

W-shaped ileal pouch–anal
    anastomosis

xanthic calculus

xanthogranulomatous
   x. cholecystitis
   x. pyelonephritis

xanthoma
   x. cell
   gastric x.
   skin x.

xanthomatosis
   biliary x.

xenogeneic transplantation

xerostomia

xiphoid
   x. appendix
   x.-to-pubis midline abdominal incision
   x.-to-umbilicus incision

X-Prep

x-ray analysis

Xylocaine topical anesthetic

xylose

xysma

Yangtze Valley fever

Yankauer esophagoscope

yeast-recombinant hepatitis B

Yellen clamp

yellow
  y. atrophy
  y. atrophy of liver
  y. fever
  y. nodule

Yersinia
  Y. enterocolitica
  Y. pseudotuberculosis

yersiniosis

yohimbine hydrochloride

yolk sac
  y. s. carcinoma
  y. s. tumor

Young
  Y. operation
  Y. syndrome
  Y.-Dees-Leadbetter proce-
    dure

Y-shaped incision

Y-V anoplasty

Zahn
   infarct of Z.

Zamboni fixation

Zantac

Zeissel layer

Zenker
   Z. diverticulum
   Z. pouch

zinc colic

Zollinger-Ellison syndrome

zona *pl.* zonae
   z. hemorrhoidalis
   z. transformans

zonal
   z. gastritis

zone
   abdominal z.
   anal transition z.

zone *(continued)*
   chemoreceptor trigger z.
   hemorrhoidal z.
   inner z. of renal medulla
   nephrogenic z.
   outer z. of renal medulla
   transformation z.
   Turck z.

Zoon erythroplasia

zoospermia

zoster
   herpes z.

Zovirax

zuckergussdarm

zuckergussleber

zymogenic
   z. cells

Drugs Used in Gastroenterology

Below are the names of generic and ℞ brand name drugs used in gastroen-
terolology, as shown in the *Saunders Pharmaceutical Xref Book*. The drugs are cate-
gorized by their "indications"—also called "designated use," "approved use," or
"therapeutic action"—which group together drugs used for a similar purpose. The
indications shown below are broad categories of therapeutic action. Individual
drugs may be placed in subcategories or have specifically targeted diseases beyond
the scope of this listing. For complete information about the drugs listed below,
including each drug's availability, specific indications, forms of administration, and
dosages, please consult the current edition of *Saunders Pharmaceutical Word Book*.

Antacids
[*see also: Peptic Ulcer and Gastric
Reflux Agents*]
aluminum hydroxide gel
calcium carbonate
Cotazym
Dialume
magaldrate
magnesia, milk of
magnesium carbonate
magnesium hydroxide
magnesium oxide
sodium bicarbonate
sodium citrate

Anthelmintics
albendazole
Albenza
Biltricide
bithionol
Bitin
diethylcarbamazine citrate
Hetrazan
ivermectin
Lorothidol
mebendazole
Mintezol
niclosamide
oxamniquine
piperazine citrate
praziquantel

Anthelmintics (continued)
pyrantel pamoate
Stromectol
thiabendazole (TBZ)
Vansil
Vermox

Antidiarrheal Agents
Antidiarrheal Agents, Antiflatulents
charcoal
simethicone
Antidiarrheal Agents, Antiperistaltics
Antispasmodic
Antrocol
Arco-Lase Plus
atropine sulfate
Barbidonna; Barbidonna No. 2
Bellacane
difenoxin HCl
diphenoxylate HCl
Donna-Sed
Donnatal
Donnatal No. 2
Hyosophen
Imodium
Logen
Lomanate
Lomotil
Lonox
loperamide HCl
Malatal

Antidiarrheal Agents, Antiperistaltics (continued)
Motofen
Sal-Tropine
Spasmolin
Susano

Antidiarrheal Agents, Intestinal Antibacterials
[see also: Antibiotics; Antifungals, Systemic]
Bactrim Pediatric
Bactrim; Bactrim DS
Bio-Tab
Cipro
ciprofloxacin
Cotrim Pediatric
Cotrim; Cotrim D.S.
Cryptosporidium parvum bovine colostrum IgG concentrate
Doryx
Doxy Caps
Doxychel Hyclate
doxycycline hyclate
Flagyl
Helidac
Immuno-C
metronidazole
Monodox
Mycostatin
Neo-fradin
neomycin sulfate
Nilstat
nystatin
Nystex
Protostat
Septra
Septra DS
Sporidin-G
Sulfatrim
Synsorb-Pk
Vancocin
vancomycin HCl
Vibra-Tabs
Vibramycin

Antidiarrheal Agents, Other
attapulgite, activated
bismuth subsalicylate (BSS)
calcium polycarbophil
dehydroemetine
Lactobacillus acidophilus

Antidiarrheal Agents, Other (continued)
Mebadin
8-methoxycarbonyloctyl oligosaccharides
polycarbophil

Antiemetics and Antinauseants
[see also: Peptic Ulcer and Gastric Reflux Agents]
alosetron HCl
Anergan 50
Antivert; Antivert/25; Antivert/50
Antrizine
Anzemet
Apo-Domperidone Ⓒ
Apo-Perphenazine Ⓒ
Apo-Trifluoperazine Ⓒ
Arrestin
chlorpromazine
chlorpromazine HCl
Clopra
Compazine
dimenhydrinate
Dimetabs
Dinate
diphenidol HCl
dolasetron mesylate
domperidone
Dramamine
Dramanate
Dramilin
Dramoject
dronabinol
droperidol
Dymenate
E-Vista
Emitasol
granisetron HCl
Hydrate
hydroxyzine HCl
Hyzine-50
Inapsine
K-Phen-50
Kytril
Marinol
Marmine
Maxolon
meclizine HCl

**Antiemetics and Antinauseants
(continued)**
Meni-D
metoclopramide HCl
metoclopramide monohydrochloride
    monohydrate
MK-869
Motilium ⓒ
Norzine
Novo-Domperidone ⓒ
Nu-Prochlor ⓒ
Octamide PFS
ondansetron HCl
Ormazine
Pentazine
perphenazine
Phenameth
Phenazine 25
Phenazine 50
Phenergan
Phenergan Fortis
Phenergan Plain
Phenoject-50
phosphorated carbohydrate solution
    (hyperosmolar solution with phos-
    phoric acid)
Pramidin
Pro-50
prochlorperazine
prochlorperazine bimaleate
prochlorperazine edisylate
prochlorperazine maleate
prochlorperazine mesylate
Prometh
Prometh-50
promethazine HCl
Prorex-25; Prorex-50
Prothazine
Prothazine Plain
Quiess
Reclomide
Reglan
Ru-Vert-M
Scopace
scopolamine hydrobromide
Stelazine
Stemetil ⓒ
T-Gen
Tebamide
thiethylperazine

**Antiemetics and Antinauseants
(continued)**
thiethylperazine malate
Thorazine
Ticon
Tigan
Torecan
Transderm Scōp
Triban; Pediatric Triban
trifluoperazine HCl
Trilafon
Trimazide
trimethobenzamide HCl
V-Gan 25; V-Gan 50
Vistacon
Vistaject-25; Vistaject-50
Vistaril
Vistazine 50
Vontrol
Zofran
Zofran ODT

Antiprotozoals
Antiprotozoals, Amebicides
dehydroemetine
diloxanide furoate
Flagyl
Flagyl IV
Flagyl IV RTU
Furamide
Humatin
iodoquinol
Mebadin
Metro I.V.
metronidazole
paromomycin sulfate
Protostat
Vytone
Yodoxin
Antiprotozoals, Antimalarials
Aralen HCl
Aralen Phosphate
Aralen Phosphate with Primaquine
    Phosphate
chloroguanide HCl
chloroquine HCl
chloroquine phosphate
Daraprim
Fansidar

Antiprotozoals, Antimalarials (continued)

Halfan
halofantrine HCl
hydroxychloroquine sulfate
Lariam
Malarone
mefloquine HCl
Mephaquin
Plaquenil Sulfate
primaquine phosphate
pyrimethamine
Quilimmune-M
Quinamm
quinidine gluconate
quinine sulfate
Quiphile

Antiprotozoals, Other

Antrypol
Arsobal
Belganyl
eflornithine HCl
Fourneau 309
Germanin
Lampit
melarsoprol
Moranyl
Naganol
Naphuride
nifurtimox
Ornidyl
Pentostam
sodium stibogluconate
suramin sodium

Antispasmodics

A-Spas S/L
Anaspaz
Antispas
Antispasmodic
Antrocol
Arco-Lase Plus
atropine sulfate
Barbidonna; Barbidonna No. 2
Bel-Phen-Ergot SR
Bellacane
Bellacane SR
belladonna extract
Bellafoline

Antispasmodics (continued)

Bellergal-S
Bentyl
Butibel
Byclomine
Cafatine-PB
Chardonna-2
clidinium bromide
Clindex
Cystospaz
Cystospaz-M
dexpanthenol
Di-Spaz
Dibent
dicyclomine HCl
Donna-Sed
Donnamar
Donnatal
Donnatal No. 2
Ed-Spaz
Enlon Plus
Folergot DF
Gastrosed
glycopyrrolate
hyoscyamine hydrobromide
hyoscyamine sulfate
Hyosophen
Ilopan
Ilopan-Choline
Kutrase
Levbid
Levsin
Levsin PB
Levsin with Phenobarbital
Levsin/SL
Levsinex
Librax
Logen
Lomanate
Lomotil
Lonox
Malatal
methscopolamine bromide
Motofen
Pamine
Phenerbel-S
Pro-Banthīne
propantheline bromide
Quarzan
Robinul

Antispasmodics (continued)
Robinul Forte
Sal-Tropine
Scopace
scopolamine hydrobromide
Spasmoject
Spasmolin
Susano
tizanidine HCl
Transderm Scōp
Zanaflex

Biliary Tract Agents
Actigall
Chenix
chenodiol
CholestaGel
colesevelam HCl
dehydrocholic acid
desoxycholic acid
Digestozyme
flumecinol
Moctanin
monoctanoin
Stanate
stannsoporfin
Urso
ursodiol
Zixoryn
Cholelithics [see: Biliary Tract Agents]
Crohn Disease: [see: Inflammatory
Bowel Disease Agents]
Enzymes, Digestive
amylase
Arco-Lase Plus
bile salts
cellulase
Cotazym
Cotazym-S
Creon
Creon 10
Creon 20
Digepepsin
Digestozyme
Donnazyme
Gustase Plus
Ilozyme
Ku-Zyme
Ku-Zyme HP

Enzymes, Digestive (continued)
Kutrase
lactase enzyme
lipase
Lipram-CR20
Lipram-PN10
Lipram-PN16
Lipram-UL12
Lipram-UL18
Lipram-UL20
Pancrease; Pancrease MT 4; Pan-
crease MT 10; Pancrease MT 16;
Pancrease MT 20
pancreatin
Pancrecarb MS-8
pancrelipase
pepsin
protease
Protilase
Ultrase; Ultrase MT 12; Ultrase MT
18; Ultrase MT 20
Viokase
Zymase
Gallbladder Disease and Gallstones
[see: Biliary Tract Agents]
**Gastroesophageal Reflux Disease
(GERD)** [see: Peptic Ulcer and Gas-
tric Reflux Agents]

Hemorrhoidal Agents
Analpram-HC
Anogesic
Anucort HC
Anumed HC
Anusol-HC
Anusol-HC 1
Cort-Dome High Potency
Dermol HC
Hemorrhoidal HC
Hemril-HC
hydrocortisone (HC)
hydrocortisone acetate (HCA)
phenol
Pramoxine HC
Proctocort
ProctoCream-HC
Proctofoam-HC
Rectacort

Inflammatory Bowel Disease Agents

[see also: Hemorrhoidal Agents]
Aliminase
alosetron HCl
aminosalicylic acid (4-aminosalicylic acid)
anakinra
Antegren
Antril
Asacol
Azulfidine
Azulfidine EN-tabs
balsalazide disodium
budesonide
Colazal
Colomed
Cortenema
Cortifoam
Dipentum
Entocort ㊎
infliximab
Lotronex
mesalamine
natalizumab
olsalazine sodium
Pamisyl
Pentasa
Remicade
Rezipas
Rowasa
Salofalk ㊎
short chain fatty acids
sulfasalazine
tegaserod
Zelmac

Intestinal Parasites [see: Anthelmintics; Antiprotozoals]

Laxatives

barley malt soup extract
bisacodyl
calcium polycarbophil
carboxymethylcellulose sodium
casanthranol
cascara fluidextract, aromatic
cascara sagrada
castor oil

Laxatives (continued)

cellulose
Chronulac
Constilac
Constulose
Duphalac
Evalose
glycerin
Heptalac
lactulose
magnesia, milk of
magnesium citrate
magnesium sulfate
methylcellulose
mineral oil
MiraLax
Osmoglyn
phenolphthalein
phenolphthalein, yellow
polycarbophil
prucalopride HCl
prucalopride succinate
psyllium husk
psyllium hydrophilic mucilloid
senna
sennosides
sodium phosphate, dibasic
sodium phosphate, monobasic

Laxatives, Pre-procedure Bowel Evacuants

bisacodyl
Clysodrast
Co-Lav
Colovage
CoLyte
Go-Evac
GoLYTELY
NuLytely
OCL
polyethylene glycol–electrolyte solution (PEG-ES)
senna

Laxatives, Stool Softeners

docusate calcium
docusate sodium

Parasites, Intestinal [see: Anthelmintics; Antiprotozoals]

Peptic Ulcer and Gastric Reflux Agents

[see also: Antacids]
Aciphex
anisotropine methylbromide
Arthrotec
Axid
Banthĩne
Cantil
Carafate
cimetidine
cimetidine HCl
cisapride
Cytotec
Daricon
enprostil
esomeprazole magnesium
famotidine
Gardrin
Gastrozepine
Hp-PAC ⓒᴬᴺ
Iamin
lansoprazole
Losec ⓒᴬᴺ
mepenzolate bromide
methantheline bromide
misoprostol
Nexium
nizatidine
omeprazole
oxyphencyclimine HCl
Panto IV ⓒᴬᴺ
pantoprazole

Peptic Ulcer and Gastric Reflux Agents (continued)

pantoprazole sodium
Pantozol
Pathilon
Pepcid
Pepcid RPD
pirenzepine HCl
PMS-Sucralfate ⓒᴬᴺ
Prepulsid ⓒᴬᴺ
Prevacid
Prevpac
Prilosec
Propulsid
Protonix
Pylorid ⓒᴬᴺ
rabeprazole sodium
ranitidine
ranitidine bismuth citrate
ranitidine HCl
roxatidine acetate HCl
Roxin
sucralfate
Tagamet
tridihexethyl chloride
Tritec
Zantac
Zantac EFFERdose
Zantac GELdose

Ulcerative Colitis [see: Inflammatory Bowel Disease Agents]

Ulcers, Gastric [see: Peptic Ulcer and Gastric Reflux Agents]